Publication Inc

# 750+ BLOCKBUSTER PROBLEMS in CHEMISTRY for NEET

AF529515

Corporate Office

DISHA PUBLICATION
45, 2nd Floor, Maharishi Dayanand Marg,
Corner Market, Malviya Nagar, New Delhi - 110017
Tel : 49842349 / 49842350



Typeset by Disha DTP Team

# Contents

## Mock Tests

# SOME BASIC CONCEPTS OF CHEMISTRY

# 1

1. A sample of pure carbon dioxide, irrespective of its source contains 27.27% carbon and 72.73% oxygen. The data supports
   (a) law of constant composition
   (b) law of conservation of mass
   (c) law of reciprocal proportions
   (d) law of multiple proportions
2. What is the mass of 1 molecule of CO?
   (a) $2.325 \times 10^{-23}$ g (b) $4.65 \times 10^{-23}$ g
   (c) $3.732 \times 10^{-23}$ g (d) $2.895 \times 10^{-23}$ g
3. Number of atoms in 558.5 gram Fe (at. wt. of Fe = 55.85 g mol$^{-1}$) is
   (a) twice that in 60 g carbon
   (b) $6.023 \times 10^{22}$
   (c) half that in 8 g He
   (d) $558.5 \times 6.023 \times 10^{23}$
4. How many moles of magnesium phosphate, $Mg_3(PO_4)_2$ will contain 0.25 mole of oxygen atoms?
   (a) $1.25 \times 10^{-2}$ (b) $2.5 \times 10^{-2}$
   (c) 0.02 (d) $3.125 \times 10^{-2}$
5. The number of molecules in 16 g of methane is
   (a) $3.0 \times 10^{23}$ (b) $\frac{16}{6.02} \times 10^{23}$
   (c) $6.023 \times 10^{23}$ (d) $\frac{16}{3.0} \times 10^{23}$
6. The number of molecules in 8.96 litre of a gas at 0ºC and 1 atm. pressure is approximately
   (a) $6.023 \times 10^{23}$ (b) $12.04 \times 10^{23}$
   (c) $18.06 \times 10^{23}$ (d) $24.09 \times 10^{22}$
7. One mole of $CO_2$ contains :
   (a) 3 g atoms of $CO_2$
   (b) $18.1 \times 10^{23}$ molecules of $CO_2$
   (c) $6.02 \times 10^{23}$ atoms of O
   (d) $6.02 \times 10^{23}$ atoms of C
8. How many atoms are contained in one mole of sucrose ($C_{12}H_{22}O_{11}$)?
   (a) $20 \times 6.02 \times 10^{23}$ atoms/mol
   (b) $45 \times 6.02 \times 10^{23}$ atoms/mol
   (c) $5 \times 6.02 \times 10^{23}$ atoms/mol
   (d) None of these
9. How many moles of helium gas occupy 22.4 litre at 0°C and 1 atm pressure ?
   (a) 0.11 (b) 1.11
   (c) 0.90 (d) 1.0
10. $O_2$, $N_2$ are present in the ratio of 1 : 4 by weight. The ratio of number of molecules is :
    (a) 7 : 32 (b) 1 : 4
    (c) 2 : 1 (d) 4 : 1
11. The number of hydrogen atoms present in 25.6 g of sucrose ($C_{12}H_{22}O_{11}$) which has a molar mass of 342.3 g is:
    (a) $22 \times 10^{23}$ (b) $9.91 \times 10^{23}$
    (c) $11 \times 10^{23}$ (d) $44 \times 10^{23}$

12. A 5 molar solution of $H_2SO_4$ is diluted from 1 litre to a volume of 10 litres, the normality of the solution will be :

(a) 1N (b) 0.1N
(c) 5N (d) 0.5N

13. With increase of temperature, which of these changes?

(a) Molality
(b) Weight fraction of solute
(c) Molarity
(d) Mole fraction

14. A metallic chloride contains 47.22% metal. Calculate the equivalent weight of metal.

(a) 39.68 (b) 31.76
(c) 36.35 (d) 33.46

15. $6.02 \times 10^{20}$ molecules of urea are present in 100 mL of its solution. The concentration of urea solution is

(a) 0.02 M (b) 0.01 M
(c) 0.001 M (d) 0.1 M

(Avogadro constant, $N_A = 6.02 \times 10^{23}$ mol$^{-1}$)

16. Density of a 2.05M solution of acetic acid in water is1.02 g/mL. The molality of the solution is

(a) 2.28 mol kg$^{-1}$ (b) 0.44 mol kg$^{-1}$
(c) 1.14 mol kg$^{-1}$ (d) 3.28 mol kg$^{-1}$

17. The density of water is 1g/mL. What is the volume occupied by 1 molecule of water?

(a) $1.44 \times 10^{-23}$ mL (b) 1 mL
(c) 18 mL (d) $2.88 \times 10^{-23}$ mL

18. The formula of an acid is $HXO_2$. The mass of 0.0242 moles of the acid is 1.657 g. What is the atomic mass of X?

(a) 35.5 (b) 28.1
(c) 128 (d) 19.0

19. The sulphate of a metal M contains 9.87% of M. This sulphate is isomorphous with $ZnSO_4.7H_2O$. The atomic mass of M is:

(a) 40.3 (b) 36.3
(c) 24.3 (d) 11.3

20. Equivalent mass of $H_3PO_2$ when it disproportionate into $PH_3$ and $H_3PO_3$ is:

(a) M (b) M/2
(c) M/4 (d) 3M/4

21. The equivalent mass of an element is 4. Its chloride has a vapour density 59.25. Then, the valency of the elements is:

(a) 4 (b) 3
(c) 2 (d) 1

22. What is the weight of oxygen required for the complete combustion of 2.8 kg of ethylene ?

(a) 2.8 kg (b) 6.4 kg
(c) 9.6 kg (d) 96 kg

23. The simplest formula of a compound containing 50% of element X (atomic mass 10) and 50% of element Y (atomic mass 20) is

(a) XY (b) $XY_3$
(c) $X_2Y$ (d) $X_2Y_3$

24. Malachite has the formula $Cu_2CO_3(OH)_2$. What percentage by mass of malachite is copper?

(a) 25% (b) 50.9%
(c) 57.5% (d) 63.5%

25. 100 mL $O_2$ and $H_2$ kept at same temperature and pressure. What is true about their number of molecules

(a) $N_{O_2} > N_{H_2}$
(b) $N_{O_2} < N_{H_2}$
(c) $N_{O_2} = N_{H_2}$
(d) $N_{O_2} + N_{H_2} = 1$ mole

**ANSWER KEY**

| | | | | | | | | | | | | | | | | | |
|---|---|---|---|---|---|---|---|---|---|---|---|---|---|---|---|---|---|
| 1 | (a) | 4 | (d) | 7 | (d) | 10 | (a) | 13 | (c) | 16 | (a) | 19 | (c) | 22 | (c) | 25 | (c) |
| 2 | (b) | 5 | (c) | 8 | (b) | 11 | (b) | 14 | (b) | 17 | (d) | 20 | (d) | 23 | (c) | | |
| 3 | (a) | 6 | (d) | 9 | (d) | 12 | (a) | 15 | (b) | 18 | (a) | 21 | (b) | 24 | (c) | | |

# STRUCTURE OF ATOM

# 2

1. Which has the highest *e*/*m* ratio ?
   (a) $He^{2+}$ (b) $H^+$
   (c) $He^+$ (d) $D^+$
2. Which of the following pairs are isosters ?
   (a) $CO_2$ and $N_2O$ (b) CaO and KF
   (c) $OF_2$ and HClO (d) All of these
3. Among the following sets which one does NOT contain isoelectronic species?
   (a) $BO_3^{3-}$, $CO_3^{2-}$, $NO_3^-$
   (b) $SO_3^{2-}$, $CO_3^{2-}$, $NO_3^-$
   (c) $CN^-$, $N_2$, $C_2^{2-}$
   (d) $PO_4^{3-}$, $SO_4^{2-}$, $ClO_4^-$
4. Which of the following statements do not form a part of Bohr's model of hydrogen atom ?
   (a) Energy of the electrons in the orbits are quantized
   (b) The electron(s) in the orbit nearest to the nucleus has the lowest energy
   (c) Electrons revolve in different orbits around the nucleus
   (d) The position and velocity of an electron in the orbit cannot be determined simultaneously.
5. When an electron of charge *e* and mass *m* moves with a velocity *v* towards the nuclear charge *Ze* in circular orbit of radius *r*, the potential energy of the electron is given by
   (a) $\frac{Ze^2}{r}$ (b) $\frac{-Ze^2}{r}$
   (c) $\frac{Ze^2}{r^2}$ (d) $\frac{mv^2}{r}$
6. The radius of hydrogen atom in the ground state is 0.53 Å. The radius of $Li^{2+}$ ion (atomic number = 3) in a similar state is
   (a) 0.17 Å (b) 0.265 Å
   (c) 0.53 Å (d) 1.06 Å
7. In a hydrogen atom, if energy of an electron in ground state is – 13.6. eV, then energy in the 2nd excited state is
   (a) – 1.51 eV (b) – 3.4 eV
   (c) – 6.04 eV (d) – 13.6 eV.

8. Zeeman effect refers to the

(a) splitting up of the lines in an emission spectrum in presence of an external electrostatic field

(b) random scattering of light by colloidal particles

(c) splitting up of the lines in an emission spectrum in a magnetic field

(d) emission of electrons from metals when light falls upon them

9. In Bohr's model, atomic radius of the first orbit is $y$, the radius of the 3rd orbit, is

(a) $y/3$ (b) $y$

(c) $3y$ (d) $9y$

10. The electron in the hydrogen atom undergoes transition from higher orbitals to orbital of radius 211.6 pm. This transition is associated with :

(a) Lyman series (b) Balmer series

(c) Paschen series (d) Brackett series

11. Number of protons, neutrons and electrons in the element $^{231}_{89}Y$ is

(a) 89, 231, 89 (b) 89, 89, 242

(c) 89, 142, 89 (d) 89, 71, 89

12. Which Bohr's orbit of $Be^{3+}$ has the same radius as that of the ground state of hydrogen atom?

(a) 3 (b) 2

(c) 4 (d) 5

13. In hydrogen atom, energy of first excited state is –3.4 eV. Find out KE of the same orbit of hydrogen atom

(a) +3.4 eV (b) +6.8 eV

(c) – 13.6 eV (d) +13.6 eV

14. Which one of the following is not the characteristic of Planck's quantum theory of radiation

(a) The energy is not absorbed or emitted in whole number or multiple of quantum.

(b) Radiation is associated with energy.

(c) Radiation energy is not emitted or absorbed continuously but in the form of small packets called quanta.

(d) This magnitude of energy associated with a quantum is proportional to the frequency.

15. The number of nodal planes in a $p_x$ orbital is

(a) one (b) two

(c) three (d) zero

16. The number of radial nodes of 3*s* and 2*p* orbitals are respectively

(a) 2, 0 (b) 0, 2

(c) 1, 2 (d) 2, 1

17. Which experimental observation given in the first column correctly accounts for the phenomenon given in the second column?

| | Column I Experimental observation | | Column II Phenomenon |
|---|---|---|---|
| (a) | X-ray spectra | p. | Charge on nucleus |
| (b) | α-particle scattering | q. | Quantised electron orbit |
| (c) | Photoelectric effect | r. | The nuclear atom |
| (d) | Emission spectra | s. | Quantisation of energy |

18. In the photoelectron emission, the energy of the emitted electron is

(a) greater than the incident photon.

(b) same as than of the incident photon.

(c) smaller than the incident photon.

(d) proportional to the intensity of incident photon.

19. Which of the following is related with both wave nature and particle nature ?

(a) Interference (b) $E = mc^2$

(c) Diffraction (d) $E = h\nu$

**20.** Which of the following sets of quantum numbers is correct for an electron in 4*f* orbital ?

(a) $n=4, \ell=3, m=+1, s=+½$

(b) $n=4, \ell=4, m=-4, s=-½$

(c) $n=4, \ell=3, m=+4, s=+½$

(d) $n=3, \ell=2, m=-2, s=+½$

**21.** Which of the following represents correct set of the four quantum numbers for an electron in a 4*d* subshell ?

(a) 4, 2, 1, 0 (b) 4, 2, 1, – 1/2

(c) 4, 3, 2, + 1/2 (d) 4, 3, – 2, – 1/2

**22.** The orbital having $m=-2$ should not be present in the following sub-shell

(a) *d* (b) *f*

(c) *g* (d) *p*

**23.** Which element's last electron in the outermost orbit has magnetic quantum number (m = 0)?

(a) Na (b) O

(c) Cl (d) N

**24.** For how many orbitals, the quantum numbers n = 3, *l* =2, m = +2 are possible?

(a) 1 (b) 2

(c) 3 (d) 4

**25.** The orbital angular momentum of 3*p* electron is:

(a) $\sqrt{3}\,h$ (b) $\sqrt{6}\,h$

(c) zero (d) $\sqrt{2}\frac{h}{2\pi}$

**ANSWER KEY**

| | | | | | | | | | | | | | | | | | |
|---|---|---|---|---|---|---|---|---|---|---|---|---|---|---|---|---|---|
| 1 | (b) | 4 | (d) | 7 | (a) | 10 | (b) | 13 | (a) | 16 | (a) | 19 | (d) | 22 | (d) | 25 | (d) |
| 2 | (d) | 5 | (b) | 8 | (c) | 11 | (c) | 14 | (a) | 17 | (d) | 20 | (a) | 23 | (a) | | |
| 3 | (b) | 6 | (a) | 9 | (d) | 12 | (b) | 15 | (a) | 18 | (c) | 21 | (b) | 24 | (a) | | |

# CLASSIFICATION OF ELEMENTS AND PERIODICITY IN PROPERTIES

# 3

1. Which is chemically most active non-metal ?
   (a) S (b) O
   (c) F (d) N
2. The elements in which $4f$ orbitals are progressively filled up are called as
   (a) Actinoids (b) Transition elements
   (c) Lanthanoids (d) Both (a) and (c)
3. The statement that is not correct for the periodic classification of elements is
   (a) the properties of elements are the periodic functions of their atomic numbers.
   (b) non-metallic elements are lesser in number than metallic elements.
   (c) the first ionisation energies of elements along a period do not vary in a regular manner with increase in atomic number.
   (d) for transition elements the $d$-subshells are filled with electrons monotonically with increase in atomic number.
4. Which of the following should be the correct order of the second ionisation potential of Li, Be, B and C ?
   (a) $Li < Be > B < C$ (b) $Be < B > C < Li$
   (c) $Be < C < B < Li$ (d) $Li < C < B < Be$
5. The order of increasing sizes of atomic radii among the elements O, S, Se and As is :
   (a) $As < S < O < Se$ (b) $Se < S < As < O$
   (c) $O < S < As < Se$ (d) $O < S < Se < As$
6. The ionization energy of boron is less than that of beryllium because
   (a) beryllium has a higher nuclear charge than boron.
   (b) beryllium has a lower nuclear charge than boron.
   (c) the outermost electron in boron occupies a $2p$-orbital.
   (d) the $2s$ and $2p$-orbitals of boron are degenerate.

7. The correct order of $IE_2$ is:

(a) Ne > F > O > N (b) O > F > Ne > N

(c) Ne > O > F > N (d) O > Ne > F > N

8. Which one of the following represents the electronic configuration of the most electropositive element ?

(a) [He] $2s^1$ (b) [Xe] $6s^1$

(c) [He] $2s^2$ (d) [Xe] $6s^2$

9. Highest energy will be absorbed to eject out the electron in the configuration

(a) $1s^2 2s^2 2p^1$ (b) $1s^2 2s^2 2p^3$

(c) $1s^2 2s^2 2p^2$ (d) $1s^2 2s^2 2p^4$

10. $Na^+, Mg^{2+}, Al^{3+}$ and $Si^{4+}$ ions are isoelectronic. The value of ionic radii of these ions would be in the order :

(a) $Na^+ > Mg^{2+} > Al^{3+} > Si^{4+}$

(b) $Na^+ < Mg^{2+} < Al^{3+} < Si^{4+}$

(c) $Na^+ > Mg^{2+} > Al^{3+} < Si^{4+}$

(d) $Na^+ < Mg^{2+} > Al^{3+} > Si^{4+}$

11. The ionisation potential order for which set is correct?

(a) Cs < Li < K (b) Cs > Li > B

(c) Li > K > Cs (d) B > Li > K

12. The valence shell of element A contains 3 electrons while the valence shell of element B contains 6 electrons . If A combines with B, the probable formula of the compound formed will be

(a) $AB_2$ (b) $A_2B$

(c) $A_2B_3$ (d) $A_3B_2$

13. Which one of these is basic?

(a) $SiO_2$ (b) $SO_2$

(c) $CO_2$ (d) $Na_2O$

14. Which of the following oxides is amphoteric in character?

(a) $SnO_2$ (b) $SiO_2$

(c) $CO_2$ (d) CaO

15. Which of the following represents correct order of electron affinity?

(a) Cl > F > S > O (b) F > O > S > Cl

(c) F > Cl > S > O (d) Cl > S > O > F

16. Which of the following order is correct for the property mentioned in brackets?

(a) $S^{2-} > Cl^- > K^+ > Ca^{2+}$ (Ionisation energy)

(b) C < N < F < O (2nd Ionisation energy)

(c) B > Al > Ga > In > Tl (Electronegativity)

(d) $Na^+ > Li^+ > Mg^{2+} > Be^{2+} > Al^{3+}$ (Ionic radius)

17. The lower electron affinity of fluorine than that of chlorine is due to

(a) Smaller size of F.

(b) Smaller nuclear charge on F.

(c) Diffrence in their electronic arrangement

(d) Highest reactivity of F.

18. Which is the correct order of electronegativity ?

(a) F > N < O > C (b) F > N > O > C

(c) F > N > O < C (d) F < N < O < C

19. Which group is called buffer group of the periodic table ?

(a) I (b) VII

(c) VIII (d) Zero

**20.** Match Column-I with Column-II and select the correct answer by the given codes.

| Columnn-I (Atoms) | Column-II (Properties) |
|---|---|
| (A) He | (p) Highly electronegative |
| (B) F | (q) Most electropositive |
| (C) Rb | (r) Strongest reducing agent |
| (D) Li | (s) Highest ionisation energy |

(a) A – (s), B – (q), C – (r), D – (p)
(b) A – (p), B – (s), C – (q), D – (r)
(c) A – (s), B – (p), C – (r), D (q)
(d) A – (s), B – (p), C – (q), D – (r)

**ANSWER KEY**

| | | | | | | | | | | | | | | | | | | | |
|---|---|---|---|---|---|---|---|---|---|---|---|---|---|---|---|---|---|---|---|
| 1 | (c) | 4 | (c) | 7 | (c) | 10 | (a) | 13 | (d) | 16 | (b) | 19 | (d) | | | | | | |
| 2 | (c) | 5 | (d) | 8 | (b) | 11 | (c) | 14 | (a) | 17 | (a) | 20 | (d) | | | | | | |
| 3 | (d) | 6 | (c) | 9 | (b) | 12 | (c) | 15 | (a) | 18 | (a) | | | | | | | | |

# CHEMICAL BONDING AND MOLECULAR STRUCTURE

# 4

1. Among the following which compound will show the highest lattice energy ?
   (a) KF (b) NaF
   (c) CsF (d) RbF
2. Which one of the following is the correct order of interactions?
   (a) covalent < hydrogen bonding < van der Waals < dipole-dipole
   (b) van der Waals < hydrogen bonding < dipole-dipole < covalent
   (c) van der Waals < dipole-dipole < hydrogen bonding < covalent
   (d) dipole-dipole < van der Waals < hydrogen bonding < covalent
3. Amongst LiCl, RbCl, $BeCl_2$ and $MgCl_2$ the compounds with the greatest and the least ionic character, respectively are:
   (a) LiCl and RbCl
   (b) RbCl and $BeCl_2$
   (c) $MgCl_2$ and $BeCl_2$
   (d) RbCl and $MgCl_2$
4. Which of the following is the electron deficient molecule?
   (a) $C_2H_6$ (b) $B_2H_6$
   (c) $SiH_4$ (d) $PH_3$
5. Which one of the following pairs of species have the same bond order?
   (a) $CN^-$ and $NO^+$ (b) $CN^-$ and $CN^+$
   (c) $O_2^-$ and $CN^-$ (d) $NO^+$ and $CN^+$
6. Which of the following would have a permanent dipole moment?
   (a) $SiF_4$ (b) $SF_4$
   (c) $XeF_4$ (d) $BF_3$
7. Pauling's electronegativity values for elements are useful in predicting
   (a) polarity of bonds in molecules
   (b) ionic and covalent nature of bonds
   (c) coordination number
   (d) both (a) and (b)
8. Polarisibility of halide ions increases in the order
   (a) $F^-, I^-, Br^-, Cl^-$ (b) $Cl^-, Br^-, I^-, F^-$
   (c) $I^-, Br^-, Cl^-, F^-$ (d) $F^-, Cl^-, Br^-, I^-$
9. $H_2O$ is polar, whereas $BeF_2$ is not. It is because
   (a) EN of F > EN of O.
   (b) $H_2O$ involves H-bonding, whereas $BeF_2$ is a discrete molecule.
   (c) $H_2O$ is linear and $BeF_2$ is angular
   (d) $H_2O$ is angular and $BeF_2$ is linear

10. In $BrF_3$ molecule, the lone pairs occupy equatorial positions to minimize
(a) lone pair - bond pair repulsion only
(b) bond pair - bond pair repulsion only
(c) lone pair - lone pair repulsion and lone pair - bond pair repulsion
(d) lone pair - lone pair repulsion only

11. Which of the following does not have a tetrahedral structure?
(a) $BH_4^-$ (b) $BH_3$
(c) $NH_4^+$ (d) $CH_4$

12. Which of the following molecules has trigonal planar geometry?
(a) $BF_3$ (b) $NH_3$
(c) $PCl_3$ (d) $IF_3$

13. How many σ- and π-bonds are there in?

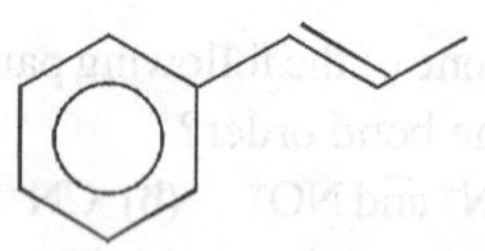

(a) 14σ, 8π (b) 18σ, 8π
(c) 19σ, 4π (d) 14σ, 2π

14. The pair of species having identical shapes for molecules of both species is
(a) $XeF_2, CO_2$ (b) $BF_3, PCl_3$
(c) $PF_5, IF_5$ (d) $CF_4, SF_4$

15. The shape of $IF_6^-$ is :
(a) Trigonally distorted octahedron
(b) Pyramidal
(c) Octahedral
(d) Square antiprism

16. The bond order in $N_2^+$ is
(a) 1.5 (b) 3.0
(c) 2.5 (d) 2.0

17. Which of the following molecule is paramagnetic?
(a) Chlorine (b) Nitrogen
(c) Oxygen (d) Hydrogen

18. Of the following hydrides which one has the lowest boiling point ?
(a) $AsH_3$ (b) $SbH_3$
(c) $PH_3$ (d) $NH_3$

19. An ether is more volatile than an alcohol having the same molecular formula. This is due to
(a) alcohols having resonance structures
(b) intermolecular hydrogen bonding in ethers
(c) intermolecular hydrogen bonding in alcohols
(d) dipolar character of ethers

20. Although $CN^-$ ion and $N_2$ molecule are isoelectronic, yet $N_2$ molecule is chemically inert because of
(a) presence of more number of electrons in bonding orbitals
(b) a bond energy
(c) absence of bond polarity
(d) uneven electron distribution.

21. The $BCl_3$ is a planar molecule whereas $NCl_3$ is pyramidal because
(a) B-Cl bond is more polar than N-Cl bond
(b) N-Cl bond is more covalent than B-Cl bond
(c) nitrogen atom is smaller than boron atom
(d) $BCl_3$ has no lone pair but $NCl_3$ has a lone pair of electrons

22. The number and type of bonds in $C_2^{2-}$ ion in $CaC_2$ are:
(a) One σ bond and one π-bond
(b) One σ bond and two π-bond
(c) Two σ bond and two π-bond
(d) Two σ bond and one π-bond

23. The boiling point of *p*-nitrophenol is higher than that of *o*-nitrophenol because
(a) $NO_2$ group at *p*-position behaves in a different way from that at *o*-position.
(b) intramolecular hydrogen bonding exists in *p*-nitrophenol
(c) there is intermolecular hydrogen bonding in *p*-nitrophenol
(d) *p*-nitrophenol has a higher molecular weight than *o*-nitrophenol.

**24.** If $N_x$ is the number of bonding orbitals of an atom and $N_y$ is the number of antibonding orbitals, then the molecule/atom will be stable if

(a) $N_x > N_y$ (b) $N_x = N_y$
(c) $N_x < N_y$ (d) $N_x \leq N_y$

**25.** Match Column-I (molecule) with Column-II (type of hybridisation) and choose the correct option from the codes given below.

| **Column-I (Molecule)** | **Column-II (Type of hybridisation)** |
|---|---|
| (A) $SF_6$ | (p) $sp^3d$ |
| (B) $PF_5$ | (q) $sp^3$ |
| (C) $BCl_3$ | (r) $sp^3d^2$ |
| (D) $C_2H_6$ | (s) $sp^2$ |

(a) A – (r), B – (p), C – (s), D – (q)
(b) A – (r), B – (p), C – (q), D – (s)
(c) A – (p), B – (r), C – (q), D – (s)
(d) A – (p), B – (r), C – (s), D – (q)

**ANSWER KEY**

| | | | | | | | | | | | | | | | | | |
|---|---|---|---|---|---|---|---|---|---|---|---|---|---|---|---|---|---|
| 1 | (c) | 4 | (c) | 7 | (c) | 10 | (a) | 13 | (d) | 16 | (b) | 19 | (d) | | | | |
| 2 | (c) | 5 | (d) | 8 | (b) | 11 | (c) | 14 | (a) | 17 | (a) | 20 | (d) | | | | |
| 3 | (d) | 6 | (c) | 9 | (b) | 12 | (c) | 15 | (a) | 18 | (a) | | | | | | |

# STATES OF MATTER

# 5

1. Air at sea level is dense. This is a practical application of
(a) Boyle's law (b) Charle's law
(c) Kelvin's law (d) Brown's law

2. The interaction energy of London force is inversely proportional to sixth power of the distance between two interacting particles but their magnitude depends upon
(a) charge of interacting particles.
(b) mass of interacting particles.
(c) polarisability of interacting particles.
(d) strength of permanent dipoles in the particles.

3. 10 g of a gas at 1 atm and 273 K occupies 5 litres. The temperature at which the volume becomes double for the same mass of gas at the same pressure is:
(a) 273 K (b) –273 °C
(c) 273 °C (d) 546 K

4. Two flasks A and B of 500 mL each are respectively filled with $O_2$ and $SO_2$ at 300 K and 1 atm pressure. The flasks will contain
(a) the same number of atoms.
(b) the same number of molecules.
(c) more number of moles of molecules in flask A as compared to flask B.
(d) the same amount of gases.

5. Which of the following gaseous mixture does not follow Dalton's law of partial pressure?
(a) $SO_2$ and $Cl_2$ (b) $CO_2$ and $N_2$
(c) CO and $CO_2$ d) CO and $N_2$

6. What is the ratio of diffusion rate of oxygen to hydrogen?
(a) 1 : 4 (b) 4 : 1
(c) 1 : 8 (d) 8 : 1

7. Among the following, the incorrect statement is:
(a) At low pressure, real gases show ideal behaviour.
(b) At very low temperature, real gases show ideal behaviour.
(c) At very large volume, real gases show ideal behaviour.
(d) At Boyle's temperature, real gases show ideal behaviour.

8. The ratio of the rate of diffusion of helium and methane under identical condition of pressure and temperature will be
(a) 4 (b) 2
(c) 1 (d) 0.5

9. The beans are cooked earlier in pressure cooker, because
   (a) boiling point increases with increasing pressure
   (b) boiling point decreases with increasing pressure
   (c) internal energy is not lost while cooking in pressure cooker
   (d) extra pressure of pressure cooker softens the beans
10. Which of the following statements about kinetic energy (K.E.) is true?
   (a) All objects moving with the same velocity have the same K.E.
   (b) The K.E. of a body will quadruple if its velocity doubles
   (c) As the velocity of a body increases, its K.E. decreases
   (d) The K.E. of a body is independent of its mass
11. Consider three one-litre flasks labelled A, B and C filled with the gases NO, $NO_2$, and $N_2O$, respectively, each at 1 atm and 273 K. In which flask do the molecules have the highest average kinetic energy?
   (a) Flask C (b) All are the same
   (c) Flask A (d) None
12. The pressure of a real gas is less than the pressure of an ideal gas because of :
   (a) increase in number of collisions
   (b) finite size of molecule
   (c) increase in KE of molecules
   (d) intermolecular forces of attraction
13. An ideal gas obeying kinetic theory of gases can be liquefied if :
   (a) its temperature is more than critical temperature $T_C$
   (b) its pressure is more than critical pressure $P_C$
   (c) its pressure is more than $P_C$ at a temperature less than $T_C$
   (d) it cannot be liquefied at any value of P and T
14. At what temperature the rms velocity of $SO_2$ be same as that of $O_2$ at 303 K ?
   (a) 273 K (b) 606 K
   (c) 303 K (d) 403 K
15. α, v and u represent most probable velocity, average velocity and root mean square velocity respectively of a gas at a particular temperature. The correct order among the following is
   (a) $u > v > \alpha$ (b) $v > u > \alpha$
   (c) $\alpha > u > v$ (d) $u > \alpha > v$
16. The root mean square velocity of a gas is doubled when the temperature is :
   (a) increased four times
   (b) increased two times
   (c) reduced to half
   (d) reduced to one fourth
17. In a closed flask of 5 litres, 1.0 g of $H_2$ is heated from 300 to 600 K. Which statement is not correct?
   (a) Pressure of the gas increases
   (b) The rate of collision increases
   (c) The number of moles of gas increases
   (d) The energy of gaseous molecules increases
18. When an ideal gas undergoes unrestrained expansion, no cooling occurs because the molecules
   (a) are above the inversion temperature
   (b) exert no attractive forces on each other
   (c) do work equal to loss in kinetic energy
   (d) collide without loss of energy
19. Consider the equation $Z = \frac{PV}{RT}$. Which of the following statements is correct?
   (a) When Z > 1, real gases are easier to compress than the ideal gas
   (b) When Z=1, real gases get compressed easily
   (c) When Z=1, real gases are difficult to compress
   (d) When Z>1, real gases are difficult to compress

**20.** The van der Waal's equation reduces itself to the ideal gas equation at
(a) high pressure and low temperature
(b) low pressure and low temperature
(c) low pressure and high temperature
(d) high pressure alone

**21.** The compressibility factor for $H_2$ and He is usually :
(a) $Z > 1$ (b) $Z = 1$
(c) $Z < 1$ (d) Either of these

**22.** In van der Waal's equation of state for a non-ideal gas, the term that accounts for intermolecular forces is
(a) $(V - b)$ (b) RT
(c) $\left(P + \frac{a}{V^2}\right)$ (d) $(RT)^{-1}$

**23.** If temperature increases, the surface tension of a liquid
(a) increases
(b) decreases
(c) remains the same
(d) increases then decreases

**24.** Select the correct order of evaporation for water, alcohol, petrol and kerosene oil
(a) water > alcohol > kerosene oil > petrol
(b) alcohol > petrol > water > kerosene oil
(c) petrol > alcohol > water > kerosene oil
(d) petrol > alcohol > kerosene oil > water

**25.** Match the columns

| Column-I | Column-II |
|---|---|
| (A) Boyle's law | (p) $V \propto n$ at constant T and P |
| (B) Charle's law | (q) $p_{total} = p_1 + p_2 + p_3 + ....$ at constant T, V |
| (C) Dalton's law | (r) $\frac{pV}{T} = \text{Constant}$ |
| (D) Avogadro law | (s) $V \propto T$ at constant $n$ and $p$ |
| | (t) $p \propto \frac{1}{V}$ at constant $n$ and T |

(a) A – (t), B – (s), C – (q), D – (p)
(b) A – (s), B – (q), C – (p), D – (t)
(c) A – (r), B – (t), C – (q), D – (p)
(d) A – (t), B – (q), C – (s), D – (r)

**ANSWER KEY**

| | | | | | | | | | | | | | | | | | |
|---|---|---|---|---|---|---|---|---|---|---|---|---|---|---|---|---|---|
| 1 | (a) | 4 | (b) | 7 | (b) | 10 | (b) | 13 | (d) | 16 | (a) | 19 | (d) | 22 | (c) | 25 | (a) |
| 2 | (c) | 5 | (a) | 8 | (b) | 11 | (b) | 14 | (b) | 17 | (c) | 20 | (c) | 23 | (b) | | |
| 3 | (d) | 6 | (a) | 9 | (a) | 12 | (d) | 15 | (a) | 18 | (b) | 21 | (a) | 24 | (d) | | |

# THERMODYNAMICS

# 6

1. For two mole of an ideal gas :
(a) $C_V - C_P = R$ (b) $C_P - C_V = 2R$
(c) $C_P - C_V = R$ (d) $C_V - C_P = 2R$
2. For the reaction;

$$FeCO_3(s) \longrightarrow FeO(s) + CO_2(g);\ \Delta H = 82.8$$

kJ at 25 °C, what is ($\Delta E$ or $\Delta U$) at 25 °C?
(a) 82.8 kJ (b) 80.32 kJ
(c) −2394.77 kJ (d) 85.28 kJ
3. Adiabatic expansions of an ideal gas is accompanied by
(a) decrease in $\Delta E$
(b) increase in temperature
(c) decrease in $\Delta S$
(d) no change in any one of the above properties
4. For the reaction

$$N_2(g) + 3H_2(g) \rightleftharpoons 2NH(g),\ \Delta H = ?$$

(a) $\Delta E + 2RT$ (b) $\Delta E - 2RT$
(c) $\Delta H = RT$ (d) $\Delta E - RT$.
5. If $\Delta H$ is the change in enthalpy and $\Delta E$ is change in internal energy accompanying a gaseous reaction, then
(a) $\Delta H$ is always greater than $\Delta E$
(b) $\Delta H < \Delta E$ only if the number of moles of the products is greater than the number of moles of the reactants
(c) $\Delta H$ is always less than $\Delta E$
(d) $\Delta H < \Delta E$ only if the number of moles of products is less than the number of moles of the reactants.
6. During isothermal expansion of an ideal gas, its
(a) internal energy increases
(b) enthalpy decreases
(c) enthalpy remains unaffected
(d) enthalpy reduces to zero.
7. When 1 mol of a gas is heated at constant volume, temperature is raised from 298 to 308 K. If heat supplied to the gas is 500 J, then which statement is correct ?
(a) $q = w = 500$ J, $\Delta U = 0$
(b) $q = \Delta U = 500$ J, $w = 0$
(c) $q = -w = 500$ J, $\Delta U = 0$
(d) $\Delta U = 0$, $q = w = -500$ J
8. A system absorbs 10 kJ of heat and does 4 kJ of work. The internal energy of the system
(a) increases by 6 kJ

(b) decreases by 6 kJ
(c) decreases by 14 kJ
(d) increases by 14 kJ

9. Use the given standard enthalpies of formation (in kJ/mol) to determine the enthalpy of reaction of the following reaction :

$NH_3(g) + 3F_2(g) \longrightarrow NF_3(g) + 3HF(g)$

$\Delta H^{\circ}_f (NH_3, (g)) = -46.2$; $\Delta H^{\circ}_f (NF_3, (g)) = -113.0$; $\Delta H^{\circ}_f (HF, (g)) = -269.0$

(a) – 335.8 kJ/mol (b) – 873.8 kJ/mol
(c) – 697.2 kJ/mol (d) – 890.4 kJ/mol

10. The values of heat of formation of $SO_2$ and $SO_3$ are –298.2kJ and –98.2 kJ. The heat of formation of the reaction $SO_2 + (1/2)O_2 \rightarrow SO_3$ will be

(a) –200kJ (b) –356.2kJ
(c) +200kJ (d) –396.2kJ

11. Which of the following equations correctly represents the standard heat of formation $(\Delta_f H^{\circ})$ of methane ?

(a) $C\,(diamond) + 4H(g) \rightarrow CH_4(g)$
(b) $C\,(diamond) + 2H_2(g) \rightarrow CH_4(g)$
(c) $C\,(graphite) + 2H_2(g) \rightarrow CH_4(g)$
(d) $C\,(graphite) + 4H(g) \rightarrow CH_4(g)$

12. Heat of neutralization of strong acid against strong base is constant and is equal to

(a) 13.7 kcal (b) 57.3 kJ
(c) $5.73 \times 10^4$ J (d) All of the above

13. The values of standard enthalpy of formation of $SF_6(g)$, S(g) and F(g) are –1100, 275 and 80 kJ $mol^{-1}$ respectively. The average S–F bond enthalpy in $SF_6$ is

(a) 57.5 kJ $mol^{-1}$ (b) 309.16 kJ $mol^{-1}$
(c) –309.16 kJ $mol^{-1}$ (d) 269.17 kJ $mol^{-1}$

14. Identify the correct statement regarding entropy

(a) At absolute zero temperature, the entropy of perfectly crystalline substances is positive.
(b) At absolute zero temperature, entropy of perfectly crystalline substance is taken to be zero.
(c) At 0°C the entropy of a perfectly crystalline substance is taken to be zero.
(d) At absolute zero temperature, the entropy of all crystalline substances is taken to be zero.

15. The entropy change during an isothermal expansion of an ideal gas from $V_1$ to $V_2$ at temperature $T$ is given by :

(a) $\Delta S = 0$
(b) $\Delta S = 2.303\, nR \log_{10} V_2/V_1$
(c) $\Delta S = 2.303\, RT \log_{10} V_2/V_1$
(d) $\Delta S = 2.303\, R \log_{10} V_1/V_2$

16. Which of the following one mole has the highest entropy?

(a) Mercury (b) Diamond
(c) Liquid nitrogen (d) Hydrogen gas

17. The process with negative entropy change is:

(a) Dissociation of $CaSO_4(s)$ to CaO(s) and $SO_3(g)$
(b) Sublimation of dry ice
(c) Dissolution of iodine in water
(d) Synthesis of ammonia from $N_2$ and $H_2$

18. At the sublimation temperature, for the process $CO_2(s) \rightleftharpoons CO_2(g)$

(a) ΔH, ΔS and ΔG are all positive
(b) $\Delta H > 0, \Delta S > 0$ and $\Delta G < 0$
(c) $\Delta H < 0, \Delta S > 0$ and $\Delta G < 0$
(d) $\Delta H > 0, \Delta S > 0$ and $\Delta G = 0$

19. The correct relationship between free energy and equilibrium constant K of a reaction is

(a) $\Delta G^{\circ} = -RT \ln K$
(b) $\Delta G = RT \ln K$
(c) $\Delta G^{\circ} = RT \ln K$
(d) $\Delta G = -RT \ln K$

**20.** Identify the correct statement for change of Gibb's energy for a system ($\Delta G_{system}$) at constant temperature and pressure?

(a) If $\Delta G_{system} = 0$, the system has attained equilibrium.

(b) If $\Delta G_{system} = 0$, the system is still moving in a particular direction.

(c) If $\Delta G_{system} < 0$, the process is not spontaneous.

(d) If $\Delta G_{system} > 0$, the process is not spontaneous.

**21.** For which of the following changes, $\Delta H \neq \Delta U$

(a) $N_2(g) + O_2(g) \rightarrow 2NO(g)$

(b) $H_2(g) + Cl_2(g) \longrightarrow 2HCl(g)$

(c) $C(s) + O_2(g) \longrightarrow CO_2(g)$

(d) $CaCO_3(s) \longrightarrow CaO(s) + CO_2(g)$

**22.** A process has $\Delta H = 200$ J mol$^{-1}$ and $\Delta S = 40$ JK$^{-1}$ mol$^{-(1)}$ Out of the values given below, choose the minimum temperature above which the process will be spontaneous:

(a) 20 K (b) 12 K

(c) 5 K (d) 4 K

**23.** Match the columns

| | Column-I | | Column-II |
|---|---|---|---|
| (A) | Exothermic | (p) | $\Delta H = 0, \Delta E = 0$ |
| (B) | Spontaneous | (q) | $\Delta G = 0$ |
| (C) | Cyclic process | (r) | $\Delta H$ is negative |
| (D) | Equilibrium | (s) | $\Delta G$ is negative |

(a) A – (q), B – (r), C – (p), D – (s)

(b) A – (s), B – (p), C – (r), D – (q)

(c) A – (p), B – (q), C – (s), D – (r)

(d) A – (r), B – (s), C – (p), D – (q)

**24.** What is the melting point of benzene if $\Delta H_{fus} = 9.95$ kJ/mol and $\Delta S_{fus} = 35.7$ J/K mol?

(a) 278.7 °C (b) 278.7 K

(c) 300 K (d) 298 K

**25.** The factor of $\Delta G$ values is important in metallurgy. The $\Delta G$ values for the following reactions at 800°C are given as :

$$S_2(s) + 2O_2(g) \longrightarrow 2SO_2(g)\ ;\ \Delta G = -544\ \text{kJ}$$

$$2Zn(s) + S_2(s) \longrightarrow 2ZnS(s)\ ;\ \Delta G = -293\ \text{kJ}$$

$$2Zn(s) + O_2(g) \longrightarrow 2ZnO(s)\ ;\ \Delta G = -480\ \text{kJ}$$

Then $\Delta G$ for the reaction :

$$2ZnS(s) + 3O_2(g) \longrightarrow 2ZnO(s) + 2SO_2(g)$$

will be :

(a) –357 kJ (b) –731 kJ

(c) –773 kJ (d) –229 kJ

**ANSWER KEY**

| | | | | | | | | | | | | | | | | | |
|---|---|---|---|---|---|---|---|---|---|---|---|---|---|---|---|---|---|
| 1 | (b) | 4 | (b) | 7 | (b) | 10 | (c) | 13 | (b) | 16 | (d) | 19 | (a) | 22 | (c) | 25 | (b) |
| 2 | (b) | 5 | (d) | 8 | (a) | 11 | (c) | 14 | (b) | 17 | (d) | 20 | (a) | 23 | (d) | | |
| 3 | (a) | 6 | (c) | 9 | (b) | 12 | (d) | 15 | (b) | 18 | (d) | 21 | (d) | 24 | (b) | | |

# 7

# EQUILIBRIUM

1. For which of the following reactions, $K_p = K_c$?

(a) $PCl_5(g) \rightleftharpoons PCl_3(g) + Cl_2(g)$

(b) $N_2(g) + O_2(g) \rightleftharpoons 2NO(g)$

(c) $N_2(g) + 3H_2(g) \rightleftharpoons 2NH_3(g)$

(d) $2SO_3(g) \rightleftharpoons 2SO_2(g) + O_2(g)$

2. At a certain temperature, only 50% HI is dissociated at equilibrium in the following reaction :

$2HI(g) \rightleftharpoons H_2(g) + I_2(g)$. The equilibrium constant for this reaction is :

(a) 0.25 (b) 1.0

(c) 3.0 (d) 0.5

3. One mole of $CH_3COOH$ and one mole of $C_2H_5OH$ react to produce $\frac{2}{3}$ mole of $CH_3COOC_2H_5$. The equilibrium constant is :

(a) 1 (b) 2

(c) 3 (d) 4

4. The equilibrium constant for the reversible reaction

$N_2 + 3H_2 \rightleftharpoons 2NH_3$ is K and for reaction

$\frac{1}{2}N_2 + \frac{3}{2}H_2 \rightleftharpoons NH_3$, the equilibrium constant is $K'$

The $K$ and $K'$ will be related as:

(a) $K \times K' = 1$ (b) $K = K'$

(c) $K' = \sqrt{K}$ (d) $K = \sqrt{K'}$

5. Some inert gas is added at constant volume to the following reaction at equilibrium

$NH_4HS(s) \rightleftharpoons NH_3(g) + H_2S(g)$

Predict the effect of adding the inert gas :

(a) The equilibrium shifts in the forward direction.

(b) The equilibrium shifts in the backward direction.

(c) The equilibrium remains unaffected.

(d) The value of $K_p$ is increased.

6. The equilibrium constant K for the reaction:

$2HI(g) \rightleftharpoons H_2(g) + I_2(g)$ at room temperature is 2.85 and that at 698 K is $1.4 \times 10^{-2}$. This implies that the forward reaction is

(a) Exothermic (b) Endothermic
(c) Exergonic (d) Unpredictable

7. According to Le Chatelier's principle, adding heat to

solid $\rightleftharpoons$ liquid equilibrium will cause the

(a) Amount of solid to decrease.
(b) Amount of liquid to decrease.
(c) Temperature to rise.
(d) Temperature to fall.

8. Which reaction is not affected by change in pressure?

(a) $H_2(g) + I_2(g) \rightleftharpoons 2HI(g)$
(b) $2C(g) + O_2(g) \rightleftharpoons 2CO(g)$
(c) $N_2(g) + 3H_2(g) \rightleftharpoons 2NH_3(g)$
(d) $PCl_5(g) \rightleftharpoons PCl_3(g) + Cl_2(g)$

9. The reaction quotient (Q) for the reaction

$N_2(g) + 3H_2(g) \rightleftharpoons 2NH_3(g)$ is given by

$Q = \dfrac{[NH_3]^2}{[N_2][H_2]^3}$. The reaction will proceed

from right to left if

(a) $Q = 0$ (b) $Q = K_c$
(c) $Q < K_c$ (d) $Q > K_c$

where $K_c$ is the equilibrium constant

10. Le-Chatelier principle is not applicable to :

(a) $H_2(g) + I_2(g) \rightleftharpoons 2HI(g)$
(b) $Fe(s) + S(s) \rightleftharpoons FeS(s)$
(c) $N_2(g) + 3H_2(g) \rightleftharpoons 2NH_3(g)$
(d) $N_2(g) + O_2(g) \rightleftharpoons 2NO(g)$

11. Conjugate acid of $NH_2^-$ is

(a) $NH_4^+$ (b) $NH_3$
(c) $NH_2^-$ (d) $NH^{2-}$

12. pH of 0.1 M $NH_3$ aqueous solution is : $(K_b = 1.8 \times 10^{-5})$

(a) 11.13 (b) 12.5
(c) 13.42 (d) 11.55

13. Which of the following is not a Lewis base ?

(a) $NH_3$ (b) $H_2O$
(c) $AlCl_3$ (d) None of these

14. pH of a 0.0001 M HCl solution is

(a) 4.0 (b) 2.0
(c) 6.0 (c) 7.0

15. The pH of $10^{-8}$M NaOH aqueous solution at 25°C is

(a) 7.04 (b) 7.0
(c) 6.89 (d) 6.0

16. Which of the following statement is correct?

(a) The pH of $1.0 \times 10^{-8}$ M solution of HCl is 8
(b) The conjugate base of $H_2PO_4^-$ is $HPO_4^{2-}$
(c) Autoprotolysis constant of water decreases with temperature
(d) When a solution of a weak monoprotic acid is titrated against a strong base, at half-neutralisation point $pH = (1/2)pK_a$.

17. The dissociation constant of two acids $HA_1$ and $HA_2$ are $3.14 \times 10^{-4}$ and $1.96 \times 10^{-5}$ respectively. The relative strength of the acids will be approximately

(a) 1 : 4 (b) 4 : 1
(c) 1 : 16 (d) 16 : 1

**18.** 0.1 M $CH_3COOH$ solution is 1.34 % ionized At 298K. The ionization constant $K_a$ for acetic acid will be

(a) $1.8 \times 10^{-5}$ (b) $18.2 \times 10^{-5}$

(c) $0.18 \times 10^{-5}$ (d) None of these

**19.** Solubility of salt $A_2B_3$ is $1 \times 10^{-4}$, its solubility product is

(a) $1.08 \times 10^{20}$ (b) $1.08 \times 10^{18}$

(c) $2.6 \times 10^{-18}$ (d) $1.08 \times 10^{-18}$

**20.** The $pK_a$ of acetylsalicylic acid (aspirin) is 3.5. The pH of gastric juice in human stomach is about 2 – 3 and the pH in the small intestine is about 8. Aspirin will be

(a) unionised in the small intestine and in the stomach

(b) completely ionised in the small intestine and in the stomach

(c) ionised in the stomach and almost unionised in the small intestine

(d) ionised in the small intestine and almost unionised in the stomach

**21.** The solubility of AgI in NaI solution is less than that in pure water because :

(a) the temperature of the solution decreases

(b) solubility product of AgI is less than that of NaI

(c) of common ion effect

(d) AgI forms complex with NaI

**22.** Solubility product of $BaCl_2$ is $4 \times 10^{-9}$ mol/L. Its solubility would be :

(a) $1 \times 10^{-27}$ (b) $1 \times 10^{-3}$

(c) $1 \times 10^{-7}$ (d) $1 \times 10^{-2}$

**23.** In qualitative analysis, in III group, $NH_4Cl$ is added before $NH_4OH$ because

(a) to increase the concentration of $NH_4^+$ ions

(b) to increase the concentration of $Cl^-$ ions

(c) to reduce the concentration of $OH^-$ ions

(d) to increase the concentration of $OH^-$ ions

**24.** Match the columns

| Column-I | Column-II |
|---|---|
| (A) $HClO_4$ | (p) Strong base |
| (B) $HNO_2$ | (q) Strong acid |
| (C) $NH_2^-$ | (r) Weak base |
| (D) $HSO_4^-$ | (s) Weak acid |

(a) A – (r), B – (q), C – (p), D – (s)

(b) A – (q), B – (s), C – (p), D – (r)

(c) A – (r), B – (p), C – (q), D – (s)

(d) A – (s), B – (q), C – (p), D – (r)

**25.** In a gaseous reversible reaction

$$N_2(g) + O_2(g) \rightleftharpoons 2NO(g) + \text{heat}$$

if pressure is increased, then the equilibrium constant would be :

(a) unchanged

(b) increased

(c) decreased

(d) sometimes increased, sometimes decreased

**ANSWER KEY**

| | | | | | | | | | | | | | | | | | |
|---|---|---|---|---|---|---|---|---|---|---|---|---|---|---|---|---|---|
| 1 | (b) | 4 | (b) | 7 | (b) | 10 | (c) | 13 | (b) | 16 | (d) | 19 | (a) | 22 | (c) | 25 | (b) |
| 2 | (b) | 5 | (d) | 8 | (a) | 11 | (c) | 14 | (b) | 17 | (d) | 20 | (a) | 23 | (d) | | |
| 3 | (a) | 6 | (c) | 9 | (b) | 12 | (d) | 15 | (b) | 18 | (d) | 21 | (d) | 24 | (b) | | |

# REDOX REACTIONS

# 8

1. Which of the following is not an intermolecular redox reaction?

(a) $MgCO_3 \longrightarrow MgO + CO_2$

(b) $O_2 + 2H_2 \longrightarrow 2H_2O$

(c) $K + H_2O \longrightarrow KOH + (1/2)H_2$

(d) $MnBr_3 \longrightarrow MnBr_2 + (1/2)Br_2$

2. Which of the following involves transfer of five electrons ?

(a) $MnO_4^- \to Mn^{2+}$

(b) $CrO_4^{2-} \to Cr^{3+}$

(c) $MnO_4^{2-} \to MnO_2$

(d) $Cr_2O_7^{2-} \to 2Cr^{3+}$

3. In the reaction

$$Cr_2O_7^{2-} + 14H^+ + 6I^- \longrightarrow 2Cr^{3+} + 7H_2O + 3I_2$$

Which element is reduced ?

(a) I (b) O

(c) H (d) Cr

4. In the reaction, $H_2S + NO_2 \to H_2O + NO + S$, $H_2S$ is

(a) oxidised (b) reduced

(c) precipitated (d) None of these

5. One gas bleaches the colour of flowers by reduction, while the other by oxidation

(a) CO and $Cl_2$ (b) $SO_2$ and $Cl_2$

(c) $H_2S$ and $Br_2$ (d) $NH_3$ and $SO_2$

6. The conversion of sugar $C_{12}H_{22}O_{11} \to CO_2$ is

(a) oxidation

(b) reduction

(c) Both oxidation and reduction

(d) Neither oxidation nor reduction

7. Which one of the following cannot act as an oxidising agent ?

(a) $I^-$ (b) S(s)

(c) $NO_3^-$(aq) (d) $Cr_2O_7^{2-}$

8. In the reaction

$$HAsO_2 + Sn^{2+} \longrightarrow As + Sn^{4+} + H_2O$$ ,

oxidising agent is

(a) $Sn^{2+}$ (b) $Sn^{4+}$

(c) As (d) $HAsO_2$

9. Which halide is not oxidised by $MnO_2$
(a) F (b) Cl
(c) Br (d) I

10. Match the columns

| Column-I | Column-II |
|---|---|
| (A) $2Mg + O_2 \longrightarrow 2MgO$ | (p) Removal of hydrogen |
| (B) $Mg + Cl_2 \longrightarrow MgCl_2$ | (q) Oxidation of Iodine |
| (C) $2H_2S + O_2 \longrightarrow 2S + 2H_2O$ | (r) Addition of oxygen |
| (D) $2KI + H_2O + O_3 \longrightarrow 2KOH + I_2 + O_2$ | (s) Addition of electronegative element, chlorine |

(a) A – (s), B – (q), C – (p), D – (r)
(b) A – (r), B – (s), C – (p), D – (q)
(c) A – (s), B – (r), C – (q), D – (p)
(d) A – (r), B – (p), C – (s), D – (q)

11. In which of the following compounds, the oxidation state of transition metal is zero?
(a) $CrO_5$ (b) $Fe_3O_4$
(c) $FeSO_4$ (d) $Fe(CO)_5$

12. Oxidation number of N in $HNO_3$ is :
(a) –3.5 (b) +3.5
(c) –5 (d) +5

13. The oxidation number of chromium in potassium dichromate is
(a) +6 (b) –5
(c) –2 (d) +2

14. Oxidation number of cobalt in $K[Co(CO)_4]$ is
(a) +1 (b) +3
(c) –1 (d) –3

15. The oxidation state of Fe in $K_4[Fe(CN)_6]$ is
(a) +2 (b) +6
(c) +3 (d) +4

16. In which of the following compounds, the oxidation number of iodine is fractional ?
(a) $IF_7$ (b) $I_3^-$
(c) $IF_5$ (d) $IF_3$

17. In the reaction
$3Br_2 + 6CO_3^{2-} + 3H_2O \longrightarrow 5Br^- + BrO_3^- + 6HCO_3^-$
(a) Bromine is oxidised and carbonate is reduced
(b) Bromine is reduced and water is oxidised
(c) Bromine is neither reduced nor oxidised
(d) Bromine is both reduced and oxidised

18. In the redox reaction,
$xKMnO_4 + NH_3 \longrightarrow yKNO_3 + 8MnO_2 + 5KOH + 2H_2O$
(a) $x = 4, y = 6$ (b) $x = 3, y = 8$
(c) $x = 8, y = 6$ (d) $x = 8, y = 3$

19. The following species will not exhibit disproportionation reaction
(a) $ClO^-$ (b) $ClO_2^-$
(c) $ClO_3^-$ (d) $ClO_4^-$

20. Number of moles of $K_2Cr_2O_7$ reduced by one mole of $Sn^{2+}$ ions is
(a) 1/3 (b) 3
(c) 1/6 (d) 6

**ANSWER KEY**

| | | | | | | | | | | | | | | | | | | | |
|---|---|---|---|---|---|---|---|---|---|---|---|---|---|---|---|---|---|---|---|
| 1 | (a) | 4 | (a) | 7 | (a) | 10 | (b) | 13 | (a) | 16 | (b) | 19 | (d) | | | | | | |
| 2 | (a) | 5 | (b) | 8 | (d) | 11 | (d) | 14 | (c) | 17 | (d) | 20 | (a) | | | | | | |
| 3 | (d) | 6 | (a) | 9 | (a) | 12 | (d) | 15 | (a) | 18 | (d) | | | | | | | | |

# HYDROGEN

# 9

1. In para-hydrogen, spins of the electrons are in the
   (a) Same direction but those of the protons in opposite directions
   (b) Opposite directions but those of the protons in same directions
   (c) Same direction and so also the spins of the protons
   (d) Opposite directions and also the spins of the protons
2. Among $CaH_2$, $NH_3$, NaH and $B_2H_6$ which are covalent hydrides?
   (a) $NH_3$ and $B_2H_6$ (b) NaH and $CaH_2$
   (c) NaH and $NH_3$ (d) $CaH_2$ and $B_2H_6$
3. Which of the following is correct for hydrogen?
   (a) It can form bonds in +1 as well as –1 oxidation state.
   (b) It is collected at cathode.
   (c) It has a very high ionisation potential.
   (d) All of the above
4. The number of protons, electrons and neutrons in tritium are
   (a) 1 : 1 : 0 (b) 1 : 1 : 1
   (c) 1 : 1 : 2 (d) 1 : 2 : 1
5. Which of the following metal evolves hydrogen on reacting with cold dilute $HNO_3$ ?
   (a) Mg (b) Al
   (c) Fe (d) Cu
6. Hydrogen can behave as a metal
   (a) at very high temperature
   (b) at very low temperature
   (c) at very high pressure
   (d) at very low pressure
7. Hydrogen at room temperature contains :
   (a) 25% ortho + 75% para
   (b) 25% para + 75% ortho
   (c) 50% ortho + 50% para
   (d) 60% ortho + 34% para
8. One part of heavy water is present in X parts of ordinary water. Here X is
   (a) 10 (b) 60
   (c) 6000 (d) 600000

9. The low density of ice compared to water is due to
   (a) weak hydrogen bonding interactions
   (b) dipole-dipole interactions
   (c) dipole-induced dipole interactions
   (d) induced dipole-induced dipole interactions
10. Which one of the following metals will not reduce water?
   (a) Ca (b) Fe
   (c) Li (d) Cu
11. The maximum possible number of hydrogen bonds a water molecule can form is
   (a) 1 (b) 2
   (c) 3 (d) 4
12. The numbers of protons, electrons and neutrons in a molecule of heavy water are respectively :
   (a) 8, 10, 11 (b) 10, 10, 10
   (c) 10, 11, 10 (d) 11, 10, 10
13. Water is :
   (a) more polar than $H_2S$
   (b) more or less identical in polarity with $H_2S$
   (c) less polar than $H_2S$
   (d) None of these
14. The process used for the removal of permanent hardness of water is
   (a) Calgon (b) Baeyer
   (c) Serpeck (d) Hoope
15. The alum used for purifying water is
   (a) ferric alum (b) chrome alum
   (c) potash alum (d) ammonium alum
16. Triple point of water is
   (a) 273 K (b) 373 K
   (c) 203 K (d) 193 K
17. Hydrogen peroxide is not stored in glass bottles because
   (a) $SiO_2$ of the glass reacts with it
   (b) glass dissolves in it
   (c) light passes through glass
   (d) alkaline oxides in glass catalyze decomposition of $H_2O_2$
18. $H_2O_2$ is
   (a) Poor polar solvent than water
   (b) Better polar solvent than $H_2O$
   (c) Both have equal polarity
   (d) Better polar solvent but its strong auto-oxidising ability limits its use as such
19. Which substance does not speed up decomposition of $H_2O_2$?
   (a) Glycerol (b) Pt
   (c) Gold (d) $MnO_2$
20. Identify the structure of water in the gaseous phase
   (a) $H - \ddot{O} - H$
   (b) $H - \overset{+}{O} - H$ (with H below O)
   (c) 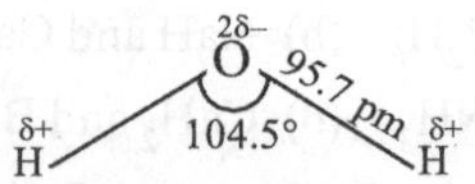

   (d) None of these

**ANSWER KEY**

| | | | | | | | | | | | | | | | |
|---|---|---|---|---|---|---|---|---|---|---|---|---|---|---|---|
| 1 | (d) | 4 | (c) | 7 | (b) | 10 | (d) | 13 | (a) | 16 | (a) | 19 | (a) | | |
| 2 | (a) | 5 | (a) | 8 | (c) | 11 | (d) | 14 | (a) | 17 | (d) | 20 | (c) | | |
| 3 | (a) | 6 | (c) | 9 | (a) | 12 | (b) | 15 | (c) | 18 | (d) | | | | |

# THE *s*-BLOCK ELEMENTS

# 10

1. Which of the following elements combines directly with nitrogen to form its nitride?
   (a) Li (b) Na
   (c) K (d) Rb
2. $KO_2$ is used in oxygen cylinders in space and submarines because it:
   (a) Absorbs $CO_2$ and increases $O_2$ content
   (b) Eliminates moisture
   (c) Absorbs $CO_2$
   (d) Produces ozone
3. Among the alkali metals cesium is the most reactive because
   (a) it has incomplete shell which is nearest to the nucleus.
   (b) it has a single electron in the valence shell.
   (c) it is the heaviest alkali metal.
   (d) the outermost electron is more loosely bounded than the outermost electron of the other alkali metals.
4. Among the carbonates of alkali metals which one has highest thermal stability?
   (a) $Cs_2CO_3$ (b) $Rb_2CO_3$
   (c) $K_2CO_3$ (d) $Na_2CO_3$
5. Metal $M + \text{air} \xrightarrow{\Delta} A \xrightarrow{H_2O} B \xrightarrow{HCl}$ White fumes; Metal M can be :
   (a) Li, Mg (b) Li, Al or K
   (c) Na, K or Mg (d) Li, Na or K
6. The correct order of the mobility of the alkali metal ions in aqueous solutions is
   (a) $Na^+ > K^+ > Rb^+ > Li^+$
   (b) $K^+ > Rb^+ > Na^+ > Li^+$
   (c) $Rb^+ > K^+ > Na^+ > Li^+$
   (d) $Li^+ > Na^+ > K^+ > Rb^+$
7. Which compound will show the highest lattice energy ?
   (a) RbF (b) CsF
   (c) NaF (d) KF
8. For which one of the following minerals, the composition given is incorrect?
   (a) Soda ash — $(Na_2CO_3)$
   (b) Carnallite — $(KCl \cdot MgCl_2 \cdot 6H_2O)$
   (c) Borax — $(Na_2B_4O_7 \cdot 7H_2O)$
   (d) Glauber's salt — $(Na_2SO_4 \cdot 10H_2O)$

**9.** Which of the following oxides is not expected to react with sodium hydroxide?

(a) CaO (b) $SiO_2$

(c) BeO (d) $B_2O_3$

**10.** Which of the following is known as fusion mixture?

(a) Mixture of $Na_2CO_3 + NaHCO_3$

(b) $Na_2CO_3.10H_2O$

(c) Mixture of $K_2CO_3 + Na_2CO_3$

(d) $NaHCO_3$

**11.** Graham's salt can be represented as

(a) $Na_2CO_3$ (b) $Ca_3(PO_4)_2$

(c) $(NaPO_3)_6$ (d) none of these

**12.** Match the following items in **column I** with the corresponding items in **column II**.

| Column-I | Column-II |
|---|---|
| (i) $Na_2CO_3.10H_2O$ | (A) Portland cement ingredient |
| (ii) $Mg(HCO_3)_2$ | (B) Castner-Kellner process |
| (iii) NaOH | (C) Solvay process |
| (iv) $Ca_3Al_2O_6$ | (D) Temporary hardness |

(a) (i) ⟶ (B); (ii) ⟶ (C); (iii) ⟶ (A); (iv) ⟶ (D)

(b) (i) ⟶ (C); (ii) ⟶ (B); (iii) ⟶ (D); (iv) ⟶ (A)

(c) (i) ⟶ (D); (ii) ⟶ (A); (iii) ⟶ (B); (iv) ⟶ (C)

(d) (i) ⟶ (C); (ii) ⟶ (D); (iii) ⟶ (B); (iv) ⟶ (A)

**13.** The metal used for making X-ray tube window is:

(a) Mg (b) Na

(c) Be (d) Ca

**14.** Which of the following bicarbonate is least soluble in water?

(a) $Mg(HCO_3)_2$ (b) $NaHCO_3$

(c) $KHCO_3$ (d) $Ca(HCO_3)_2$

**15.** Mg burns in air to give

(a) $Mg_3N_2$

(b) MgO

(c) MgO and $Mg_3N_2$

(d) $MgCO_3$

**16.** Which is not obtained when metal carbides react with $H_2O$?

(a) $Al_4C_3 + H_2O \longrightarrow CH \equiv CH$

(b) $CaC_2 + H_2O \longrightarrow CH \equiv CH$

(c) $Mg_4C_3 + H_2O \longrightarrow CH_3C \equiv CH$

(d) $Be_2C + H_2O \longrightarrow CH_4$

**17.** The correct order of thermal stability of hydroxides is:

(a) $Ba(OH)_2 < Ca(OH)_2 < Sr(OH)_2 < Mg(OH)_2$

(b) $Mg(OH)_2 < Sr(OH)_2 < Ca(OH)_2 < Ba(OH)_2$

(c) $Mg(OH)_2 < Ca(OH)_2 < Sr(OH)_2 < Ba(OH)_2$

(d) $Ba(OH)_2 < Sr(OH)_2 < Ca(OH)_2 < Mg(OH)_2$

**18.** Which of the following has maximum lattice energy?

(a) $Li_2O$ (b) $Na_2O$

(c) MgO (d) $K_2O$

**19.** Colemanite is

(a) $Ca[B_3O_4(OH)_2].2H_2O$

(b) $Ca_2B_6O_{11}.5H_2O$

(c) $Ca(OH)_2$

(d) $Na_2B_4O_7.2H_2O$

**20.** Which one of the following is flourspar?

(a) $CaF_2$ (b) CaO

(c) $H_2F_2$ (d) $CaCO_3$

**ANSWER KEY**

| 1 | (a) | 3 | (d) | 5 | (a) | 7 | (c) | 9 | (a) | 11 | (c) | 13 | (c) | 15 | (c) | 17 | (d) | 19 | (b) |
|---|---|---|---|---|---|---|---|---|---|---|---|---|---|---|---|---|---|---|---|
| 2 | (a) | 4 | (a) | 6 | (c) | 8 | (c) | 10 | (c) | 12 | (d) | 14 | (a) | 16 | (a) | 18 | (c) | 20 | (a) |

# 11 THE *p*-BLOCK ELEMENTS (GROUP 13 AND GROUP 14)

1. $Na_2B_4O_7 . 10H_2O$ is correctly represented as
   (a) $2NaBO_2 . Na_2B_2O_2 . 10H_2O$
   (b) $Na_2[B_4O_5(OH)_4] . 8H_2O$
   (c) $Na_2[B_4(H_2O)_4O_7] . 6H_2O$
   (d) All of the above

2. $AlCl_3$ is an electron-deficient compound but $AlF_3$ is not, because
   (a) Atomic size of F is smaller than Cl, which makes $AlF_3$ more covalent.
   (b) $AlCl_3$ is a covalent compound while $AlF_3$ is an ionic compound.
   (c) Al in $AlCl_3$ is $sp^3$ hybridised but in $AlF_3$, Al is $sp^2$ hybridised.
   (d) $AlCl_3$ exists as a dimer but $AlF_3$ does not.

3. Aluminium chloride exists as a dimer because aluminium has:
   (a) Greater ionisation enthalpy
   (b) Incomplete *p*-orbital
   (c) High nuclear charge
   (d) Larger radius

4. In the commercial electrochemical process for aluminium extraction, the electrolyte used is
   (a) $Al(OH)_3$ in NaOH solution
   (b) An aqueous solution of $Al_2(SO_4)_3$.
   (c) A molten mixture of $Al_2O_3$ and $Na_3AlF_6$
   (d) A molten mixture of AlO(OH) and $Al(OH)_3$

5. Thermite is a mixture of :
   (a) $Cr_2O_3 + Al_2O_3$ (b) $Fe_2O_3 + Al$
   (c) $Fe_2O_3 + Al_2O_3$ (d) $Al_2O_2 + 2\,Cr$

6. Which of the following method is not used for extraction of Al?
   (a) van Arkel
   (b) Serpeck's process
   (c) Baeyer's process
   (d) Hall-Heroult's process

7. Amphoteric oxide among the following is –
   (a) $B_2O_3$ (b) $Ga_2O_3$
   (c) $In_2O_3$ (d) $Tl_2O_3$

8. In the electrolytic extraction of aluminium, cryolite is used
   (a) to obtain more aluminium
   (b) to decrease temperature to dissolve bauxite
   (c) to protect the anode
   (d) as reducing agent

9. In aqueous solution GaCl disproportionates to
(a) $GaCl_2$ and $GaCl_3$
(b) Ga and $GaCl_3$
(c) $GaCl_2$ and Ga
(d) $GaCl_3$ and $GaCl_5$

10. Which of the following statement is false about carbon?
(a) $C_{60}$ is also one of the allotrope of carbon.
(b) It has crystalline as well as amorphous allotropes.
(c) It can form $p_\pi - p_\pi$ bond with other C-atoms.
(d) It cannot form $p_\pi - p_\pi$ bond with atoms such as N and O.

11. 'Softening of lead' means :
(a) Conversion of lead to PbO.
(b) Conversion of lead to $Pb_3O_4$.
(c) Removal of impurities (metallic) from lead.
(d) Washing lead with $HNO_3$ followed by a dilute alkali solution.

12. Structure of silicates in which three oxygen atoms of $[SiO_4]^{4-}$ are shared is :
(a) Pyrosilicate
(b) Sheet silicate
(c) Linear chain silicate
(d) Three dimensional silicate

13. Lead pipes are not suitable for drinking water because
(a) Lead forms basic lead carbonate
(b) Lead reacts with water containing air to form $Pb(OH)_2$
(c) A layer of lead dioxide is deposited over pipes
(d) Lead reacts with air to form litharge

14. The element that shows greater ability to form $p_\pi - p_\pi$ multiple bonds, is :
(a) Sn (b) C
(c) Ge (d) Si

15. The reducing power of divalent species decreases in the order
(a) Ge > Sn > Pb (b) Sn > Ge > Pb
(c) Pb > Sn > Ge (d) None of these

16. Glass is a
(a) liquid
(b) solid
(c) supercooled liquid
(d) transparent organic polymer

17. Red lead is:
(a) $Pb_3O_4$ (b) $Pb_2O_3$
(c) $Pb_2O$ (d) PbO

18. Litharge is chemically
(a) PbO (b) $PbO_2$
(c) $Pb_3O_4$ (d) $Pb(CH_3COO)_2$

19. Graphite conducts electricity because of :
(a) Weak van der Waal's forces between layers
(b) Covalent bonding between carbon atoms of layers
(c) Delocalized electrons in each layer
(d) $sp^2$ hybridisation of carbon atoms in a layer

20. When tin is treated with concentrated nitric acid:
(a) It is converted into stannous nitrate.
(b) It becomes passive.
(c) It converted into stannic nitrate.
(d) It is converted into metastannic acid.

21. White lead is
(a) $PbCO_3$
(b) $PbCO_3 . PbO$
(c) $2PbCO_3 . Pb(OH)_2$
(d) $2PbSO_4 . PbO$

22. The element that does NOT show catenation is:
(a) Ge (b) Si
(c) Sn (d) Pb

23. Match the columns

| Column-I | Column-II |
|---|---|
| (A) Borazine | (p) $CaSO_4 \cdot \frac{1}{2} H_2O$ |
| (B) Plaster of Paris | (q) $C_{60}$ |
| (C) Boric acid | (r) $SiO_2$ |
| (D) Quartz | (s) $B_3N_3H_6$ |
| (E) Buckminsterfullerene | (t) $H_3BO_3$ |

(a) A – (r); B – (p); C – (q); D – (t); E – (s)
(b) A – (p); B – (t); C – (r); D – (s); E – (q)
(c) A – (t); B – (q); C – (p); D – (r); E – (s)
(d) A – (s); B – (p); C – (t); D – (r); E – (q)

24. Which of the following metals burn in air at high temperature with the evolution of heat ?

(a) Cu (b) Hg
(c) Pb (d) Al

25. In the reaction $B_2O_3 + C + Cl_2 \rightarrow A + CO$. The A is

(a) $BCl_3$ (b) $BCl_2$
(c) $B_2Cl_2$ (d) $CCl_2$

**ANSWER KEY**

| | | | | | | | | | | | | | | | | | |
|---|---|---|---|---|---|---|---|---|---|---|---|---|---|---|---|---|---|
| 1 | (b) | 4 | (c) | 7 | (b) | 10 | (d) | 13 | (b) | 16 | (c) | 19 | (c) | 22 | (d) | 25 | (a) |
| 2 | (b) | 5 | (b) | 8 | (b) | 11 | (c) | 14 | (b) | 17 | (a) | 20 | (d) | 23 | (d) | | |
| 3 | (b) | 6 | (a) | 9 | (b) | 12 | (b) | 15 | (a) | 18 | (a) | 21 | (c) | 24 | (d) | | |

# 12

# ORGANIC CHEMISTRY – SOME BASIC PRINCIPLES AND TECHNIQUES

1. What is the IUPAC name of the compound ?

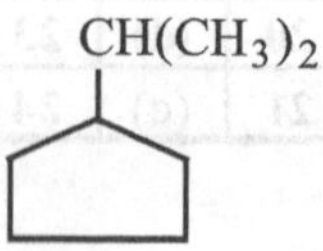


(a) 1, 1 - Dimethyl - 1 - cyclopentyl methane
(b) 2 - Cyclopentyl propane
(c) 1 - (1 - Methyl) ethyl cyclopentane
(d) Cumene

2. The number of secondary hydrogens in 2, 2-dimethylbutane is :
(a) 8 (b) 6
(c) 4 (d) 2

3. Maleic acid and fumaric acids are
(a) Chain isomers (b) Functional isomers
(c) Tautomers (d) Geometrical isomers

4. Which of the following is optically active
(a) *n* - Propanol (b) 2 - Chlorobutane
(c) *n* - Butanol (d) 3 - Hydroxy pentane

5. Ethoxy ethane and methoxy propane are
(a) geometrical isomers
(b) optical isomers
(c) functional group isomers
(d) metamers

6. An important chemical method to resolve a racemic mixture makes use of the formation of
(a) a meso compound
(b) enantiomers
(c) diasteromers
(d) racemates

7. Tautomerism will be exhibited by
(a) $(CH_3)_2NH$ (b) $(CH_3)_3CNO$
(c) $R_3CNO_2$ (d) $RCH_2NO_2$

8. Number of chiral carbons in

$\beta - D - (+) -$ glucose is
(a) five (b) six
(c) three (d) four

9. Which one of the following pairs represents stereoisomerism?
(a) Structural isomerism and geometrical isomerism
(b) Optical isomerism and geometrical isomerism
(c) Chain isomerism and rotational isomerism.
(d) Linkage isomerism and geometrical isomerism

**10.** How many optically active stereoisomers are possible for lactic acid ?

(a) 1 (b) 2

(c) 4 (d) 3

**11.** Keto-enol tautomerism is observed in :

(a) $H_5C_6-\overset{\overset{O}{\|}}{C}-CH_2-\overset{\overset{O}{\|}}{C}-C_6H_5$

(b) $H_5C_6-\overset{\overset{O}{\|}}{C}-CH_3$

(c) $H_5C_6-\overset{\overset{O}{\|}}{C}-H$

(d) Both (a) and (b)

**12.** The correct statement about the compounds (A), (B) and (C) is :

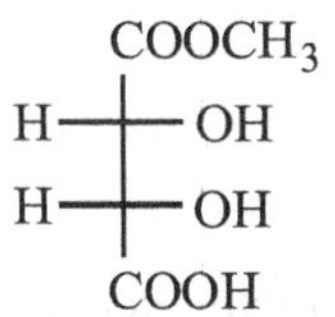

(A)

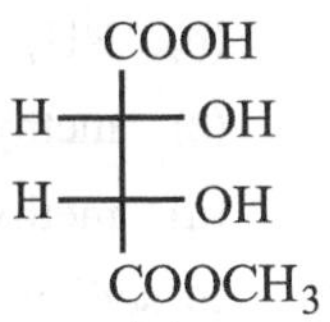

(B)

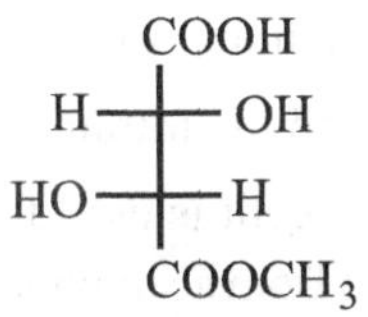

(C)

(a) (A) and (B) are identical

(b) (A) and (B) are diastereomers

(c) (A) and (C) are enantiomers

(d) (A) and (B) are enantiomers

**13.** The molecular formula of diphenylmethane,

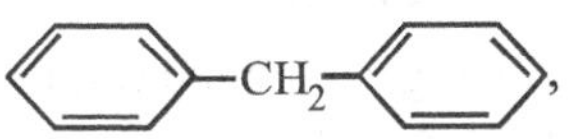

, is $C_{13}H_{12}$.

How many structural isomers are possible when one of the hydrogens is replaced by a chlorine atom?

(a) 6 (b) 4

(c) 8 (d) 7

**14.** Dipole moment is shown by

(a) 1, 2-dichlorobenzene

(b) *trans*- 2, 3-dichloro-2-butene

(c) 1, 4-chlorobenzene

(d) *trans*-1, 2-dinitroethene

**15.** $CH_3-\overset{\overset{O}{\|}}{C}\underset{a}{-}O\underset{b}{-}CH_3$;

The correct relation between the bond lengths *a* and *b* is:

(a) $a = b$ (b) $b > a$

(c) $b < a$ (d) Impossible to predict

**16.** One among the following compounds will not give effervescence with sodium carbonate:

(a) $C_6H_5CO_2H$ (b) 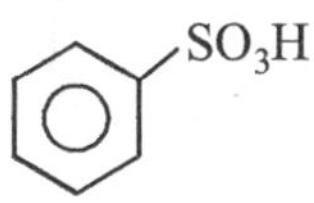

(c) $C_6H_5OH$ (d) 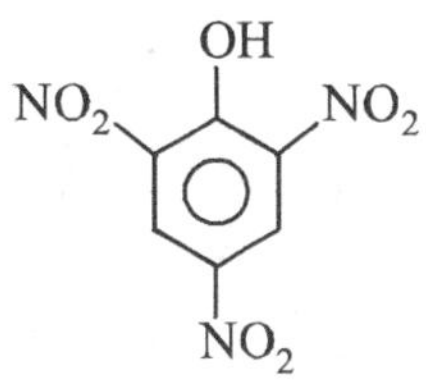

**17.** Which of the following alkenes is the most stable?

(a) 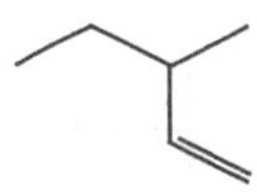 (b) 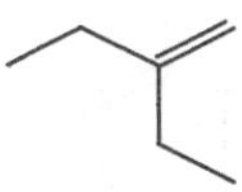

(c) 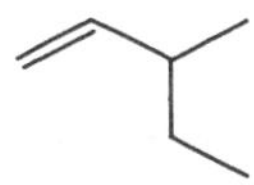 (d) 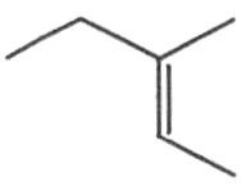

**18.** The addition of HBr on but-2-ene in presence of peroxide follows the

(a) electrophilic addition

(b) free radical addition

(c) nucleophilic addition

(d) None of these

**19.** Of the following compounds which will have a zero dipole moment

(a) 1, 1 - Dichloroethylene

(b) *trans* -1, 2 - Dichloroethylene

(c) *cis* - 1 , 2 - Dichloroethylene

(d) None of these

**20.** Which of the following will show aromatic behaviour ?

(a) 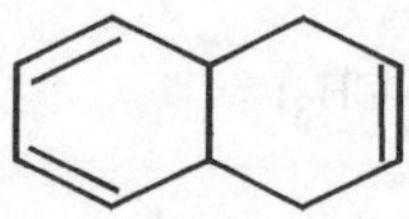

(b) 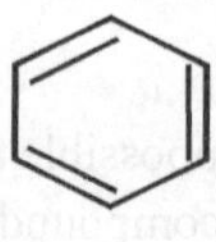

(c) 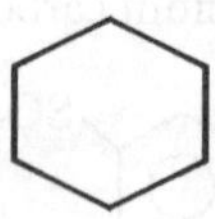

(d) 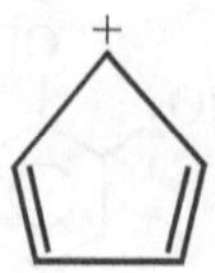

**21.** Which of the following reactions cannot proceed by $S_N1$ mechanism ?

(a) 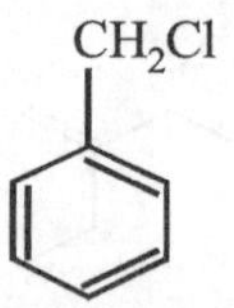
(b) 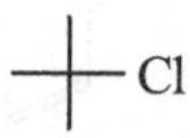

(c) 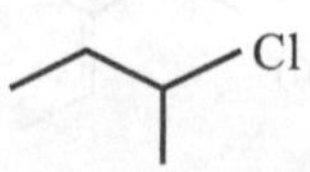
(d) 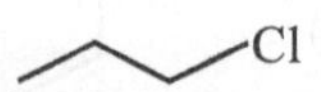

**22.** The correct order regarding the electronegativity of hybrid orbitals of carbon is

(a) $sp > sp^2 > sp^3$ (b) $sp < sp^2 > sp^3$

(c) $sp < sp^2 < sp^3$ (d) $sp > sp^2 < sp^3$

**23.** The increasing order of stability of the following free radicals is

(a) $(C_6H_5)_2\dot{C}H < (C_6H_5)_3\dot{C} < (CH_3)_3\dot{C} < (CH_3)_2\dot{C}H$

(b) $(CH_3)_2\dot{C}H < (CH_3)_3\dot{C} < (C_6H_5)_2\dot{C}H < (C_6H_5)_3\dot{C}$

(c) $(CH_3)_3\dot{C} < (CH_3)_2\dot{C}H < (C_6H_5)_2\dot{C}H < (C_6H_5)_3\dot{C}$

(d) $(C_6H_5)_3\dot{C} < (C_6H_5)_2\dot{C}H < (CH_3)_3\dot{C} < (CH_3)_2\dot{C}H$

**24.** The number of σ and π bonds in a molecule of acetonitrile are respectively

(a) 2, 5 (b) 3, 4

(c) 4, 3 (d) 5, 2

**25.** The shape of methyl carbanion is similar to that of –

(a) $BF_3$

(b) $NH_3$

(c) methyl free radical

(d) methyl carbocation

**26.** In sodium fusion test of organic compounds, the nitrogen of the organic compound is converted into

(a) sodamide (b) sodium cyanide

(c) sodium nitrite (d) sodium nitrate

**27.** Which of the following reagent is used for the separation of acetaldehyde from acetophenone?

(a) $NH_2OH$ (b) NaOI

(c) Tollen's reagent (d) $C_6H_5NHNH_2$

**28.** The Beilstein test for organic compounds is used to detect

(a) nitrogen (b) sulphur

(c) carbon (d) halogens

**29.** Which of the following compound cannot used in preparation of iodoform?

(a) $CH_3CHO$ (b) $CH_3COCH_3$

(c) HCHO (d) 2- Propanol

**30.** Lassaigne's test for the detection of nitrogen fails in

(a) $NH_2CONHNH_2.HCl$

(b) $NH_2NH_2.HCl$

(c) $NH_2CONH_2$

(d) $C_6H_5NHNH_2.HCl$

| ANSWER KEY | | | | | | | | | | | | | | | | | |
|---|---|---|---|---|---|---|---|---|---|---|---|---|---|---|---|---|---|
| **1** | (c) | **5** | (d) | **9** | (b) | **13** | (b) | **17** | (d) | **21** | (d) | **25** | (b) | **29** | (c) | | |
| **2** | (d) | **6** | (c) | **10** | (b) | **14** | (a) | **18** | (b) | **22** | (a) | **26** | (b) | **30** | (b) | | |
| **3** | (d) | **7** | (d) | **11** | (d) | **15** | (b) | **19** | (b) | **23** | (b) | **27** | (c) | | | | |
| **4** | (b) | **8** | (a) | **12** | (d) | **16** | (c) | **20** | (b) | **24** | (d) | **28** | (d) | | | | |

# 13

# HYDROCARBONS

1. Which of the following compounds can best be prepared by Wurtz reaction?
   (a) Iso-butane (b) *n*-butane
   (c) *n*-Pentane (d) Iso-pentane
2. The highest boiling point is expected for :
   (a) iso-octane
   (b) *n*-octane
   (c) 2, 2, 3, 3-tetramethylbutane
   (d) *n*-butane
3. The major product obtained in the photo catalysed bromination of 2-methylbutane is
   (a) 1-bromo-2-methylbutane
   (b) 1-bromo-3-methylbutane
   (c) 2-bromo-3-methylbutane
   (d) 2-bromo-2-methylbutane
4. Which of the following is the least stable conformer of cyclohexane?

   (a) 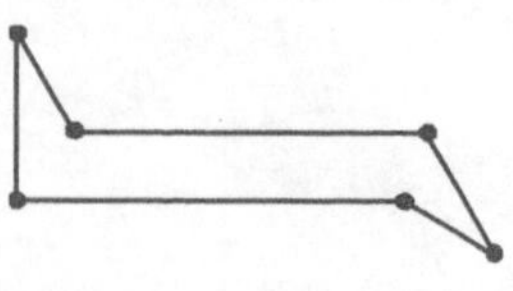

   (Chair)

   (b) 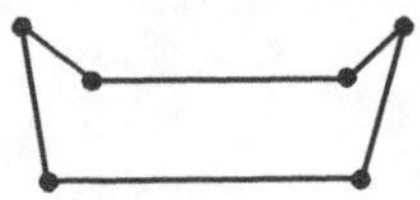

   (Boat)

   (c) 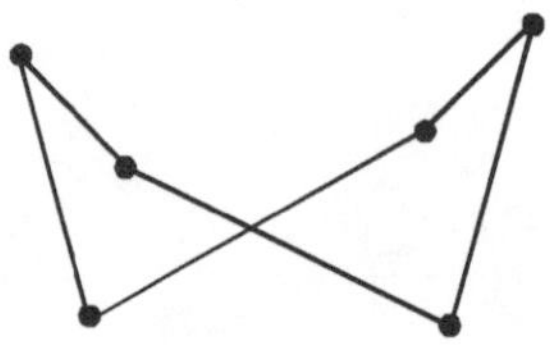

   (d) 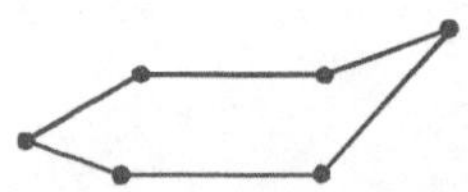
5. The addition of HBr is easiest with :
   (a) $(CH_3)_2C=CH_2$ (b) $CH_3-CH=CH_2$
   (c) $ClCH=CHCl$ (d) $CH_2=CH-Cl$
6. Anti-Markovnikoff addition of HBr is not observed in :
   (a) propene (b) 1-butene
   (c) but-2-ene (d) pent-2-ene

7. Butene-1 may be converted to butane by reaction with
   (a) Sn – HCl (b) Zn – Hg
   (c) $Pd/H_2$ (d) Zn – HCl

8. The most reactive hydrocarbon towards electrophiles is :
   (a) ethane (b) methane
   (c) acetylene (d) ethylene

9. Which of the following has highest knocking ?
   (a) Olefins
   (b) Branched chain olefins
   (c) Straight chain olefins
   (d) Aromatic hydrocarbons

10. The compound most likely to decolourise a solution of alkaline $KMnO_4$ is :
   (a) $CH_3CH = CHCH_2CH_2CH_3$
   (b) $C_{10}H_{22}$
   (c) $CH_3 - CH_3$
   (d) $(CH_3)_4C$

11. Which one of the following compounds gives acetone $(CH_3)_2C{=}O$ as one of the products of its ozonolysis?

(a) 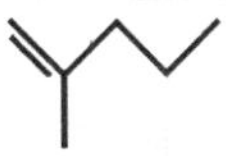 (b) 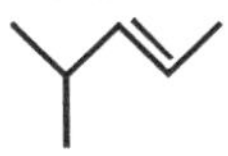

(c) 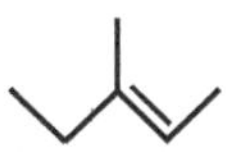 (d) 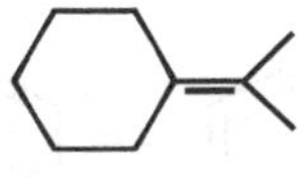

12. Acetylenic hydrogens are acidic because
   (a) sigma electron density of C – H bond in acetylene is nearer to carbon, which has 50% *s*-character
   (b) acetylene has only open hydrogen in each carbon
   (c) acetylene contains least number of hydrogens among the possible hydrocarbons having two carbons
   (d) acetylene belongs to the class of alkynes with molecular formula, $C_nH_{2n-2}$.

13. $R - CH_2 - CCl_2 - R \xrightarrow{\text{Reagent}} R - C \equiv C - R$
   The reagent is
   (a) Na
   (b) $NaNH_2$
   (c) KOH in $C_2H_5OH$
   (d) both (b) and (c)

14. Which of these will not react with acetylene?
   (a) NaOH (b) Ammonical $AgNO_3$
   (c) Na (d) HCl.

15. Ammonical silver nitrate forms a white precipitate easily with
   (a) $CH_3C \equiv CH$ (b) $CH_3C \equiv CCH_3$
   (c) $CH_3CH = CH_2$ (d) $CH_2 = CH_2$

16. What is the end product of the following sequence of operations?

$$CaC_2 \xrightarrow{H_2O} A \xrightarrow[Hg^{++}]{dil.H_2SO_4} B \xrightarrow[H_2]{Ni} C$$

   (a) Methyl alcohol (b) Acetaldehyde
   (c) $C_2H_5OH$ (d) $C_2H_4$

17. Which of the following is not an aromatic compound?

(a) 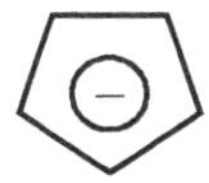 (b) 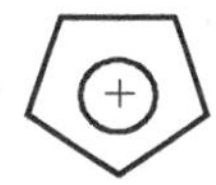

(c) 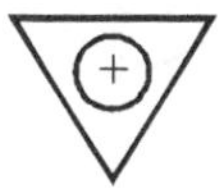 (d) 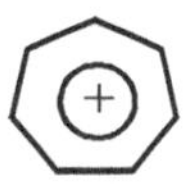

18. The compound X in the reaction.

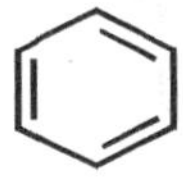 $+ ICl \xrightarrow{\text{anhydrous } AlCl_3} X$

(a) 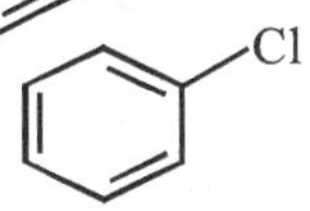 (b) 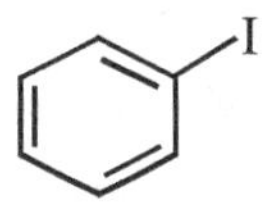

(c) 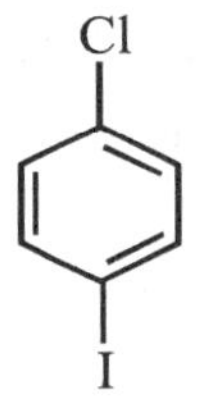 (d) 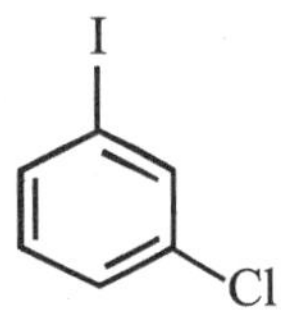

**19.** Which of the following would not give 2-phenylbutane as the major product in a Friedal-Craft's alkylation of benzene?

(a) 1-butene + HF

(b) 2-butanol + $H_2SO_4$

(c) Butanoyl chloride + $AlCl_3$ then Zn, HCl

(d) Butyl chloride + $AlCl_3$

**20.** The product of the reaction between ethyl benzene and N-bromosuccinimide is

(a) 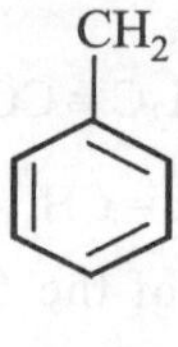

(b) 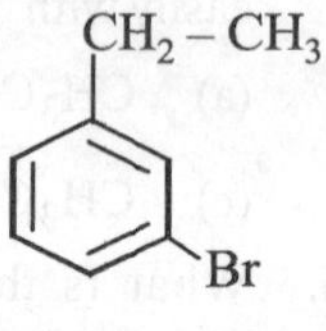

(c) 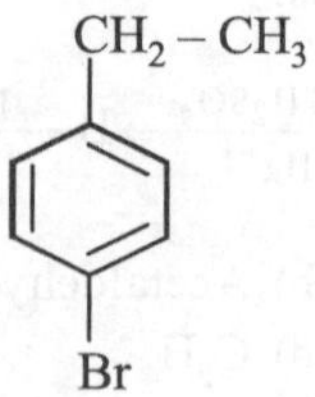

(d) 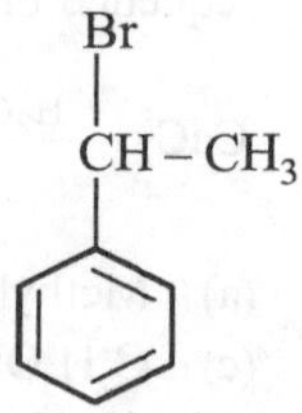

**21.** Which of the following will have fastest rate of reaction with $Br_2/FeBr_3$?

(a) 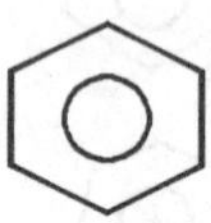

(b) 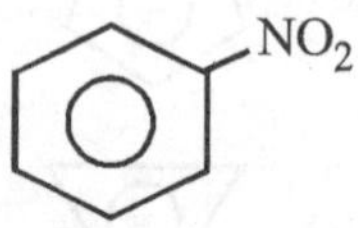

(c) 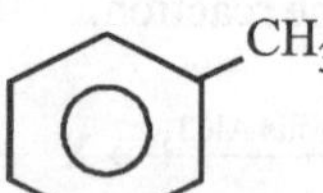

(d) 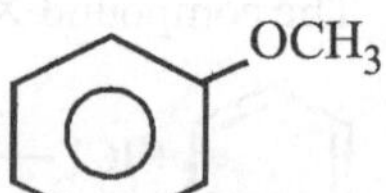

**22.** *n*-Butylbenzene on oxidation will give

(a) benzoic acid (b) butanoic acid

(c) benzyl alcohol (d) benzaldehyde

**23.** During nitration of benzene with nitrating mixture, $HNO_3$ acts as

(a) an acid (b) a base

(c) catalyst (d) reducing agent.

**24.** Nitration of toluene using fuming sulphuric and nitric acid gives :

(a) *p*-nitrotoluene (b) *o*-nitrotoluene

(c) *m*-nitrotoluene (d) *tri*-nitrotoluene

**25.** Resonance energy of benzene represents :

(a) stability of benzene

(b) energy required to break C – C bond

(c) energy required to break C – H bond

(d) energy for 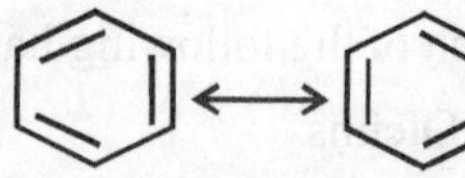

**26.** Toluene on treatment with $CrO_3$ and $(CH_3CO)_2O$ followed by hydrolysis with dil.HCl gives

(a) benzaldehyde (b) benzoic acid

(c) phenol (d) phenylacetaldehyde

**27.** Aromatic compounds burn with sooty flame because

(a) they have a ring structure of carbon atoms

(b) they have relatively high percentage of hydrogen

(c) they have relatively high percentage of carbon

(d) they resist reaction with oxygen of air

**28.** Match the columns

| Column-I | Column-II |
|---|---|
| (A) 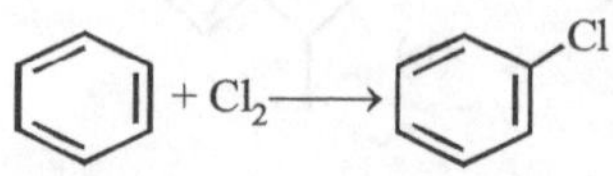 | (p) $Cl_2$, uv, 500 K |
| (B) 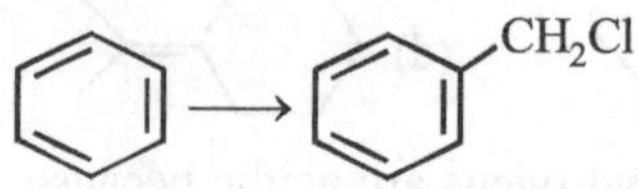 | (q) anhy. $AlCl_3$ |
| (C) 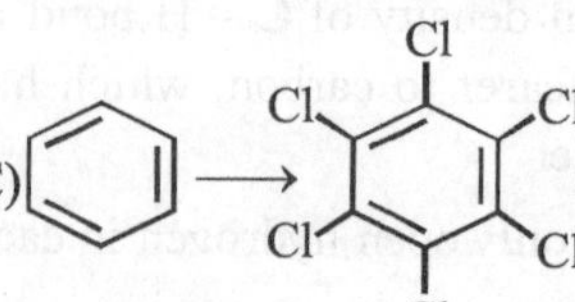 | (r) $CH_2Cl_2$, anhy. $AlCl_3$ |
| (D) 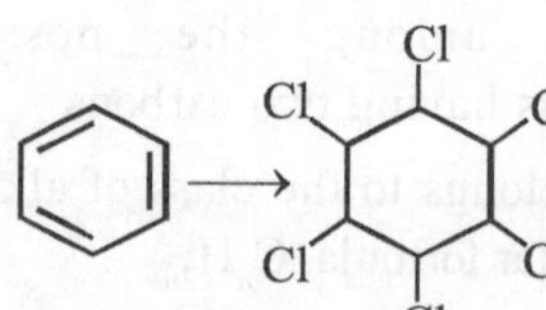 | (s) $Cl_2$, anhy. $AlCl_3$, |

(a) A – (s), B – (r), C – (q), D – (p)

(b) A – (q), B – (r), C – (s), D – (p)

(c) A – (r), B – (p), C – (q), D – (s)

(d) A – (q), B – (p), C – (s), D – (r)

**29.** In the reaction

$$CH_3C \equiv C^-Na^+ + (CH_3)_2CH - Cl \longrightarrow ?$$

the product formed is :

(a) propene

(b) propyne

(c) propyne and propene

(d) 4-methylpentyne-2

**30.** The correct order for acid strength of compounds $CH{\equiv}CH_2$, $CH_3{-}C{\equiv}CH$ and $CH_2{=}CH_2$ is as follows:

(a) $CH{\equiv}CH > CH_2{=}CH_2 > CH_3{-}C{\equiv}CH$

(b) $CH_3{-}C{\equiv}CH > CH{\equiv}CH > CH_2{=}CH_2$

(c) $CH_3{-}C{\equiv}CH > CH_2{=}CH_2 > HC{\equiv}CH$

(d) $HC{\equiv}CH > CH_3{-}C{\equiv}CH > CH_2{=}CH_2$

## ANSWER KEY

| | | | | | | | | | | | | | | | | | |
|---|---|---|---|---|---|---|---|---|---|---|---|---|---|---|---|---|---|
| 1 | (b) | 5 | (a) | 9 | (c) | 13 | (d) | 17 | (b) | 21 | (d) | 25 | (a) | 29 | (c) | | |
| 2 | (b) | 6 | (c) | 10 | (a) | 14 | (a) | 18 | (b) | 22 | (a) | 26 | (a) | 30 | (d) | | |
| 3 | (d) | 7 | (c) | 11 | (d) | 15 | (a) | 19 | (c) | 23 | (b) | 27 | (c) | | | | |
| 4 | (d) | 8 | (d) | 12 | (a) | 16 | (c) | 20 | (d) | 24 | (d) | 28 | (b) | | | | |

# 14

# ENVIRONMENTAL CHEMISTRY

1. An increase in $CO_2$ concentration in the atmosphere will result in
   (a) adverse effects of natural vegetation
   (b) global warming
   (c) temperature decrease in global atmosphere
   (d) genetic disorders in plants and animals
2. Which one is not main pollutant from automobile exhaust?
   (a) CO (b) Acrolin
   (c) NO (d) hydrocarbons
3. Ultraviolet radiation is absorbed by
   (a) exosphere (b) ionosphere
   (c) mesosphere (d) stratosphere
4. Persons working in cement plants and lime stone quarries are more prone to disease like:
   (a) asthma (b) cancer
   (c) silicosis (d) pneumoconiosis
5. Peroxyacetyl nitrate (PAN), an eye irritant is produced by :
   (a) classical smog (b) acid rain
   (c) organic waste (d) photochemical smog
6. Identify the pollutant gases largely responsible for the discoloured and lustreless nature of marble of the Taj Mahal.
   (a) $O_3$ and $CO_2$ (b) $CO_2$ and $NO_2$
   (c) $SO_2$ and $NO_2$ (d) $SO_2$ and $O_3$
7. Which of the following is a set of green house gases ?
   (a) $CH_4, O_3, N_2, SO_2$
   (b) $O_3, N_2, CO_2, NO_2$
   (c) $O_3, NO_2, SO_2, Cl_2$
   (d) $CO_2, CH_4, N_2O, O_3$
8. High concentration of which of the following in atmosphere leads to stiffness of flower buds which eventually fall off from plants?
   (a) $NO_2$ (b) $SO_2$
   (c) CFC (d) Smog
9. Which is related to 'Green House Effect'?
   (a) Farming of green plants
   (b) Farming of vegetables in houses
   (c) Global warming
   (d) Biodegradable pollutant
10. Which of the following strategy is not a correct approach to reduce global warming ?
    (a) Reducing the green house gas emission by limiting the use of fossil fuels.
    (b) Increase the vegetation cover particularly the forest for photosynthetic utilization of $CO_2$.
    (c) Minimizing the use of nitrogen fertilizers in agriculture for reducing $N_2O$ emission.
    (d) Increasing the use of air conditioners, refrigeration unit and production of plastic foams and propellants in aerosal spray cans.

11. Photochemical smog formed in congested metropolitan cities mainly consists of
    (a) ozone, peroxyacetyl nitrate and $NO_x$
    (b) smoke, peroxyacetyl nitrate and $SO_2$
    (c) hydrocarbons, $SO_2$ and $CO_2$
    (d) hydrocarbons, ozone and $SO_x$

12. Which of the following is the major cause of global warming?
    (a) Re-radiation of U.V. rays by $CO_2$ and $H_2O$
    (b) Re-radiation of I.R. rays by $CO_2$ and $H_2O$
    (c) Re-radiation of I.R. rays by $O_2$ and $N_2$
    (d) Re-radiation of U.V. rays by $O_2$ and $N_2$

13. Green chemistry means such reactions which
    (a) produce colour during reactions.
    (b) reduce the use and production of hazardous chemicals.
    (c) are related to the depletion of ozone layer.
    (d) study the reactions in plants.

14. BHC and DDT act as:
    (a) carcinogens (b) allergens
    (c) asthmatic agents (d) all of these

15. Biochemical Oxygen Demand, (BOD) is a measure of organic material present in water. BOD value less than 5 ppm indicates a water sample to be
    (a) rich in dissolved oxygen
    (b) poor in dissolved oxygen
    (c) highly polluted
    (d) not suitable for aquatic life

16. Addition of phosphate fertilisers to water bodies causes:
    (a) increase in amount of dissolved oxygen in water
    (b) deposition of calcium phosphate
    (c) increase in fish population
    (d) enhanced growth of algae

17. Brewery and sugar factory waste alters the quality of a water body by increasing
    (a) temperature (b) turbidity
    (c) pH (d) COD and BOD

18. Excess nitrate in drinking water can cause
    (a) methemoglobinemia
    (b) kidney damage
    (c) liver damage
    (d) laxative effect

19. Match the columns

| Column-I | Column-II |
|---|---|
| (A) Nitrous oxide | (p) Secondary pollutant from car exhausts |
| (B) Chlorofluorocarbon | (q) Combustion of fossil (CFCs) fuels, wood, etc |
| (C) Methane | (r) Denitrification |
| (D) Ozone ($O_3$) | (s) Refrigerators, aerosol, sprays |
| (E) Carbon dioxide | (t) Cattle, rice fields, toilets. |

    (a) A – (r), B – (s), C – (t), D – (p), E – (q)
    (b) A – (t), B – (p), C – (r), D – (s), E – (q)
    (c) A – (s), B – (t), C – (p), D – (q), E – (r)
    (d) A – (p), B – (r), C – (s), D – (t), E – (q)

20. Synthesis of ethanal commercially from which of the following reagent is the part of green chemistry ?
    (a) $CH_3CH_2OH$ (b) $CH_2=CH_2$
    (c) $HC \equiv CH$ (d) All of these

**ANSWER KEY**

| | | | | | | | | | | | | | | | | | |
|---|---|---|---|---|---|---|---|---|---|---|---|---|---|---|---|---|---|
| 1 | (b) | 4 | (c) | 7 | (d) | 10 | (d) | 13 | (b) | 16 | (d) | 19 | (d) | | | | |
| 2 | (b) | 5 | (d) | 8 | (b) | 11 | (a) | 14 | (a) | 17 | (d) | 20 | (b) | | | | |
| 3 | (d) | 6 | (c) | 9 | (c) | 12 | (b) | 15 | (a) | 18 | (a) | | | | | | |

# THE SOLID STATE

# 15

1. Most crystals show good cleavage because their atoms, ions or molecules are
   (a) weakly bonded together.
   (b) strongly bonded together.
   (c) spherically symmetrical.
   (d) arranged in planes.
2. In which of the following pairs of structures, tetrahedral as well as octahedral holes are found?
   (a) *bcc* and *fcc* (b) *hcp* and simple cubic
   (c) *hcp* and *ccp* (d) *bcc* and *hcp*
3. The most unsymmetrical and symmetrical systems are, respectively :
   (a) Tetragonal, Cubic
   (b) Triclinic, Cubic
   (c) Rhombohedral, Hexagonal
   (d) Orthorhombic, Cubic
4. In which of the following crystals alternate tetrahedral voids are occupied?
   (a) NaCl (b) ZnS
   (c) $CaF_2$ (d) $Na_2O$
5. In a solid '*AB*' having the NaCl structure, '*A*' atoms occupy the corners of the cubic unit cell. If all the face-centred atoms along one of the axes are removed, then the resultant stoichiometry of the solid is
   (a) $AB_2$ (b) $A_2B$
   (c) $A_4B_3$ (d) $A_3B_4$
6. For orthorhombic system axial ratios are $a \neq b \neq c$ and the axial angles are
   (a) $\alpha = \beta = \gamma \neq 90°$ (b) $\alpha = \beta = \gamma = 90°$
   (c) $\alpha = \beta = \gamma = 90°, \beta = 90°$
   (d) $\alpha \neq \beta \neq \gamma = 90°$
7. If the ratio of coordination no. of A to that of B is x : y, then the ratio of no. of atoms of A to that no. of atoms of B in unit cell is:
   (a) x : y (b) y : x
   (c) $x^2 : y$ (d) $y : x^2$
8. Which of the following is the incorrect statement?
   (a) NaCl has 6 : 6 coordination and CsCl has 8 : 8 coordination.
   (b) In $Na_2O$ each oxide ion is coordinated by $8Na^+$ ions and each $Na^+$ ion by 4 oxide ions
   (c) NaCl structure transform to CsCl structure on heating
   (d) In $CaF_2$ structure each $F^-$ ion is coordinated by 4 $Ca^{2+}$

9. For an ionic crystal of the general formula AX and coordination number 6, the radius ratio value will be
(a) greater than 0.73
(b) between 0.73 and 0.41
(c) between 0.41 & 0.22
(d) Less than 0.22

10. The total number of Bravais lattice in a crystal is
(a) 7 (b) 14
(c) 230 (d) 32

11. In the body centred cubic unit cell and simple cubic unit cell, the radius of atom in terms of edge length (a) of the unit cell is respectively:
(a) $\frac{a}{2}, \frac{a}{2\sqrt{2}}$ (b) $\frac{a}{\sqrt{2}}, \frac{a}{2}$
(c) $\frac{a}{2\sqrt{2}}, \frac{a}{2}$ (d) $\frac{\sqrt{3}\,a}{4}, \frac{a}{2}$

12. Edge length of a cube is 400 pm. Its body diagonal would be
(a) 500 pm (b) 566 pm
(c) 600 pm (d) 693 pm

13. Each edge of a cubic unit cell is 400 pm long. If atomic mass of the element is 120 and its density is 6.25 g/cm$^3$, the crystal lattice is :
(use $N_A = 6 \times 10^{23}$)
(a) primitive (b) body centred
(c) face centred (d) end centred

14. An element (atomic mass = 100 g / mol) having *bcc* structure has unit cell edge 400 pm. Then, density of the element is
(a) 10.376 g/cm$^3$ (b) 5.188 g/cm$^3$
(c) 7.289 g/cm$^3$ (d) 2.144 g/cm$^3$

15. A solid has a '*bcc*' structure. If the distance of nearest approach between two atoms is 1.73Å, the edge length of the cell is
(a) 314.20 pm (b) 1.41 pm
(c) 200 pm (d) 216 pm

16. Potassium fluoride has NaCl type structure. What is the distance between $K^+$ and $F^-$ ions if cell edge is 'a' cm?
(a) 2a cm (b) a/2 cm
(c) 4a cm (d) a/4 cm

17. Doping of silicon (Si) with boron (B) leads to :
(a) *n*-type semiconductor
(b) *p*-type semiconductor
(c) metal
(d) insulator

18. Which of the following structure represents ferrimagnetism?
(a) ↑↓↑↓↑↓ (b) ↑↑↑↑↑
(c) ↓↓↓↓↓ (d) ↑↑↓↑↑↓

19. Dopping of AgCl crystals with $CdCl_2$ results in:
(a) Schottky defect
(b) Frenkel defect
(c) Substitutional cation vacancy
(d) Formation of F-centres

20. The electrical conductivity of semiconductor is:
(a) $10^8$ ohm$^{-1}$ cm$^{-1}$
(b) $10^{-22}$ ohm$^{-1}$ cm$^{-1}$
(c) In the range of $10^{-8}$ to $10^2$ ohm$^{-1}$ cm$^{-1}$
(d) None of the above

21. Each of the following solids show, the Frenkel defect except
(a) ZnS (b) AgBr
(c) AgI (d) KCl

22. Crystal defect indicated in the diagram below is

$Na^+Cl^-Na^+Cl^-Na^+Cl^-$
$Cl^-$ □ $Cl^-Na^+$ □ $Na^+$
$Na^+Cl^-$ □ $Cl^-Na^+Cl^-$
$Cl^-Na^+Cl^-Na^+$ □ $Na^+$

(a) Interstitial defect
(b) Schottky defect
(c) Frenkel defect
(d) Frenkel and Schottky defects

**23.** A metal crystallizes in *bcc* lattice. The percent fraction of edge length not covered by atom is

(a) 10.4% (b) 13.4%
(c) 12.4% (d) 11.4%

**24.** A compound of formula $A_2B_3$ has the hcp lattice. Which atom forms the hcp lattice and what fraction of tetrahedral voids is occupied by the other atoms:

(a) *hcp* lattice – A, $\frac{2}{3}$ Tetrahedral voids – B
(b) *hcp* lattice – A, $\frac{1}{3}$ Tetrahedral voids – B
(c) *hcp* lattice – B, $\frac{2}{3}$ Tetrahedral voids – A
(d) *hcp* lattice – B, $\frac{1}{3}$ Tetrahedral voids – A

**25.** Molecules/ions and their magnetic properties are given below

| | Molecule/ion | Magnetic property |
|---|---|---|
| (i) | $C_6H_6$ | (1) Antiferromagnetic |
| (ii) | $CrO_2$ | (2) Ferrimagnetic |
| (iii) | MnO | (3) Ferromagnetic |
| (iv) | $Fe_3O_4$ | (4) Paramagnetic |
| (v) | $Fe^{3+}$ | (5) Diamagnetic |

The correctly matched pairs in the above is:

(a) i-5, ii-3, iii-2, iv-1, v-4
(b) i-3, ii-5, iii-1, iv-4, v-2
(c) i-5, ii-3, iii-1, iv-2, v-4
(d) i-5, ii-3, iii-1, iv-4, v-2

## ANSWER KEY

| | | | | | | | | | | | | | | | | | |
|---|---|---|---|---|---|---|---|---|---|---|---|---|---|---|---|---|---|
| 1 | (d) | 4 | (b) | 7 | (b) | 10 | (b) | 13 | (b) | 16 | (b) | 19 | (c) | 22 | (b) | 25 | (c) |
| 2 | (c) | 5 | (d) | 8 | (c) | 11 | (d) | 14 | (b) | 17 | (b) | 20 | (c) | 23 | (b) | | |
| 3 | (b) | 6 | (b) | 9 | (b) | 12 | (d) | 15 | (c) | 18 | (d) | 21 | (d) | 24 | (d) | | |

# SOLUTIONS

# 16

1. The solubility of $N_2$ in water at 300 K and 500 torr partial pressure is 0.01 g $L^{-1}$. The solubility (in g $L^{-1}$) at 750 torr partial pressure is :
   (a) 0.0075 (b) 0.005
   (c) 0.02 (d) 0.015
2. Molarity of liquid HCl will be, if density of solution is 1.17 g/cc
   (a) 36.5 (b) 32.05
   (c) 18.25 (d) 42.10
3. Which of the following concentration terms is/are independent of temperature?
   (a) Molality only
   (b) Molality and mole fraction
   (c) Molarity and mole fraction
   (d) Molality and normality
4. In a mixture of A and B, components show positive deviation when:
   (a) A – B interaction is stronger than A – A and B – B interaction
   (b) A – B interaction is weaker than A – A and B – B interaction
   (c) $\Delta V_{mix} < 0, \Delta S_{mix} > 0$
   (d) $\Delta V_{mix} = 0, \Delta S_{mix} > 0$
5. A mixture of volatile components A and B has total vapour pressure (in torr)
   $P = 254 - 119x_A$
   where $x_A$ is the mole fraction of A in mixture.
   Hence, $P_A^\circ$ and $P_B^\circ$ are (in torr)
   (a) 254, 119 (b) 119, 254
   (c) 135, 254 (d) 154, 119
6. Which of the following liquid pairs shows a positive deviation from Raoult's law ?
   (a) Water - Nitric acid
   (b) Benzene - Methanol
   (c) Water - Hydrochloric acid
   (d) Acetone - Chloroform
7. 18 g of glucose ($C_6H_{12}O_6$) is added to 178.2 g of water. The vapour pressure of water for this aqueous solution is
   (a) 76.00 torr (b) 752.40 torr
   (c) 759.00 torr (d) 7.60 torr
8. $K_2HgI_4$ is 40% ionised in aqueous solution. The value of its van't Hoff factor (i) is :
   (a) 1.6 (b) 1.8
   (c) 2.0 (d) 2.2

**9.** Four solutions of $K_2SO_4$ with the concentrations 0.1 *m*, 0.01 *m*, 0.001 *m* and 0.0001 *m* are available. The maximum value of colligative property corresponds to :

(a) 0.0001 m solution
(b) 0.001 m solution
(c) 0.01 m solution
(d) 0.1 m solution

**10.** Calculate the percentage degree of dissociation of an electrolyte $XY_2$ (Normal molar mass = 164) in water if the observed molar mass by measuring elevation in boiling point is 65.6:

(a) 75% (b) 25%
(c) 65% (d) None of these

**11.** Elevation in the boiling point for 1 molal solution of glucose is 2 K. The depression in the freezing point for 2 molal solution of glucose in the same solvent is 2 K. The relation between $K_b$ and $K_f$ is:

(a) $K_b = 1.5\ K_f$ (b) $K_b = K_f$
(c) $K_b = 0.5\ K_f$ (d) $K_b = 2\ K_f$

**12.** 1.00 g of a non-volatile solute (molar mass 250 g $mol^{-1}$) was dissolved in 51.2 g of benzene. If the freezing point depression constant, $K_f$ of benzene is 5.12 K kg $mol^{-1}$, the freezing point of benzene will be lowered by

(a) 0.3 K (b) 0.5 K
(c) 0.4 K (d) 0.2 K

**13.** Which one of the following aqueous solutions will exihibit highest boiling point ?

(a) 0.015 M urea (b) 0.01 M $KNO_3$
(c) 0.01 M $Na_2SO_4$ (d) 0.015 M glucose

**14.** The elevation in boiling point of a solution of 13.44 g of $CuCl_2$ in 1 kg of water using the following information will be (Molecular weight of $CuCl_2$= 134.4 g and $K_b$= 0.52 K kg $mol^{-1}$)

(a) 0.16 (b) 0.05
(c) 0.1 (d) 0.2

**15.** The temperature at which 10% aqueous solution (*w*/*v*) of glucose will exhibit the osmotic pressure of 14 bar is –

(a) 307.3 °C (b) 307.3 K
(c) 34 K (d) – 34 °C

**16.** The correct order of osmotic pressure of 0.01M aqueous solution of the following is

(a) Sucrose > $CH_3COOH$ > KCl
(b) $CH_3COOH$ > Sucrose > KCl
(c) Sucrose > KCl > $CH_3COOH$
(d) KCl > $CH_3COOH$ > Sucrose

**17.** An aqueous solution of a salt $MX_2$ at certain temperature has a van't Hoff factor of 2. The degree of dissociation for this solution of the salt is :

(a) 0.50 (b) 0.33
(c) 0.67 (d) 0.80

**18.** An aqueous solution freezes at –0.186°C ($K_f$= 1.86K kg $mol^{-1}$; $K_b$ = 0.512 K kg $mol^{-}$). What is the elevation in boiling point?

(a) 0.186 (b) 0.512
(c) $\frac{0.512}{1.86}$ (d) 0.0512

**19.** The value of P° for benzene is 640 mm of Hg. The vapour pressure of solution containing 2.5g substance in 39g benzene is 600mm of Hg. The molecular mass of *X* is –

(a) 65.25 (b) 130
(c) 40 (d) 80

**20.** The volume of 4 N HCl and 10 N HCl required to make 1 litre of 6 N HCl are

(a) 0.75 litre of 10 N HCl and 0.25 litre of 4 N HCl
(b) 0.50 litre of 4 N HCl and 0.50 litre of 10 N HCl
(c) 0.67 litre of 4 N HCl and 0.33 litre of 10 N HCl
(d) 0.80 litre of 4 N HCl and 0.20 litre of 10 N HCl

**21.** A 10 mg effervescent tablet containing sodium bicarbonate and oxalic acid releases 0.25 mL of $CO_2$ at T = 298.15K and P = 1 bar. If molar volume of $CO_2$ is 25.0 L under such condition, what is the percentage of sodium bicarbonate in each tablet? [Molar mass of $NaHCO_3$ = 84 g $mol^{-1}$]

(a) 0.84 (b) 33.6
(c) 16.8 (d) 8.4

**22.** Liquid 'M' and liquid 'N' form an ideal solution. The vapour pressures of pure liquids 'M' and 'N' are 450 and 700 mmHg, respectively, at the same temperature. Then correct statement is:
($x_M$ = Mole fraction of 'M' in solution;
$x_N$ = Mole fraction of 'N' in solution;
$y_M$ = Mole fraction of 'M' in vapour phase;
$y_N$ = Mole fraction of 'N' in vapour phase)

(a) $\frac{x_M}{x_N} = \frac{y_M}{y_N}$

(b) $(x_M - y_M) < (x_N - y_N)$

(c) $\frac{x_M}{x_N} < \frac{y_M}{y_N}$

(d) $\frac{x_M}{x_N} > \frac{y_M}{y_N}$

**23.** Liquids $A$ and $B$ form an ideal solution and the former has stronger intermolecular forces. If $x_A$ and $x'_A$ are the mole fractions of $A$ in the solution and vapour in equilibrium, then

(a) $\frac{x'_A}{x_A}=1$ (b) $\frac{x'_A}{x_A}>1$

(c) $\frac{x'_A}{x_A}<1$ (d) $x'_A+x_A=1$

**24.** Two liquids $X$ and $Y$ form an ideal solution. At 300 K, vapour pressure of the solution containing 1 mol of $X$ and 3 mol of $Y$ is 550 $mm$Hg. At the same temperature, if 1 mol of $Y$ is further added to this solution, vapour pressure of the solution increases by 10 $mm$Hg. Vapour pressure (in $mm$Hg) of $X$ and $Y$ in their pure states will be, respectively:

(a) 300 and 400 (b) 400 and 600
(c) 500 and 600 (d) 200 and 300

**25.** $\Delta H_1$ and $\Delta H_2$ are molar enthalpies of vaporisation of solvent from pure state and solution containing non-volatile solute respectively. Corresponding entropy changes are $\Delta S_1$ and $\Delta S_2$. Select the correct of the following

(a) $\Delta H_1 < \Delta H_2$; $\Delta S_1 > \Delta S_2$

(b) $\Delta H_1 = \Delta H_2$; $\Delta S_1 > \Delta S_2$

(c) $\Delta H_1 > \Delta H_2$; $\Delta S_1 = \Delta S_2$

(d) $\Delta H_1 > \Delta H_2$; $\Delta S_1 < \Delta S_2$

**26.** The mole fraction of the solute in one molal aqueous solution is:

(a) 0.009 (b) 0.018
(c) 0.027 (d) 0.036

**27.** If $M_{normal}$ is the normal molecular mass and $\alpha$ is the degree of ionization of $K_3[Fe(CN)_6]$, then the abnormal molecular mass of the complex in the solution will be:

(a) $M_{normal}(1+2\alpha)^{-1}$
(b) $M_{normal}(1+3\alpha)^{-1}$
(c) $M_{normal}(1+\alpha)^{-1}$
(d) equal to $M_{normal}$

**28.** Freezing point of a 4% aqueous solution of X is equal to freezing point of 12% aqueous salution of Y. If molecular weight of X is A, then molecular weight of Y is:

(a) 3A (b) 2A
(c) A (d) 4A

**29.** If the various terms in the expressions given below have usual meanings, the van't Hoff factor ($i$) cannot be calculated by which one of the following expressions

(a) $\pi V = \sqrt{inRT}$

(b) $\Delta T_f = iK_f.m$

(c) $\Delta T_b = iK_b.m$

(d) $\frac{P^\circ_{solvent} - P_{solution}}{P^\circ_{solvent}} = i\left(\frac{n}{N+n}\right)$

**30.** The vapour pressure of water at 20 °C is 17.5 mm Hg. If 18 g of glucose ($C_6H_{12}O_6$) is added to 178.2 g of water at 20 °C, the vapour pressure of the resulting solution will be

(a) 17.323 mm Hg (b) 15.750 mm Hg

(c) 16.500 mm Hg (d) 17.500 mm Hg

**ANSWER KEY**

| | | | | | | | | | | | | | | | | | | | |
|---|---|---|---|---|---|---|---|---|---|---|---|---|---|---|---|---|---|---|---|
| 1 | (d) | 5 | (c) | 9 | (d) | 13 | (c) | 17 | (a) | 21 | (d) | 25 | (b) | 29 | (a) | | | | |
| 2 | (b) | 6 | (b) | 10 | (a) | 14 | (a) | 18 | (d) | 22 | (d) | 26 | (b) | 30 | (a) | | | | |
| 3 | (b) | 7 | (b) | 11 | (d) | 15 | (b) | 19 | (d) | 23 | (c) | 27 | (b) | | | | | | |
| 4 | (b) | 8 | (b) | 12 | (c) | 16 | (d) | 20 | (c) | 24 | (b) | 28 | (a) | | | | | | |

# ELECTROCHEMISTRY

# 17

1. The E° at 25° C for the following reaction is 0.22 V. Calculate the equilibrium constant at 25° C

$$H_2(g)+2AgCl(s)\longrightarrow 2Ag(s)+2HCl(aq)$$

(a) $2.8\times10^7$ (b) $5.2\times10^8$

(c) $5.2\times10^6$ (d) $5.2\times10^3$

2. Which of the following will form a cell with the highest voltage?

(a) $1\,M\,Ag^+, 1\,M\,Co^{2+}$

(b) $2\,M\,Ag^+, 2\,M\,Co^{2+}$

(c) $0.1\,M\,Ag^+, 2\,M\,Co^{2+}$

(d) $2\,M\,Ag^+, 0.1\,M\,Co^{2+}$

3. The EMF of the cell

$Ni\,|\,Ni^{2+}\,(1.0\,M)\,||\,Au^{3+}\,(1.0M)|\,Au$ is

[Given $E^0_{Ni^{2+}/Ni} = -0.25$ V and $E^0_{Au^{3+}/Au} = +1.5$ V]

(a) 2.00 V (b) 1.25 V

(c) −1.25 V (d) 1.75 V

4. The standard cell potential of

$Zn\,|\,Zn^{2+}(aq)\,||\,Cu^{2+}(aq)\,|\,Cu$ cell is 1.10 V. The maximum work obtained by this cell will be

(a) 106.15 kJ (b) −212.30 kJ

(c) −318.45 kJ (d) −424.60 kJ

5. If the following half cells have $E^0$ values as

$$A^{3+}+e^-\longrightarrow A^{2+},\ E^0=y_2V$$

$$A^{2+}+2e^-\longrightarrow A,\ E^0=-y_1V$$

The $E^0$ of the half cell $A^{3+}+3e^-\longrightarrow A$ will be

(a) $\frac{2y_1-y_2}{3}$ (b) $\frac{y_2-2y_1}{3}$

(c) $2y_1-3y_2$ (d) $y_2-2y_1$

6. The ionic conductivity of $Ba^{2+}$ and $Cl^-$ at infinite dilution are 127 and 76 $ohm^{-1}\,cm^2\,eq^{-1}$ respectively. The equivalent conductivity of $BaCl_2$ at infinity dilution (in $ohm^{-1}cm^2\,eq^{-1}$) would be

(a) 203 (b) 279

(c) 101.5 (d) 139.5

7. Which of the following when dissolved in water forms a non-conducting solution ?

(a) Chile salt petre (b) Potash alum

(c) Green vitriol (d) Ethyl alcohol

**8.** The resistance of 0.01 N solution of an electrolyte was found to be 220 ohm at 298 K using a conductivity cell with a cell constant of $0.88 cm^{-1}$. The value of equivalent conductance of solution is –

(a) 400 mho $cm^2$ g $eq^{-1}$

(b) 295 mho $cm^2$ g $eq^{-1}$

(c) 419 mho $cm^2$ g $eq^{-1}$

(d) 425 mho $cm^2$ g $eq^{-1}$

**9.** Calculate the current (in mA) required to deposit 0.195 g of platinum metal in 5.0 hours from a solution of $[PtCl_6]^{2-}$ : (Atomic mass: Pt = 195)

(a) 310 (b) 31

(c) 21.44 (d) 5.36

**10.** How many Faradays are required to reduce 0.25 g of Nb (V) to the metal? (Atomic mass : Nb = 93)

(a) $2.7 \times 10^{-3}$ (b) $1.3 \times 10^{-2}$

(c) $2.7 \times 10^{-2}$ (d) $7.8 \times 10^{-3}$

**11.** In passing 3 F of electricity through three electrolytic cells connected in series containing $Ag^+$, $Ca^{2+}$, and $Al^{3+}$ ions, respectively. The molar ratio in which the three metal ions are liberated at the electrodes is

(a) 1 : 2 : 3 (b) 2 : 3 : 1

(c) 6 : 3 : 2 (d) 3 : 4 : 2

**12.** 10800 C of electricity passed through the electrolyte deposited 2.977 g of metal with atomic mass 106.4 g $mol^{-1}$. The charge on the metal cation is

(a) +4 (b) +3

(c) +2 (d) +1

**13.** If 0.5 amp. current is passed through acidified silver nitrate solution for 100 minutes. The mass of silver deposited on cathode, is (eq.wt.of silver = 108)

(a) 2.3523 g (b) 3.3575 g

(c) 5.3578 g (d) 6.3575 g

**14.** The number of coulombs required to reduce 12.3 g of nitrobenzene to aniline is :

(a) 115800 C (b) 5790 C

(c) 28950 C (d) 57900 C

**15.** The best way to prevent rusting of iron is

(a) making it cathode

(b) putting in saline water

(c) both of these

(d) None of these

**16.** During the charging of lead storage battery, the reaction at anode is represented by :

(a) $Pb^{2+} + SO_4^{2-} \longrightarrow PbSO_4$

(b) $PbSO_4 + 2H_2O \longrightarrow PbO_2 + SO_4^{2-} + 4H^+ + 2e^-$

(c) $Pb \longrightarrow Pb^{2+} + 2e^-$

(d) $Pb^{2+} + 2e^- \longrightarrow Pb$

**17.** A gas X at 1 atm is bubbled through a solution containing a mixture of 1 M$Y^-$ and 1 M$Z^-$ at 25°C. If the reduction potential of Z > Y > X, then

(a) Y will oxidize X and not Z

(b) Y will oxidize Z and not X

(c) Y will oxidize both X and Z

(d) Y will reduce both X and Z

**18.** Consider an electrochemical cell in which the following reaction occurs and predict which changes will decrease the cell voltage :

$$Fe^{2+} (aq) + Ag^+ (aq) \rightarrow Ag (s) + Fe^{3+} (aq)$$

(I) decrease the $[Ag^+]$

(II) increase in $[Fe^{3+}]$

(III) increase the amount of Ag

(a) I (b) II and III

(c) II (d) I and II

19. To find the standard potential of $M^{3+}/M$ electrode, the following cell is constituted :

$Pt|M|M^{3+}(0.001\ mol\ L^{-1})|Ag^+(0.01\ mol\ L^{-1})|Ag$

The emf of the cell is found to be 0.421 volt at 298 K. The standard potential of half reaction $M^{3+} + 3e \rightarrow M$ at 298 K will be : (Given $E^0_{Ag^+/Ag}$ at 298 K = 0.80 Volt)

(a) 0.38 Volt (b) 0.32 Volt

(c) 1.28 Volt (d) 0.66 Volt

20. On the basis of the information available from the reaction

$$\frac{4}{3}Al + O_2 \rightarrow \frac{2}{3}Al_2O_3, \Delta G = -827\ kJ\ mol^{-1},$$

the minimum E.M.F required to carry out an electrolysis of $Al_2O_3$ is (F = 96500 C $mol^{-1}$)

(a) 8.56V (b) 2.14V

(c) 4.28V (d) 6.42V

21. The specific conductance of a saturated solution of silver bromide is κ S $cm^{-1}$. The limiting ionic conductivity of $Ag^+$ and $Br^-$ ions are x and y, respectively. The solubility of silver bromide in g $L^{-1}$ is : (molar mass of AgBr = 188)

(a) $\frac{\kappa \times 1000}{x - y}$ (b) $\frac{\kappa}{x + y} \times 188$

(c) $\frac{\kappa \times 1000 \times 188}{x + y}$ (d) $\frac{x + y}{\kappa} \times \frac{1000}{188}$

22. The conductance of a salt solution (AB) measured by two parallel electrodes of area 100 $cm^2$ separated by 10 cm was found to be 0.0001 $\Omega^{-1}$. If volume enclosed between two electrode contain 0.1 mole of salt, what is the molar conductivity (S $cm^2\ mol^{-1}$) of salt at same concentration :

(a) 10 (b) 0.1

(c) 1 (d) None of these

23.

| Electrolyte: | KCl | $KNO_3$ | HCl | NaOAc | NaCl |
|---|---|---|---|---|---|
| $\Lambda^\infty(S\ cm^2\ mol^{-1})$: | 150 | 145 | 426 | 91 | 127 |

Calculate $\Lambda^\infty_{HOAc}$ using appropriate molar conductances of the electrolytes listed above at infinite dilution in $H_2O$ at 25°C

(a) 217.5 (b) 390.7

(c) 552.7 (d) 517.2

24. Aluminium oxide may be electrolysed at 1000 °C to furnish aluminium metal (At. Mass = 27 amu; 1 Faraday = 96,500 Coulombs). The cathode reaction is $Al^{3+} + 3e^- \rightarrow Al$

To prepare 5.12kg of aluminium metal by this method would require

(a) $5.49 \times 10^7$ C of electricity

(b) $1.83 \times 10^7$ C of electricity

(c) $5.49 \times 10^4$ C of electricity

(d) $5.49 \times 10^1$ C of electricity

25. Given the ionic conductance of $\begin{matrix} COO^- \\ | \\ COO^- \end{matrix}$, $K^+$, and $Na^+$ are 74, 50 and 73 $cm^2\ ohm^{-1}\ eq^{-1}$, respectively. The equivalent conductance at infinite dilution of the salt $\begin{matrix} COONa \\ | \\ COOK \end{matrix}$ is

(a) 197 $cm^2\ ohm^{-1}\ eq^{-1}$

(b) 172 $cm^2\ ohm^{-1}\ eq^{-1}$

(c) 135.5 $cm^2\ ohm^{-1}\ eq^{-1}$

(d) 160.5 $cm^2\ ohm^{-1}\ eq^{-1}$

26. The equation that is incorrect is:

(a) $(\Lambda^0_m)_{NaBr} - (\Lambda^0_m)_{NaCl} = (\Lambda^0_m)_{KBr} - (\Lambda^0_m)_{KCl}$

(b) $(\Lambda^0_m)_{KCl} - (\Lambda^0_m)_{NaCl} = (\Lambda^0_m)_{KBr} - (\Lambda^0_m)_{NaBr}$

(c) $(\Lambda^0_m)_{H_2O} = (\Lambda^0_m)_{HCl} + (\Lambda^0_m)_{NaOH} - (\Lambda^0_m)_{NaCl}$

(d) $(\Lambda^0_m)_{NaBr} - (\Lambda^0_m)_{NaI} = (\Lambda^0_m)_{KBr} - (\Lambda^0_m)_{NaBr}$

**27.** 250 mL of a waste solution obtained from the workshop of a goldsmith contains 0.1 M $AgNO_3$ and 0.1 M AuCl. The solution was electrolyzed at 2 V by passing a current of 1 A for 15 minutes. The metal/metals electrodeposited will be :

$\left(E^0_{Ag^+/Ag} = 0.80 \text{ V}, E^0_{Au^+/Au} = 1.69 \text{ V}\right)$

(a) only gold
(b) silver and gold in proportion to their atomic weights
(c) only silver
(d) silver and gold in equal mass proportion

**28.** For the given cell;

$Cu(s)|Cu^{2+}(C_1M)||Cu^{2+}(C_2M)|Cu(s)$

change in Gibbs energy ($\Delta G$) is negative, if :

(a) $C_1 = C_2$ (b) $C_2 = \frac{C_1}{\sqrt{2}}$

(c) $C_1 = 2C_2$ (d) $C_2 = \sqrt{2}C_1$

**29.** Given that the standard potentials ($E^0$) of $Cu^{2+}$/Cu and $Cu^+$/Cu are 0.34 V and 0.522 V respectively, the $E^0$ of $Cu^{2+}/Cu^+$ is:

(a) +0.182 V (b) +0.158 V
(c) – 0.182 V (d) – 0.158 V

**30.** Calculate the standard cell potential (in V) of the cell in which following reaction takes place : $Fe^{2+}$ (aq) + $Ag^+$ (aq) → $Fe^{3+}$ (aq) + Ag(s)

Given that

$E^0_{Ag^+/Ag} = x \text{ V}; \ E^0_{Fe^{2+}/Fe} = y \text{ V}; \ E^0_{Fe^{3+}/Fe} = z \text{ V}$

(a) $x - z$ (b) $x - y$
(c) $x + 2y - 3z$ (d) $x + y - z$

## ANSWER KEY

| | | | | | | | | | | | | | | | | | |
|---|---|---|---|---|---|---|---|---|---|---|---|---|---|---|---|---|---|
| 1 | (a) | 5 | (b) | 9 | (c) | 13 | (b) | 17 | (a) | 21 | (c) | 25 | (c) | 29 | (b) | | |
| 2 | (d) | 6 | (b) | 10 | (b) | 14 | (d) | 18 | (d) | 22 | (b) | 26 | (d) | 30 | (c) | | |
| 3 | (d) | 7 | (d) | 11 | (c) | 15 | (a) | 19 | (b) | 23 | (b) | 27 | (a) | | | | |
| 4 | (b) | 8 | (a) | 12 | (a) | 16 | (b) | 20 | (b) | 24 | (a) | 28 | (d) | | | | |

# 18

# CHEMICAL KINETICS

1. For the reaction $2A + B \rightarrow 3C + D$
Which of the following does not express the reaction rate ?
(a) $-\frac{d[B]}{dt}$ (b) $\frac{d[D]}{dt}$
(c) $-\frac{1}{2}\frac{d[A]}{dt}$ (d) $-\frac{1}{3}\frac{d[C]}{dt}$

2. In the reaction $2A + B \rightarrow A_2B$, if the concentration of A is doubled and that of B is halved, then the rate of the reaction will
(a) increase 2 times
(b) increase 4 times
(c) decrease 2 times
(d) remain the same

3. For an elementary chemical reaction, $A_2 \underset{k_{-1}}{\overset{k_1}{\rightleftharpoons}} 2A$, the expression for $\frac{d[A]}{dt}$ is:
(a) $k_1[A_2] - k_{-1}[A]^2$
(b) $2k_1[A_2] - k_{-1}[A]^2$
(c) $k_1[A_2] + k_{-1}[A]^2$
(d) $2k_1[A_2] - 2k_{-1}[A]^2$

4. The reaction $2X \rightarrow B$ is a zeroth order reaction. If the initial concentration of X is 0.2 M, the half-life is 6 h. When the initial concentration of X is 0.5 M, the time required to reach its final concentration of 0.2 M will be :
(a) 9.0 h (b) 12.0 h
(c) 18.0 h (d) 7.2 h

5. For the reaction $3A(g) \xrightarrow{k} B(g) + C(g)$, $k$ is $10^{-4}$ L mol$^{-1}$ min$^{-1}$. If $[A] = 0.5$ M then the value of $-\frac{d[A]}{dt}$ (in $Ms^{-1}$) is:
(a) $7.5 \times 10^{-5}$ (b) $3 \times 10^{-4}$
(c) $2.5 \times 10^{-5}$ (d) $1.25 \times 10^{-6}$

6. The reaction $A \rightarrow B$ follows first order kinetics. The time taken for 0.8 mole of A to produce 0.6 mole of B is 1 hour. What is the time taken for conversion of 0.9 mole of A to produce 0.675 mole of B?
(a) 2 hours (b) 1 hour
(c) 0.5 hour (d) 0.25 hour

7. Decomposition of X exhibits a rate constant of 0.05 μg/year. How many years are required for the decomposition of 5 μg of x into 2.5 μg?

(a) 50 (b) 25
(c) 20 (d) 40

8. The rate constant of a reaction is $3.00 \times 10^3$ L $mol^{-1}$ $sec^{-1}$. The order of this reaction will be:
(a) 0 (b) 1
(c) 2 (d) 3

9. Ethylene is produced by $C_4H_8 \xrightarrow{\Delta} 2C_2H_4$
The rate constant is $2.3 \times 10^{-4}$ $sec^{-1}$. Approximately in what time will the molar ratio of ethylene to cyclobutane in mixture attain the value equal to one ? ($\log 2 = 0.3, \log 3 = 0.47$)
(a) 1760 sec (b) 1600 sec
(c) 2000 sec (d) 1200 sec

10. $t_{1/4}$ can be taken as the time taken for the concentration of a reactant to drop to $\frac{3}{4}$ of its initial value. If the rate constant for a first order reaction is $k$, the $t_{1/4}$ can be written as
(a) $0.75/k$ (b) $0.69/k$
(c) $0.29/k$ (d) $0.10/k$

11. What is the half life of a radioactive substance if 87.5% of any given amount of the substance disintegrates in 40 minutes ?
(a) 20 minutes (b) 10 minutes
(c) 13 minutes 32 sec (d) 160 minutes

12. An exothermic reaction $A \rightarrow B$ has an activation energy of 17 kJ per mole of A. The heat of the reaction is 40 kJ. Calculate the activation energy for the reverse reaction $B \rightarrow A$.
(a) 60 kJ (b) 57 kJ
(c) 75 kJ (d) 90 kJ

13. If a reaction follows the Arrhenius equation, the plot lnk vs $\frac{1}{(RT)}$ gives straight line with a gradient (– y) unit. The energy required to activate the reactant is:
(a) y/R unit (b) y unit
(c) yR unit (d) – y unit

14. A catalyst lowers the activation energy of a certain reaction from 83.314 to 75 kJ $mol^{-1}$ at 500 K. What will be the rate of reaction as compared to uncatalysed reaction? Assume other things being equal.
(a) Double (b) 28 times
(c) 7.38 times (d) $7.38 \times 10^3$ times

15. In a reversible reaction the energy of activation of the forward reaction is 50 kcal. The energy of activation for the reverse reaction will be
(a) < 50 kcal
(b) either greater than or less than 50 kcal
(c) 50 kcal
(d) > 50 kcal

16. Activation energy of a chemical reaction can be determined by
(a) evaluating rate constant at standard temperature
(b) evaluating velocities of reaction at two different temperatures
(c) evaluating rate constants at two different temperatures
(d) changing concentration of reactants

17. Consider the reaction :
$$Cl_2(aq) + H_2S(aq) \rightarrow S(s) + 2H^+(aq) + 2Cl^-(aq)$$
The rate equation for this reaction is
rate = $k[Cl_2][H_2S]$
Which of these mechanisms is/are consistent with this rate equation?
A. $Cl_2 + H_2S \rightarrow H^+ + Cl^- + Cl^+ + HS^-$ (slow)
$Cl^+ + HS^- \rightarrow H^+ + Cl^- + S$ (fast)
B. $H_2S \rightleftharpoons H^+ + HS^-$ (fast equilibrium)
$Cl_2 + HS^- \rightarrow 2Cl^- + H^+ + S$ (Slow)
(a) B only (b) Both A and B
(c) Neither A nor B (d) A only

18. In the reversible reaction

$$2\,NO_2 \underset{k_2}{\overset{k_1}{\rightleftharpoons}} N_2O_4,$$

the rate of disappearance of $NO_2$ is equal to

(a) $\frac{2k_1}{k_2}[NO_2]^2$

(b) $2k_1[NO_2]^2 - 2k_2[N_2O_4]$

(c) $2k_1[NO_2]^2 - k_2[N_2O_4]$

(d) $(2k_1 - k_2)\,[NO_2]$

19. For the reaction $N_2 + 3H_2 \rightarrow 2NH_3$

if $\frac{\Delta[NH_3]}{\Delta t} = 2 \times 10^{-4}$ mol $L^{-1}$ $s^{-1}$, the value of $\frac{-\Delta[H_2]}{\Delta t}$ would be

(a) $1 \times 10^{-4}$ mol $L^{-1}$ $s^{-1}$
(b) $3 \times 10^{-4}$ mol $L^{-1}$ $s^{-1}$
(c) $4 \times 10^{-4}$ mol $L^{-1}$ $s^{-1}$
(d) $6 \times 10^{-4}$ mol $L^{-1}$ $s^{-1}$

20. The mechanism of the reaction

$2NO + O_2 \longrightarrow 2NO_2$ is

$$NO + NO \underset{k_{-1}}{\overset{k_1}{\rightleftharpoons}} N_2O_2 \text{ (fast)};$$

$$N_2O_2 + O_2 \xrightarrow{k_2} 2NO_2 \text{ (slow)}$$

The rate constant of the reaction is

(a) $k_2$ (b) $k_2k_1(k_{-1})$

(c) $k_2k_1$ (d) $k_2\left(\frac{k_1}{k_{-1}}\right)$

21. The rate constant for a chemical reaction has units L $mol^{-1}s^{-1}$, order of the reaction will be

(a) 0 (b) 1
(c) 2 (d) 3

22. The dissociation of nitrogen pentaoxide is a first order reaction. In first 24 min, 75% of nitrogen pentaoxide is dissociated. What amount of nitrogen pentaoxide will be left behind after one hour of the start of reaction?

(a) Approximately 1%
(b) Approximately 2%
(c) Approximately 3%
(d) None of these

23. The value of $\frac{t_{0.875}}{t_{0.50}}$ for $n^{th}$ order reaction is

(a) $2^{(2n-2)}$ (b) $2^{(2n-2)-1}$

(c) $\frac{8^{n-1}-1}{2^{n-1}-1}$ (d) None of these

24. For a first order reaction the rate constant is 6.909 $min^{-1}$. The time taken for 75% conversion in minutes is

(a) $\frac{3}{2}\log 2$ (b) $\frac{2}{3}\log 3$

(c) $\frac{2}{3}\log 2$ (d) $\frac{3}{2}\log\left(\frac{3}{4}\right)$

25. The initial rates of reaction

$3A + 2B + C \longrightarrow$ Products, at different initial concentrations are given below:

| Initial rate | $[A]_0$ | $[B]_0$ | $[C]_0$ |
|---|---|---|---|
| $5.0 \times 10^{-3}$ | 0.010 | 0.005 | 0.010 |
| $5.0 \times 10^{-3}$ | 0.010 | 0.005 | 0.015 |
| $1.0 \times 10^{-2}$ | 0.010 | 0.010 | 0.010 |
| $1.25 \times 10^{-3}$ | 0.005 | 0.005 | 0.010 |

The order with respect to the reactants, A, B and C are respectively

(a) 3, 2, 0 (b) 3, 2, 1
(c) 2, 2, 0 (d) 2, 1, 0

26. A first order reaction is half completed in 45 minutes. How long does it need for 99.9% of the reaction to be completed?

(a) 5 hours (b) 7.5 hours
(c) 10 hours (d) 20 hours

**27.** The rate constants $k_1$ and $k_2$ for two different reactions are $10^{16} . e^{-2000/T}$ and $10^{15} . e^{-1000/T}$, respectively. The temperature at which $k_1 = k_2$ is:

(a) 1000K (b) $\frac{2000}{2.303}$K

(c) 2000K (d) $\frac{1000}{2.303}$K

**28.** For the reaction:

$[Cr(H_2O)_6]^{3+} + [SCN^-]$

$\rightarrow [Cr(H_2O)_5NCS]^{2+} + H_2O$

The rate law is: $r = k[Cr(H_2O)_6]^{3+} + [SCN^-]$.

The value of $k$ is $2.0 \times 10^{-6}$ L mol$^{-1}$ s$^{-1}$ at 14 °C and $2.2 \times 10^{-5}$ L mol$^{-1}$ s$^{-1}$ at 30 °C. What is the value of $E_a$?

(a) 26 kcal mol$^{-1}$ (b) 2.6 kcal mol$^{-1}$

(c) 2600 kcal mol$^{-1}$ (d) 260 kcal mol$^{-1}$

**29.** For reaction A → B, the rate constant $k_1 = A_1\left(e^{-E_{a_1}/RT}\right)$ and for the reaction X → Y, the rate constant $k_2 = A_2\left(e^{-E_{a_2}/RT}\right)$. If $A_1 = 10^9$, $A_2 = 10^{10}$ and $E_{a_1} = 1200$ cal/mol and $E_{a_2} = 1800$ cal/mol, then the temperature at which $k_1 = k_2$ is : (Given; R = 2 cal/Kmol)

(a) 300 K (b) 300 × 2.303 K

(c) $\frac{303}{2.303}$K (d) None of these

**30.** For the equilibrium, A(g) ⇌ B(g), ΔH is –40 kJ/mol. If the ratio of the activation energies of the forward ($E_f$) and reverse ($E_b$) reactions is $\frac{2}{3}$ then :

(a) $E_f$ = 80 kJ/mol; $E_b$ = 120 kJ/mol

(b) $E_f$ = 60 kJ/mol; $E_b$ = 100 kJ/mol

(c) $E_f$ = 30 kJ/mol; $E_b$ = 70 kJ/mol

(d) $E_f$ = 70 kJ/mol; $E_b$ = 30 kJ/mol

## ANSWER KEY

| | | | | | | | | | | | | | | | | | | | |
|---|---|---|---|---|---|---|---|---|---|---|---|---|---|---|---|---|---|---|---|
| 1 | (d) | 5 | (d) | 9 | (a) | 13 | (b) | 17 | (d) | 21 | (c) | 25 | (d) | 29 | (c) | | | | |
| 2 | (a) | 6 | (b) | 10 | (c) | 14 | (c) | 18 | (b) | 22 | (c) | 26 | (b) | 30 | (a) | | | | |
| 3 | (d) | 7 | (a) | 11 | (c) | 15 | (b) | 19 | (b) | 23 | (c) | 27 | (d) | | | | | | |
| 4 | (c) | 8 | (c) | 12 | (b) | 16 | (c) | 20 | (d) | 24 | (c) | 28 | (a) | | | | | | |

# SURFACE CHEMISTRY

19

1. The volume of gases $NH_3$, $CO_2$ and $H_2$ adsorbed by one gram of charcoal at 300 K are in order of:
   (a) $H_2 > CO_2 > NH_3$ (b) $NH_3 > H_2 > CO_2$
   (c) $NH_3 > CO_2 > H_2$ (d) $CO_2 > NH_3 > H_2$
2. Which among the following statements is false?
   (a) Increase of pressure increases the amount of adsorption
   (b) Increase of temperature may decrease the amount of adsorption
   (c) Adsorption may be monolayered or multilyered
   (d) Particle size of the adsorbent will no affect the amount of adsorption
3. Softening of hard water is done using sodium aluminium silicate (zeolite). This causes
   (a) Adsorption of $Ca^{2+}$ and $Mg^{2+}$ ions of hard water replacing $Na^+$ ions.
   (b) Adsorption of $Ca^{2+}$ and $Mg^{2+}$ ions of hard water replacing $Al^{3+}$ ions.
   (c) Both (a) and (b) are true
   (d) None is true
4. A particular adsorption process has the following characteristics : (i) It arises due to van der Waals forces and (ii) it is reversile. Identify the correct statement that describes the above adsorption process :
   (a) Adsorption is monolayer.
   (b) Adsorption increases with increase in temperature.
   (c) Enthalpy of adsorption is greater than 100 kJ $mol^{-1}$
   (d) Energy of activation is required.
5. Which of the following is not an example of heterogeneous catalytic reaction?
   (a) Ostwald's process
   (b) Combustion of coal
   (c) Hydrogenatoin of vegetable oils
   (d) Haber's process
6. The size of particles in suspension, true solution and colloidal solution varies in the order
   (a) suspension > colloidal > true solution
   (b) true solution > suspension > colloidal
   (c) suspension > colloidal = true solution
   (d) none of these

7. Among the colloids cheese (C), milk (M) and smoke (S), the correct combination of the dispersed phase and dispersion medium, respectively is :
(a) C : liquid in solid; M : liquid in solid; S : solid in gas
(b) C : liquid in solid; M : liquid in liquid; S : solid in gas
(c) C : solid in liquid; M : liquid in liquid; S : gas in solid
(d) C : solid in liquid; M : solid in liquid; S : solid in gas

8. Hardy-Schulze rule explains the effect of electrolytes on the coagulation of colloidal solution. According to this rule, coagulation power of cations follow the order
(a) $Ba^{2+} > Na^{+} > Al^{3+}$
(b) $Al^{3+} > Na^{+} > Ba^{2+}$
(c) $Al^{3+} > Ba^{2+} > Na^{+}$
(d) $Ba^{2+} > Al^{3+} > Na^{+}$

9. Which of the following is the best protective colloid?
(a) Gelatin (Gold No. = 0.005)
(b) Gum arabic (Gold No. = 0.15)
(c) Egg albumin (Gold No. = 0.08)
(d) All possess same protective power

10. Aluminium hydroxide forms a positively charged sol. Which of the following ionic substances should be most effective in coagulating the sol?
(a) NaCl (b) $CaCl_2$
(c) $Fe_2(SO_4)_3$ (d) $K_3PO_4$

11. For the graph below, select correct order of temperature?

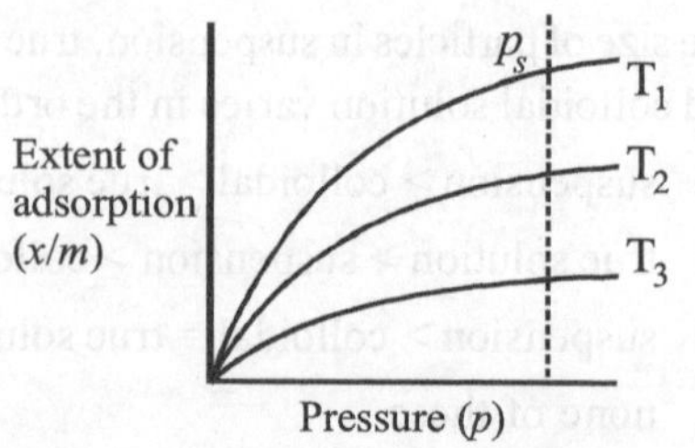


(a) $T_1 > T_2 > T_3$ (b) $T_2 > T_3 > T_1$
(c) $T_3 > T_2 > T_1$ (d) $T_1 = T_2 = T_3$

12. 100 mL of 0.6 M acetic acid is shaken with 2 g activated carbon. The final concentration of the solution after adsorption is 0.5 M. What is the amount of acetic acid adsorbed per gram of carbon?
(a) 0.6 g (b) 0.3 g
(c) 1.2 g (d) None of these

13. Which of the following statements is incorrect regarding physisorption?
(a) More easily liquefiable gases are adsorbed readily.
(b) Under high pressure it results into multi layer on adsorbent surface.
(c) Enthalpy of adsorption ($\Delta H_{adsorption}$) is low and positive.
(d) It occurs because of van der Waal's forces.

14. In the titration of $Cl^-$ ions in solution with $AgNO_3$, sodium salt of fluorescein is used as an indicator. The equivalence point is marked with the appearance of reddish pink colour. This is due to
(a) adsorption of $Cl^-$ ions by AgCl precipitate particles
(b) adsorption of $NO_3^-$ ions by AgCl precipitate particles
(c) adsorption of $Ag^+$ ions by AgCl particles followed by adsorption of fluorescein anion.
(d) reaction of fluorescein anion with $Ag^+$ ions in the solution

15. Hydrolysis of urea is an example of
(a) homogenous catalysis
(b) heterogenous catalysis
(c) biochemical catalysis
(d) zeolite catalysis

16. On adding $AgNO_3$ solution into KI solution, a negatively charged colloidal sol is obtained when they are in
(a) 50 mL of 0.1 M $AgNO_3$ + 50 mL of 0.1 M KI
(b) 50 mL of 0.1 M $AgNO_3$ + 50 mL of 0.2 M KI
(c) 50 mL of 0.2 M $AgNO_3$ + 50 mL of 0.1 M KI
(d) none of these

17. Equal volume each of two sols of AgI, one obtained by adding $AgNO_3$ to slight excess of KI and another obtained by adding KI to slight excess of $AgNO_3$, are mixed together. Then
(a) the two sols will stabilize each other
(b) the sol particles will acquire more electric charge
(c) the sols will coagulate each other mutually
(d) a true solution will be obtained

18. Which of the following statements is not true about the oil-in-water type emulsion?
(a) Addition of small amount of water, no separate layer of water is formed
(b) Addition of a small amount of oil soluble dye renders the entire emulsion coloured
(c) Addition of oil results in the formation of two layers
(d) Addition of a small amount of an electrolyte increases the conductivity of the emulsion

19. Select incorrect statement :
(a) Gold sol is multimolecular colloid
(b) Large number of particles of a substance aggregate together and formed multimolecular colloids
(c) Metal sulphides are lyophobic colloids
(d) Sulphur sol is multimolecular colloid and hydrophilic in nature

20. Which of the following is most powerful to coagulate the negative colloid?
(a) $ZnSO_4$ (b) $Na_3PO_4$
(c) $AlCl_3$ (d) $K_4[Fe(CN)_6]$

21. The disperse phase in colloidal iron (III) hydroxide and colloidal gold is positively and negatively charged, respectively. Which of the following statements is NOT correct?
(a) Coagulation in both sols can be brought about by electrophoresis
(b) Mixing the sols has no effect
(c) Sodium sulphate solution causes coagulation in both sols
(d) Magnesium chloride solution coagulates, the gold sol more readily than the iron (III) hydroxide sol

22. Match the columns

| | Column-I | Column-II |
|---|---|---|
| (A) | $\frac{x}{m} = kc^{1/n}$ | (p) Adsorption varies directly with pressure |
| (B) | $\log\frac{x}{m} = \log k + \frac{1}{n}\log p$ $\left(\frac{1}{n} = 0\right)$ | (q) Adsorption from solution phase |
| (C) | $\log\frac{x}{m} = \log k + \frac{1}{n}\log p$ $\left(\frac{1}{n} = 1\right)$ | (r) Freudlich isotherm cannot be explained |
| (D) | $\frac{x}{m} = kp^{1/n}$ (high pressure) | (s) Adsorption is independent of pressure |

(a) A – (q), B – (s), C – (p), D – (r)
(b) A – (q), B – (p), C – (s), D – (r)
(c) A – (r), B – (p), C – (s), D – (q)
(d) A – (r), B – (s), C – (p), D – (q)

23. Coagulation value of the electrolytes $AlCl_3$ and NaCl for $As_2S_3$ sol are 0.093 and 52 respectively. How many times $AlCl_3$ has greater coagulating power than NaCl ?
(a) 930 (b) 520
(c) 560 (d) None of these

24. Point out the false statement
(a) The colloidal solution of a liquid in liquid is called gel
(b) Hardy Schulze rule is related with coagulation

(c) Brownian movement and Tyndall effect are shown by colloidal system
(d) Gold number is a measure of the protective power of lyophilic colloid

**25.** Match the columns

| Column-I | Column-II |
|---|---|
| (A) $As_2S_3$ sol | (p) Bredig's Arc method |
| (B) $Fe(OH)_3$ sol | (q) Double decomposition |
| (C) Colloidal sols of metals like Au, Ag, Pt, etc. | (r) Peptization |
| (D) Conversion of freshly prepared precipitate into a colloidal sol | (s) Hydrolysis |

(a) A – (q), B – (s), C – (r), D – (p)
(b) A – (q), B – (p), C – (s), D – (r)
(c) A – (s), B – (q), C – (p), D – (r)
(d) A – (q), B – (s), C – (p), D – (r)

**ANSWER KEY**

| 1 | (c) | 4 | (d) | 7 | (b) | 10 | (d) | 13 | (c) | 16 | (b) | 19 | (d) | 22 | (a) | 25 | (d) |
|---|---|---|---|---|---|---|---|---|---|---|---|---|---|---|---|---|---|
| 2 | (d) | 5 | (b) | 8 | (c) | 11 | (c) | 14 | (c) | 17 | (c) | 20 | (c) | 23 | (c) | | |
| 3 | (a) | 6 | (a) | 9 | (a) | 12 | (b) | 15 | (c) | 18 | (b) | 21 | (b) | 24 | (a) | | |

# GENERAL PRINCIPLES AND PROCESSES OF ISOLATION OF ELEMENTS

# 20

1. Which ore contains both iron and copper?
   (a) Cuprite (b) Chalcocite
   (c) Chalcopyrite (d) Malachite
2. Calamine is an ore of :
   (a) zinc (b) aluminium
   (c) iron (d) copper
3. Which of the following is an ore of tin ?
   (a) Carborundum (b) Epsomite
   (c) Cassiterite (d) Spodumene
4. Chromium is obtained by reducing concentrated chromite ore with:
   (a) red hot cake
   (b) gaseous hydrogen
   (c) aluminium powder
   (d) carbon monoxide
5. Highly electropositive metal(s) can not be commercially extracted by carbon reduction process at high temperature because these
   (a) metals combine with carbon to form covalent carbide
   (b) metals combine with carbon to form ionic carbide
   (c) $\Delta G_f$ of highly electropositive metal oxide is having low negative value
   (d) metal oxides are not reduced by carbon
6. The electrolysis of pure alumina is not feasible because
   (a) it is bad conductor of electricity and its fusion temperature is high
   (b) it is volatile in nature
   (c) it is decomposed when fused
   (d) it is amphoteric
7. In the froth floatation process for beneficiation of ores, the ore particles float because
   (a) they are light
   (b) their surface is not easily wetted by water
   (c) they bear electrostatic charge
   (d) they are insoluble
8. Electric furnaces are lined with magnesia because
   (a) It melts at a very high temperature
   (b) It is not affected by acids
   (c) It has no effect of electricity
   (d) It liberates oxygen on heating
9. In the Hall-Heroult process, aluminium is formed at the cathode. The cathode is made out of:
   (a) Pure aluminium (b) Carbon
   (c) Copper (d) Platinum

10. The electrolytic reduction technique is used in the extraction of
(a) highly electronegative elements
(b) highly electropositive elements
(c) metalloids
(d) transition metals.

11. Which one of the furnaces among the following can produce the highest temperature?
(a) muffle furnace
(b) blast furnace
(c) reverberatory furnace
(d) electric furnace

12. Which of the following process is used in the extraction of magnesium?
(a) Fused salt electrolysis
(b) Self reduction
(c) Aqueous solution electrolysis
(d) Thermite reduction

13. Poling process is used for
(a) The removal of $Cu_2O$ from Cu
(b) The removal of $Al_2O_3$ from Al
(c) The removal of $Fe_2O_3$ from Fe
(d) All of these

14. van Arkel method of purification of metals involves converting the metal to a
(a) volatile stable compound
(b) volatile unstable compound
(c) non volatile stable compound
(d) None of the above

15. If the impurities in a metal has a greater affinity for oxygen and is more easily oxidised than the metal, then the purification of metal may be carried out by
(a) distillation
(b) zone refining
(c) electrolytic refining
(d) cupellation

16. Extraction of zinc from zinc blende is achieved by
(a) roasting followed by self-reduction
(b) electrolytic reduction
(c) roasting followed by reduction with carbon
(d) roasting followed by reduction with another metal

17. Carbon and CO gas are used to reduce which of the following pairs of metal oxides for extraction of metals ?
(a) FeO, SnO (b) SnO, ZnO
(c) BaO, $Na_2O_2$ (d) FeO, ZnO

18. Refractory materials are generally used in furnaces because
(a) they possess great structural strength
(b) they can withstand high temperature
(c) they are chemically inert
(d) they do not require replacement

19. Match the columns.

| Column-I | Column-II |
|---|---|
| (A) Coloured bands | (p) Zone refining |
| (B) Impure metal to volatile complex | (q) Fractional distillation |
| (C) Purification of Ge and Si | (r) Mond Process |
| (D) Purification of mercury | (s) Chromatography |
| | (t) Liquation |

(a) A – (p), B – (q), C – (s), D – (t)
(b) A – (s), B – (r), C – (p), D – (q)
(c) A – (r), B – (s), C – (p), D – (q)
(d) A – (t), B – (s), C – (r), D – (q)

20. Match the columns

| Column-I | Column-II |
|---|---|
| (A) Distillation | (p) Zr |
| (B) Electrolytic refining | (q) Cu |
| (C) Liquation | (r) Hg |
| (D) Vapour phase refining | (s) Sn |

(a) A – (q), B – (r), C – (s), D – (p)
(b) A – (r), B – (q), C – (s), D – (p)
(c) A – (r), B – (s), C – (q), D – (p)
(d) A – (r), B – (q), C – (p), D – (s)

**ANSWER KEY**

| | | | | | | | | | | | | | | | | | | | |
|---|---|---|---|---|---|---|---|---|---|---|---|---|---|---|---|---|---|---|---|
| 1 | (c) | 4 | (c) | 7 | (b) | 10 | (b) | 13 | (a) | 16 | (c) | 19 | (b) | | | | | | |
| 2 | (a) | 5 | (b) | 8 | (a) | 11 | (d) | 14 | (a) | 17 | (d) | 20 | (b) | | | | | | |
| 3 | (c) | 6 | (a) | 9 | (b) | 12 | (a) | 15 | (d) | 18 | (b) | | | | | | | | |

# 21

# THE *p*-BLOCK ELEMENTS (GROUP 15, 16, 17 & 18)

1. Which one of the following halide does not get hydrolysed?
   (a) $SbCl_3$ (b) $AsCl_3$
   (c) $PCl_3$ (d) $NF_3$
2. Catalytic oxidation of $NH_3$ (passing a mixture of $NH_3$ and air over heated Pt gauze) gives
   (a) NO (b) $N_2O$
   (c) $N_2O_3$ (d) $N_2O_5$
3. Which of the following orders regarding thermal stability of hydrides $MH_3$ of group 15 is correct?
   (a) $NH_3 > PH_3 > AsH_3$
   (b) $NH_3 < PH_3 < AsH_3$
   (c) $NH_3 > PH_3 < AsH_3$
   (d) $NH_3 < PH_3 > AsH_3$
4. Which of the following fertilizers has the highest nitrogen percentage?
   (a) Ammonium sulphate
   (b) Calcium cyanamide
   (c) Urea
   (d) Ammonium nitrate
5. $PCl_3$ reacts with excess of water to form
   (a) $PH_3$ (b) $H_3PO_4$ and HCl
   (c) $POCl_3$ (d) $H_3PO_4$
6. Most acidic oxide among the following is –
   (a) $N_2O_5$ (b) $P_2O_5$
   (c) $N_2O_4$ (d) $As_2O_3$
7. $PH_4I + NaOH$ forms
   (a) $PH_3$ (b) $NH_3$
   (c) $P_4O_6$ (d) $P_4O_{10}$
8. $P_2O_5$ is heated with water to give
   (a) hypophosphorous acid
   (b) phosphorous acid
   (c) hypophosphoric acid
   (d) orthophosphoric acid
9. Which of the following oxides of nitrogen is a coloured gas?
   (a) $N_2O$ (b) NO
   (c) $N_2O_5$ (d) $NO_2$
10. The number of P – O – P bonds in cyclic metaphosphoric acid is
    (a) zero (b) two
    (c) three (d) four
11. Producer gas is a mixture of :
    (a) CO and $N_2$ (b) $CO_2$ and $H_2$
    (c) $N_2$ and $O_2$ (d) $CH_4$ and $N_2$

12. Which is the most thermodynamically stable allotropic form of phosphorus?
(a) Red (b) White
(c) Black (d) Yellow

13. The product formed in the reaction of $SOCl_2$ with white phosphorous is
(a) $PCl_3$ (b) $SO_2Cl_2$
(c) $SCl_2$ (d) $POCl_3$

14. It is possible to obtain oxygen from air by fractional distillation because
(a) oxygen is in a different group of the periodic table from nitrogen.
(b) oxygen is more reactive than nitrogen.
(c) oxygen has higher b.p. than nitrogen.
(d) oxygen has a lower density than nitrogen.

15. Oxidation of thiosulphate by iodine gives
(a) tetrathionate ion
(b) sulphide ion
(c) sulphate ion
(d) sulphite ion

16. Which compound is used in photography?
(a) $Na_2SO_5$ (b) $Na_2S_2O_8$
(c) $Na_2S_2O_6$ (d) $Na_2S_2O_3$

17. A gas that cannot be collected over water is
(a) $N_2$ (b) $O_2$
(c) $SO_2$ (d) $PH_3$

18. Which of the following is not oxidized by $O_3$ ?
(a) KI (b) $FeSO_4$
(c) $KMnO_4$ (d) $K_2MnO_4$

19. Of the interhalogen $AX_3$ compounds, $ClF_3$ is most reactive but $BrF_3$ has higher conductance in liquid state. This is because
(a) $BrF_3$ has higher molecular mass
(b) $ClF_3$ is more volatile
(c) $BrF_3$ dissociates into $BrF_2^+$ and $BrF_4^-$ most easily
(d) Electrical conductance does not depend on concentration

20. Interhalogen compounds are more reactive than the individual halogen because
(a) two halogens are present in place of one.
(b) they are more ionic.
(c) their bond energy is less than the bond energy of the halogen molecule.
(d) they carry more energy.

21. Which one of the following oxides of chlorine is obtained by passing dry chlorine over silver chlorate at 90 °C ?
(a) $Cl_2O$ (b) $ClO_3$
(c) $ClO_2$ (d) $ClO_4$

22. Which of the following xenon-oxo compounds may not be obtained by hydrolysis of xenon fluorides?
(a) $XeO_2F_2$ (b) $XeOF_4$
(c) $XeO_3$ (d) $XeO_4$

23. Total number of lone pair of electrons in $XeOF_4$ is
(a) 0 (b) 1
(c) 2 (d) 3

24. Which one of the following noble gases is not found in the atmosphere?
(a) Rn (b) Kr
(c) Ne (d) Ar

25. The shape of $XeO_2F_2$ molecule is
(a) trigonal bipyramidal
(b) square planar
(c) tetrahedral
(d) see-saw

**ANSWER KEY**

| 1 | (d) | 4 | (c) | 7 | (a) | 10 | (c) | 13 | (a) | 16 | (d) | 19 | (c) | 22 | (d) | 25 | (d) |
|---|---|---|---|---|---|---|---|---|---|---|---|---|---|---|---|---|---|
| 2 | (a) | 5 | (b) | 8 | (d) | 11 | (a) | 14 | (c) | 17 | (c) | 20 | (c) | 23 | (b) | | |
| 3 | (a) | 6 | (a) | 9 | (d) | 12 | (c) | 15 | (a) | 18 | (c) | 21 | (c) | 24 | (a) | | |

# THE *d*- AND *f*-BLOCK ELEMENTS

# 22

1. The element that usually does **NOT** show variable oxidation states is:
(a) Cu (b) Ti
(c) Sc (d) V

2. In which of the following pairs both the ions are coloured in aqueous solutions?
(a) $Sc^{3+}$, $Ti^{3+}$ (b) $Sc^{3+}$, $Co^{2+}$
(c) $Ni^{2+}$, $Cu^{+}$ (d) $Ni^{2+}$, $Ti^{3+}$

3. The transition metal ions responsible for colour in ruby and emerald are, respectively :
(a) $Co^{3+}$ and $Cr^{3+}$ (b) $Co^{3+}$ and $Co^{3+}$
(c) $Cr^{3+}$ and $Cr^{3+}$ (d) $Cr^{3+}$ and $Co^{3+}$

4. Which one of the following exhibits the large number of oxidation states?
(a) Ti (22) (b) V (23)
(c) Cr (24) (d) Mn (25)

5. Titanium shows magnetic moment of 1.73 B.M. in itscompound. What is the oxidation number of Ti in the compound?
(a) +1 (b) +4
(c) +3 (d) +2

6. Which of the following ions has the maximum magnetic moment?
(a) $Mn^{2+}$ (b) $Fe^{2+}$
(c) $Ti^{2+}$ (d) $Cr^{2+}$.

7. The atomic number of V, Cr, Mn and Fe are respectively 23, 24, 25 and 26. Which one of these may be expected to have the highest second ionisation enthalpy?
(a) V (b) Cr
(c) Mn (d) Fe

8. Which of the following statements is incorrect ?
(a) Across a period from Sc to Cu the densities increase with increasing atomic number.
(b) The melting point of transition elements rise to a maximum from Sc to Cr and then decreases from Fe to Zn.
(c) Transition elements have high enthalpies of atomization and in 3*d* series increase regularly from Sc to Cu.
(d) On going down a group from 3*d* to 6*d* series the stability of higher oxidation state increases with increasing atomic number.

9. Among the following pairs of ions, lower oxidation state in aqueous solution is more stable than the other in
(a) $Ti^{+}$, $Ti^{3+}$ (b) $Cu^{+}$, $Cu^{2+}$
(c) $Cr^{2+}$, $Cr^{3+}$ (d) $V^{2+}$, $VO^{2+}$

10. Which of the following cannot reduce the acidified solution of permaganate?
(a) $(COOH)_2$
(b) $H_2$
(c) Nascent hydrogen
(d) $Fe^{2+}$ ions

11. Which of the following is known as WORM SILVER?
(a) AgCl
(b) A specific horn, type article made of silver
(c) $Ag_2S$
(d) PbS containing traces of $Ag_2S$

12. $KMnO_4$ acts as an oxidising agent in alkaline medium. When alkaline $KMnO_4$ is treated with KI, iodide ion is oxidised to ________.
(a) $I_2$ (b) $IO^-$
(c) $IO_3^-$ (d) $IO_4^-$

13. Mercury is the only metal which is liquid at 0°C. This is due to its
(a) very high ionisation energy and weakly metallic bond.
(b) low ionisation potential.
(c) high atomic weight.
(d) high vapour pressure.

14. Which of the following is called Wilkinson's catalyst?
(a) $[(Ph_3P)_3RhCl]$ (b) $TiCl_4 + (C_2H_5)_3Al$
(c) $(C_2H_5)_4Pb$ (d) $[PtCl_2(NH_3)_2]$

15. Which compound is formed when iron reacts with carbon?
(a) $FeC_2$ (b) $Fe_3C$
(c) $FeC_3$ (d) $Fe_2C$

16. Potassium dichromate when heated with concentrated sulphuric acid and a soluble chloride, gives brown-red vapours of :
(a) $CrO_3$ (b) $CrCl_3$
(c) $CrO_2Cl_2$ (d) $Cr_2O_3$

17. The correct statement of the following is:
(a) $FeI_3$ is stable in aqueous solution.
(b) An acidified solution of $K_2CrO_4$ gives green precipitate on mixing with lead acetate.
(c) The species $[CuCl_4]^{2-}$ exists but $[CuI_4]^{2-}$ does not.
(d) Both copper (I) and copper (II) salts are known in aqueous solution.

18. $K_2Cr_2O_7$ on heating with aqueous NaOH gives
(a) $CrO_4^{2-}$ (b) $Cr(OH)_3$
(c) $Cr_2O_7^{2-}$ (d) $Cr(OH)_2$

19. What would happen when a solution of potassium chromate is treated with an excess of dilute nitric acid?
(a) $Cr_2O_7^{2-}$ and $H_2O$ are formed
(b) $CrO_4^{2-}$ is reduced to +3 state of Cr
(c) $CrO_4^{2-}$ is oxidized to +7 state of Cr
(d) $Cr^{3+}$ and $Cr_2O_7^{2-}$ are formed

20. Copper becomes green when exposed to moist air for longer period –
(a) because of the formation of a layer of cupric oxide on the surface of copper
(b) because of the formation of a layer of basic carbonate of copper on the surface of copper
(c) because of the formation of a layer of cupric hydroxide on the surface of copper
(d) because of the formation of a layer of cupric acetate on the surface of copper

21. Gun metal is an alloy of :
(a) Cu and Al (b) Cu and Sn
(c) Cu, Zn and Sn (d) Cu, Zn and Ni

22. The treatment of Cu with dilute $HNO_3$ gives :
(a) $N_2O$ (b) NO
(c) $NH_4^+$ (d) $NO_2$

23. The chief ore of Hg is:
(a) Pyrolusite (b) Bauxite
(c) Galena (d) Cinnabar

24. Which one of the following species is stable in aqueous solution ?
(a) $Cr^{2+}$ (b) $MnO_4^{2-}$
(c) $MnO_4^{3-}$ (d) $Cu^{+}$

25. Arrange (I) $Ce^{3+}$, (II) $La^{3+}$ (III) $Pm^{3+}$ and (IV) $Yb^{3+}$ in increasing order of their ionic radii.
(a) IV < III < I < II (b) I < IV < III < II
(c) IV < III < II < I (d) III < II < I < IV

26. In aqueous solutions $Eu^{2+}$ acts as
(a) an oxidising agent
(b) a reducing agent
(c) can act either of these
(d) can act as redox agent

27. What is the percentage of lanthanoid metal in mischmetall?
(a) 90% (b) 20%
(c) 5% (d) 95%

28. Among the lanthanoids, the one obtained by synthetic method is
(a) Lu (b) Pm
(c) Pr (d) Gd

29. Which one of the following elements shows maximum number of different oxidation states in its compounds?
(a) Eu (b) La
(c) Gd (d) Am

30. The correct order of atomic radii is :
(a) Ce > Eu > Ho (b) Ho > Eu > Ce
(c) Ce > Eu < Ho (d) Eu > Ce > Ho

**ANSWER KEY**

| | | | | | | | | | | | | | | | | | |
|---|---|---|---|---|---|---|---|---|---|---|---|---|---|---|---|---|---|
| 1 | (c) | 5 | (c) | 9 | (d) | 13 | (a) | 17 | (c) | 21 | (c) | 25 | (a) | 29 | (d) | | |
| 2 | (d) | 6 | (a) | 10 | (b) | 14 | (a) | 18 | (a) | 22 | (b) | 26 | (b) | 30 | (d) | | |
| 3 | (c) | 7 | (b) | 11 | (a) | 15 | (b) | 19 | (a) | 23 | (d) | 27 | (d) | | | | |
| 4 | (d) | 8 | (c) | 12 | (c) | 16 | (c) | 20 | (b) | 24 | (b) | 28 | (b) | | | | |

# 23

# COORDINATION COMPOUNDS

1. The IUPAC name for the complex $[Co(NO_2)(NH_3)_5]Cl_2$ is :
   (a) Pentaammine nitrito-N-cobalt(II) chloride
   (b) Pentaammine nitrito-N-cobalt(III) chloride
   (c) Nitrito-N-pentaamminecobalt(III) chloride
   (d) Nitrito-N-pentaamminecobalt(II) chloride

2. Which one of the following will be able to show geometrical isomerism if complexes are square planar?
   (a) $Ma_4$ (b) $Ma_3b$
   (c) Mabcd (d) $[M(aa)_2]$

3. Which one of the following complexes will consume more equivalents of aqueous solution of $AgNO_3$?
   (a) $Na_2[CrCl_5(H_2O)]$ (b) $Na_3[CrCl_6]$
   (c) $[Cr(H_2O)_5Cl]Cl_2$ (d) $[Cr(H_2O)_6]Cl_3$

4. The geometry of $Ni(CO)_4$ and $[Ni(ph_3)_2]Cl_2$ are
   (a) both square planar
   (b) tetrahedral and square planar
   (c) both tetrahedral
   (d) None of these

5. Which of the following co-ordination ion/ compound does not exhibit structural isomerism?
   (a) $[PtBrCl(H_2O)_4]SO_4$
   (b) $[Co(NH_3)_6][Cr(CN)_6]$
   (c) $[Co(ox)(H_2O)_4]Br$
   (d) $[Ir(ONO)_3(H_2O)_3]$

6. Complexes $[Co(NH_3)_5SO_4]Br$ and $[Co(NH_3)_5Br]SO_4$ can be distinguished by
   (a) conductance measurement
   (b) using $BaCl_2$
   (c) using $AgNO_3$
   (d) Both (b) and (c)

7. Which of the following statements is not true about the complex ion $[Cr(en)_2Cl_2]^+$ (en = ethylene diamine)
   (a) It has two geometrical isomers - *cis* and *trans*.
   (b) Both the *cis* and *trans* isomers display optical activity.
   (c) Only the *cis* isomer displays optical activity.
   (d) Only the *cis* isomer has non-superimposable mirror image.

8. Which of the following complexes will not show geometrical isomerism ?
(a) $[Pt(NH_3)_2Cl_2]$
(b) $[Pt(NH_3)(NH_2OH)(NO_2)(C_6H_5N)]\ NO_2$
(c) $[Pt(NH_2CH_2COO)_2]$
(d) $[Cu(NH_3)_4]Cl_2$

9. Select correct match :
(a) $[Co(ox)(H_2O)_3(NH_3)]$ Br : Optical isomerism
(b) $[Cr(SCN)(H_2O)_3(en)](C_2O_4)$ : Ionization isomerism
(c) $[ZnBr(CN)(SCN)(NH_3)]^-$ : Geometrical isomerism
(d) $[CoBrCl(H_2O)_4][Ag(CN)_2]$ : Coordination isomerism

10. Type of isomerism which exists between $[Pd(C_6H_5)_2(SCN)_2]$ and $[Pd(C_6H_5)_2(NCS)_2]$ is :
(a) Linkage isomerism
(b) Coordination isomerism
(c) Ionisation isomerism
(d) Solvate isomerism

11. Which of the following complex ions will exhibit optical isomerism? (en = 1, 2-diamine ethane).
(a) $[Cr(NH_3)_2Cl_2]^+$ (b) $[Co(en)_2Cl_2]^+$
(c) $[Co(NH_3)_4Cl_2]^+$ (d) $[Zn(en)_2]^{2+}$

12. Which one of the following octahedral complexes will not show geometric isomerism? (A and B are monodentate ligands)
(a) $[MA_5B]$ (b) $[MA_2B_4]$
(c) $[MA_3B_3]$ (d) $[MA_4B_2]$

13. Which of the following is considered to be an anticancer species?

(a) 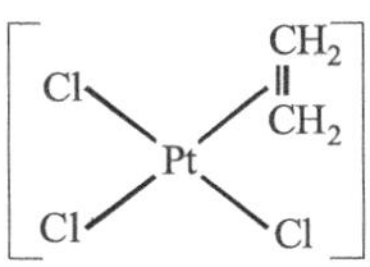


(b) 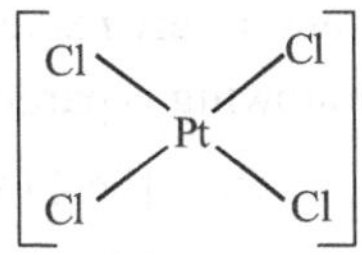


(c) 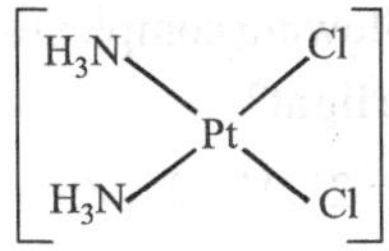


(d) 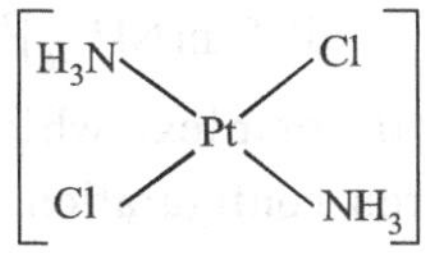


14. Which of the following has five donor (coordinating) sites?
(a) Triethylene tetramine
(b) Ethylenediamine tetracetate ion
(c) Ethylenediamine triacetate ion
(d) Diethylene triamine

15. The ionisation isomer of $[Cr(H_2O)_4Cl(NO_2)]Cl$ is
(a) $[Cr(H_2O)_4(O_2N)]Cl_2$
(b) $[Cr(H_2O)_4Cl_2](NO_2)$
(c) $[Cr(H_2O)_4Cl(ONO)]Cl$
(d) $[Cr(H_2O)_4Cl_2(NO_2)].H_2O$

16. Which of the following complexes have a maximum number of unpaired electrons?
(a) $[Ni(CO)_4]$
(b) $[Co(NH_3)_4(NO_2)_2]^+$
(c) $[Ag(CN)_2]^-$
(d) $[CuBr_4]^{2-}$

17. Relative to the average energy in the spherical crystal field, the $t_2$ orbitals in tetrahedral field is
(a) Raised by (2/5) $\Delta_t$
(b) Lowered by (2/5) $\Delta_t$
(c) Raised by (3/5) $\Delta_t$
(d) Lowered by (1/5) $\Delta_t$

**18.** Atomic number of Cr and Fe are respectively 25 and 26, which of the following is paramagnetic?

(a) $[Cr(CO)_6]$ (b) $[Fe(CO)_5]$

(c) $[Fe(CN)_6]^{4-}$ (d) $[Cr(NH_3)_6]^{3+}$

**19.** Which one of the following complexes will most likely absorb visible light?

(At nos. Sc = 21, Ti = 22, V = 23, Zn = 30)

(a) $[Sc(H_2O)_6]^{3+}$ (b) $[Ti(NH_3)_6]^{4+}$

(c) $[V(NH_3)_6]^{3+}$ (d) $[Zn(NH_3)_6]^{2+}$

**20.** For an octahedral complex, which of the following *d*-electron configuration will give maximum CFSE?

(a) High spin with $d^6$ configuration

(b) Low spin with $d^4$ configuration

(c) Low spin with $d^5$ configuration

(d) High spin with $d^7$ configuration

**21.** Which of the following complex is diamagnetic?

(a) $[Mn(H_2O)_6]^{2+}$ (b) $[Cu(H_2O)_6]^{3+}$

(c) $[Co(NH_3)_6]^{3+}$ (d) $[Co(H_2O)_6]^{2+}$

**22.** The correct order of ligands in the spectrochemical series is

(a) $Cl^- > en > CN^- > NCS^-$

(b) $CN^- > en > NCS^- > Cl^-$

(c) $NCS^- > CN^- > Cl^- > en$

(d) $en > CN^- > Cl^- > NCS^-$

**23.** Incorrect match is :

(a) $[Rh(PPh_3)_3Cl]$ : Wilkinson's catalyst

(b) $[Co(CO)_4]^-$ : Bond order of Co—CO bond is greater than one

(c) $[Zn(NH_3)_4]^{2+}$ : colorless complex

(d) $[Cr(CN)_6]^{3-}$ : Inner orbital low spin complex

**24.** $[Cr(H_2O)_6]Cl_3$ (at. no. of Cr = 24) has a magnetic moment of 3.83 B. M. The correct distribution of 3*d* electrons in the chromium of the complex is

(a) $3d^1_{xy}, (3d_{x^2-y^2})^1, 3d^1_{yz}$

(b) $3d^1_{xy}, 3d^1_{yz}, 3d^1_{xz}$

(c) $3d^1_{xy}, 3d^1_{yz}, 3d^1_{z^2}$

(d) $(3d_{x^2-y^2})^1, 3d^1_{z^2}, 3d^1_{xz}$

**25.** $[Sc(H_2O)_6]^{3+}$ ion is :

(a) colourless and diamagnetic

(b) coloured and octahedral

(c) colourless and paramagnetic

(d) coloured and paramagnetic

**26.** Which complex of $Co^{2+}$ will have the weakest crystal field splitting –

(a) $[CoCl_6]^{4-}$ (b) $[Co(CN)_6]^{4-}$

(c) $[Co(NH_3)_6]^{2+}$ (d) $[Co(en)_3]^{2+}$

**27.** The complex showing a spin-only magnetic moment of 2.82 B.M. is :

(a) $Ni(CO)_4$ (b) $[NiCl_4]^{2-}$

(c) $Ni(PPh_3)_4$ (d) $[Ni(CN)_4]^{2-}$

**28.** Which one of the following complexes is an outer orbital complex ?

(a) $[Co(NH_3)_6]^{3+}$ (b) $[Mn(CN)_6]^{4-}$

(c) $[Fe(CN)_6]^{4-}$ (d) $[Ni(NH_3)_6]^{2+}$

(Atomic nos. : Mn = 25; Fe = 26; Co = 27, Ni = 28)

**29.** A square planar complex is formed by hybridisation of which atomic orbitals?

(a) $s, p_x, p_y, d_{yz}$ (b) $s, p_x, p_y, d_{x^2-y^2}$

(c) $s, p_x, p_y, d_{z^2}$ (d) $s, p_y, p_z, d_{xy}$

**30.** Match the columns.

| Column-I (Coordination compound) | Column-II (Central metal atom) |
|---|---|
| (A) Chlorophyll | (p) Rhodium |
| (B) Blood pigment | (q) Cobalt |
| (C) Wilkinson catalyst | (r) Calcium |
| (D) Vitamin $B_{12}$ | (s) Iron |
| | (t) Magnesium |

(a) A – (t), B – (s), C – (p), D – (q)
(b) A – (s), B – (q), C – (p), D – (r)
(c) A – (p), B – (q), C – (r), D – (s)
(d) A – (r), B – (t), C – (p), D – (q)

**ANSWER KEY**

| | | | | | | | | | | | | | | | | | | | |
|---|---|---|---|---|---|---|---|---|---|---|---|---|---|---|---|---|---|---|---|
| **1** | (b) | **4** | (b) | **7** | (b) | **10** | (a) | **13** | (c) | **16** | (d) | **19** | (c) | **22** | (b) | **25** | (a) | **28** | (d) |
| **2** | (c) | **5** | (c) | **8** | (d) | **11** | (b) | **14** | (c) | **17** | (a) | **20** | (c) | **23** | (d) | **26** | (a) | **29** | (b) |
| **3** | (d) | **6** | (d) | **9** | (d) | **12** | (a) | **15** | (b) | **18** | (d) | **21** | (c) | **24** | (b) | **27** | (b) | **30** | (b) |

# 24

# HALOALKANES AND HALOARENES

1. The total number of acyclic isomers including the stereoisomers with the molecular formula $C_4H_7Cl$
   (a) 11 (b) 12
   (c) 9 (d) 10
2. Which of the following is most reactive toward $S_N2$ reaction?
   (a) $CH_2{=}CH—CH_2—Cl$
   (b) $Ph—CH_2—Cl$
   (c) Me—O⌒Cl
   (d) $Ph—C(=O)—CH_2—Cl$
3. The major product formed when 1, 1, 1-trichloropropane is treated with aqueous potassium hydroxide is:
   (a) Propyne (b) 1-Propanol
   (c) 2-Propanol (d) Propionic acid
4. Among the following, the molecule with the lowest dipole moment is
   (a) $CHCl_3$ (b) $CH_3Cl$
   (c) $CH_2Cl_2$ (d) $CCl_4$
5. When chlorine is passed through propene at 400°C, which of the following is formed ?
   (a) PVC (b) Allyl chloride
   (c) Alkyl chloride (d) 1, 2-Dichloroethane
6. 2-Bromopentane is heated with potassium ethoxide in ethanol. The major product obtained is
   (a) 2-ethoxypentane
   (b) pentene-1
   (c) *trans*-2-pentene
   (d) *cis*-pentene-2
7. In the following sequence of reactions

   $$C_2H_5Br \xrightarrow{AgCN} X(major) \xrightarrow{Reduction} Y;$$

   Y is
   (a) *n*-propyl amine (b) isopropylamine
   (c) ethylamine (d) ethylmethyl amine
8. The organic chloro compound, which shows complete stereochemical inversion during $S_N2$ reaction is
   (a) $(C_2H_5)_2CHCl$ (b) $(CH_3)_3CCl$
   (c) $(CH_3)_2CHCl$ (d) $CH_3Cl$

**9.** In a nucleophilic substitution reaction:

$$R-Br+Cl^- \xrightarrow{DMF} R-Cl+Br^-,$$

which one of the following undergoes complete inversion of configuration?

(a) $C_6H_5CHC_6H_5Br$ (b) $C_6H_5CH_2Br$

(c) $C_6H_5CHCH_3Br$ (d) $C_6H_5CCH_3C_6H_5Br$

**10.** The major product of the following reaction is :

$$CH_3\underset{\displaystyle Br}{\underset{|}{C}}HCH_2\underset{\displaystyle Br}{\underset{|}{C}}HCH_2CH_3 \xrightarrow[heat]{KOH,CH_3OH}$$

(a) $CH_2=CHCH_2CH=CHCH_3$

(b) $CH_2=CHCH=CHCH_2CH_3$

(c) $CH_3CH=C=CHCH_2CH_3$

(d) $CH_3CH=CH-CH=CHCH_3$

**11.** Identify Z in the following series

$$C_2H_5I \xrightarrow{Alc.\ KOH} X \xrightarrow{Br_2} Y \xrightarrow{KCN} Z$$

(a) $CH_3CH_2CN$ (b) $NCCH_2-CH_2CN$

(c) $BrCH_2-CH_2CN$ (d) $BrCH=CHCN$

**12.** Benzene reacts with *n*-propyl chloride in the presence of anhydrous $AlCl_3$ to give

(a) 3 – Propyl – 1 – chlorobenzene

(b) *n*-Propylbenzene

(c) Isopropylbenzene

(d) No reaction occurs

**13.** Silver benzoate reacts with bromine to form

(a) 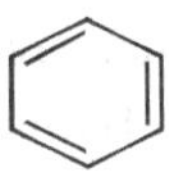

(b) 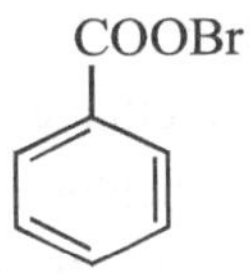


(c) 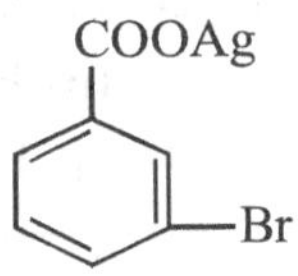


(d) $C_6H_5Br$

**14.** The Wurtz-Fittig reaction involves condensation of :

(a) two molecules of aryl halides

(b) one molecule each of aryl halide and alkyl halide.

(c) one molecule each of aryl halide and phenol.

(d) two molecules of aralkyl halides.

**15.** The correct kinetic rate equation for the addition-elimination mechanism of nucleophilic aromatic substitution is:

(a) rate = $k$ [aryl halide] [nucleophile]

(b) rate = $k$ [aryl halide]

(c) rate = $k$ [aryl halide] [nucleophile]$^2$

(d) rate = $k$ [ nucleophile]

**16.** Freon used as refrigerant is

(a) $CF_2=CF_2$ (b) $CH_2F_2$

(c) $CCl_2F_2$ (d) $CF_4$

**17.** Phosgene is a common name for

(a) phosphoryl chloride

(b) thionyl chloride

(c) carbon dioxide and phosphine

(d) carbonyl dichloride.

**18.** The order of reactivity of the given haloalkanes towards nucleophile is :

(a) RI > RBr > KCl (b) RCl > RBr > RI

(c) RBr > RCl > RI (d) RBr > RI > RCl

**19.** In the following groups :

–OAc (I) –OMe (II)

$-OSO_2Me$ (III) $-OSO_2CF_3$ (IV)

the order of leaving group ability is

(a) I > II > III > IV (b) IV > III > I > II

(c) III > II > I > IV (d) II > III > IV > I

**20.** Elimination of bromine from 2-bromobutane results in the formation of –

(a) predominantly 2-butyne

(b) predominantly 1-butene

(c) predominantly 2-butene

(d) equimolar mixture of 1- and 2-butenes

**21.** The reaction of tert-butyl bromide with sodium methoxide produces mainly–

(a) iso-butane

(b) iso-butylene

(c) tert-butyl methyl ether

(d) sodium tert butoxide

**22.** Ethylidene bromide on heating with metallic sodium in ether solution yields :

(a) ethene (b) ethyne

(c) 2-butene (d) 1-butene

**23.** The product of reaction between alcoholic silver nitrite with ethyl bromide is :

(a) ethene (b) ethane

(c) ethyl nitrile (d) nitroethane

**24.** The reaction conditions leading to the best yields of $C_2H_5Cl$ are :

(a) $C_2H_6 \text{ (excess)} + Cl_2 \xrightarrow{\text{UV light}}$

(b) $C_2H_6 + Cl_2 \xrightarrow[\text{room temperature}]{\text{dark}}$

(c) $C_2H_6 + Cl_2 \text{ (excess)} \xrightarrow{\text{UV light}}$

(d) $C_2H_6 + Cl_2 \xrightarrow{\text{UV light}}$

**25.** Halogenation of alkanes is

(a) a reductive process

(b) an oxidative process

(c) an isothermal process

(d) an endothermal process

**26.** A compound is formed by substitution of two chlorine for two hydrogens in propane. The number of possible isomeric compounds is

(a) 4 (b) 3

(c) 5 (d) 2

**27.** The chief reaction product of reaction between *n*-butane and bromine at 573K is :

(a) $CH_3CH_2CH_2CH_2Br$

(b) $CH_3CH_2CHBr$ with $CH_3$ on the CHBr carbon

(c) $CH_3-CH_2CHBr$ with $CH_2Br$ on the CHBr carbon

(d) $CH_3CH_2CBr_2$ with $CH_3$ on the $CBr_2$ carbon

**28.** Aryl fluoride may be prepared from arene diazonium chloride using :

(a) $HBF_4/\Delta$ (b) $HBF_4/NaNO_2, Cu, \Delta$

(c) CuF/HF (d) Cu/HF

**29.** How many isomeric naphthylamines are expected in the following reaction ?

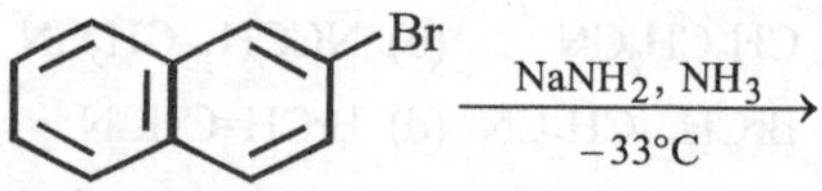


(a) two (b) only single product

(c) four (d) three

**30.** Match the columns

| Column - I (Haloalkane/arene) | Column - II (Applications) |
|---|---|
| (A) Iodoform | (p) $CF_4$ |
| (B) BHC | (q) Antiseptic |
| (C) Freon - 14 | (r) Moth repellant |
| (D) Halothanes | (s) Inhalative anaesthetic |
| (E) *p*-Dichlorobenzene | (t) Termite pesticide |

(a) A – (q), B – (s), C – (t), D – (r), E – (p)

(b) A – (q), B – (t), C – (p), D – (s), E – (r)

(c) A – (r), B – (s), C – (q), D – (p), E – (t)

(d) A – (p), B – (r), C – (t), D – (q), E – (s)

**ANSWER KEY**

| | | | | | | | | | | | | | | | | | | | |
|---|---|---|---|---|---|---|---|---|---|---|---|---|---|---|---|---|---|---|---|
| 1 | (a) | 4 | (d) | 7 | (d) | 10 | (d) | 13 | (d) | 16 | (c) | 19 | (b) | 22 | (c) | 25 | (b) | 28 | (a) |
| 2 | (d) | 5 | (b) | 8 | (d) | 11 | (b) | 14 | (b) | 17 | (d) | 20 | (c) | 23 | (d) | 26 | (c) | 29 | (a) |
| 3 | (d) | 6 | (c) | 9 | (c) | 12 | (c) | 15 | (a) | 18 | (a) | 21 | (b) | 24 | (a) | 27 | (b) | 30 | (b) |

# 25 ALCOHOLS, PHENOLS AND ETHERS

1. Which is oxidized most easily?

(a) $CH_3 - CHOH - CH_3$

(b) 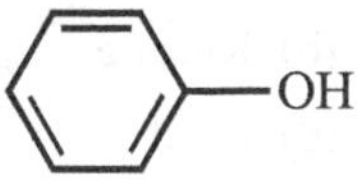

(c) $CH_3 - CH_2 - O - CH_2 - CH_3$

(d) 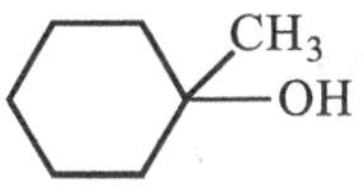

2. Consider the following alcohols,

(I) 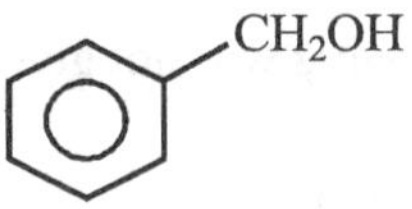

(II) 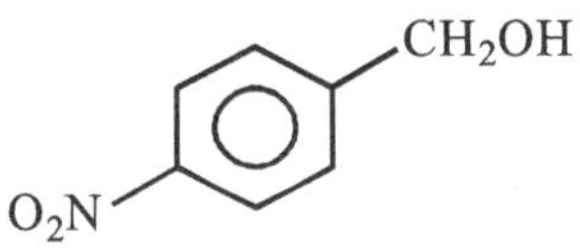

(III) 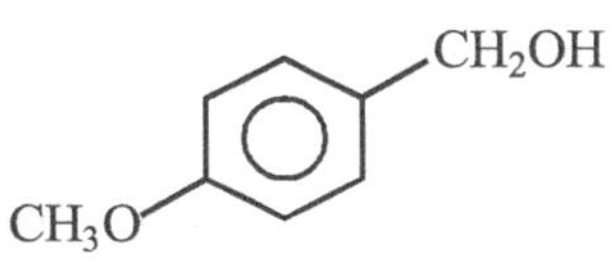

(IV) 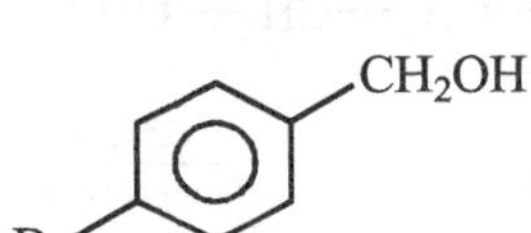

The order of decreasing reactivities of these alcohols towards nucleophilic substitution with HBr is:

(a) III > I > IV > II (b) III > I > II > IV

(c) I > III > IV > II (d) I > III > II > IV

3. Which of the following reagents would carry out the following transformation? ($D = {}^2H$)

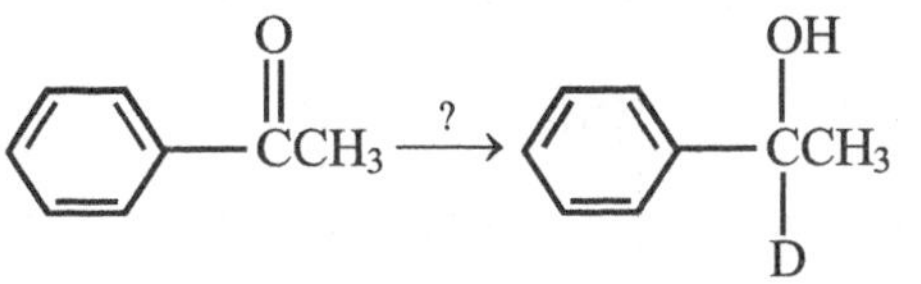

(a) $NaBD_4$ in $CH_3OH$

(b) $LiAlH_4$, then $D_2O$

(c) $NaBD_4$ in $CH_3OD$

(d) $LiAlD_4$, then $D_2O$

**4.** In which of the following reactions hydrogen gas will not be evolved?

(a) $CH_3CH_2OH \xrightarrow{Na}$

(b) $CH_3CH_2OH \xrightarrow{K}$

(c) $CH_3CH(CH_3)OH \xrightarrow{Al}$ (i.e. $CH_3\underset{\displaystyle CH_3}{\underset{|}{C}}HOH$)

(d) $CH_3CH(CH_3)OH \xrightarrow{CH_3MgBr}$

**5.** What is the major product of the following reaction?

$$CH_3-\overset{\displaystyle OH}{\overset{|}{C}H}-CH_2-CH_2-OH \xrightarrow[\text{Pyridine cold}]{CrO_3} \text{Product}$$

(a) $CH_3-\overset{\displaystyle OH}{\overset{|}{C}H}-CH_2-\overset{\displaystyle O}{\overset{\|}{C}}-H$

(b) $CH_3-\overset{\displaystyle O}{\overset{\|}{C}}-CH_2-\overset{\displaystyle O}{\overset{\|}{C}}-H$

(c) $CH_3-\overset{\displaystyle O}{\overset{\|}{C}}-CH_2-\overset{\displaystyle O}{\overset{\|}{C}}-OH$

(d) $CH_3-\overset{\displaystyle OH}{\overset{|}{C}H}-CH_2-\overset{\displaystyle O}{\overset{\|}{C}}-OH$

**6.** 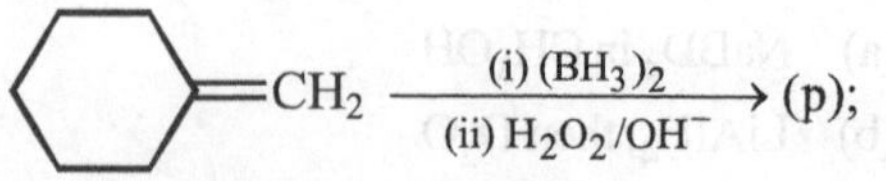


Product (P) in the reaction is:

(a) 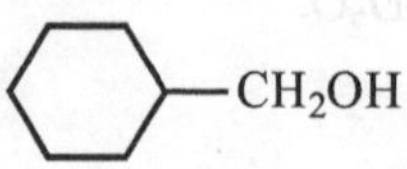


(b) 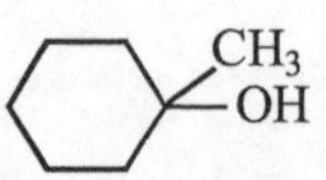


(c) 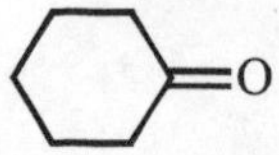


(d) 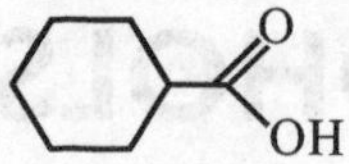


**7.** Rate of dehydration of alcohols follows the order:

(a) $2° > 1° > CH_3OH > 3°$

(b) $3° > 2° > 1° > CH_3OH$

(c) $2° > 3° > 1° > CH_3OH$

(d) $CH_3OH > 1° > 2° > 3°$

**8.** HBr reacts fastest with

(a) 2-methylpropan-1-ol

(b) 2-methylpropan-2-ol

(c) propan-2-ol

(d) propan-1-ol.

**9.** What is formed when a primary alcohol undergoes catalytic dehydrogenation ?

(a) Aldehyde (b) Ketone

(c) Alkene (d) Acid

**10.** The best method to prepare cyclohexene from cyclohexanol is by using

(a) Conc. $HCl + ZnCl_2$

(b) Conc. $H_3PO_4$

(c) HBr

(d) Conc. HCl

**11.** Which of the following will not give iodoform test?

(a) Isopropyl alcohol

(b) Ethanol

(c) Ethanal

(d) Benzyl alcohol

**12.** Glycerol is more viscous than ethanol due to

(a) high molecular weight

(b) high boiling point

(c) many hydrogen bonds per molecule

(d) Fajan's rule

13. 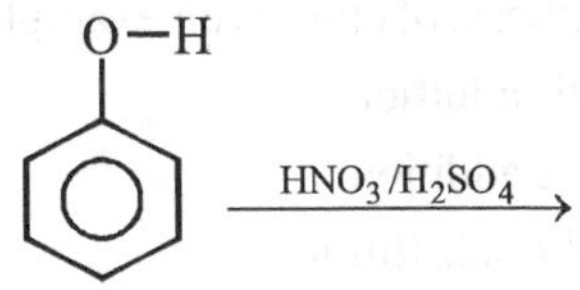

(A) + (B)
(more volatile) (less volatile)

Product (A) of the above reaction is:

(a) 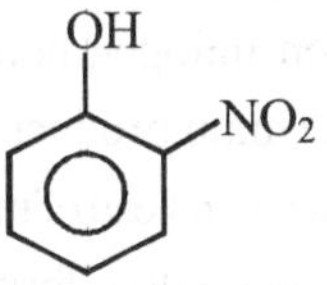 (b) 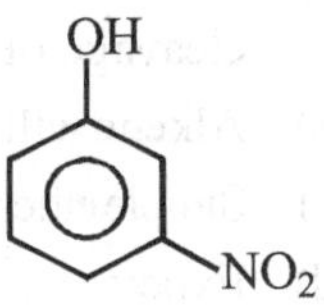

(c) 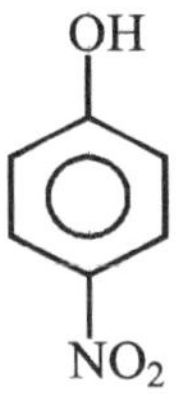 (d) 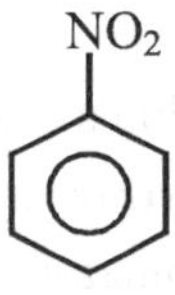

14. Which of the following is the correct order of the acidity of the three compounds ?

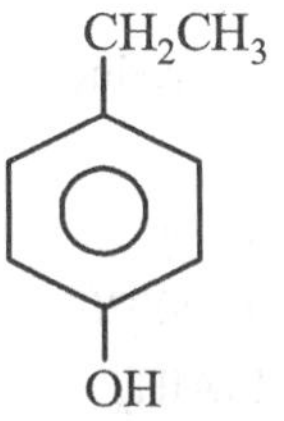
I

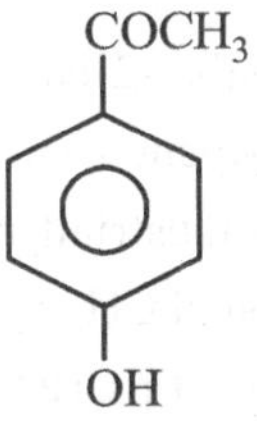
II

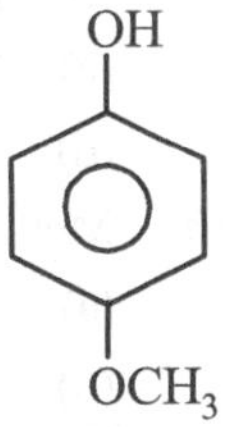
III

(a) II > III > I (b) III > II > I
(c) II > I > III (d) III > I > II

15. Phenol on heating with $CHCl_3$ and NaOH gives salicylaldehyde. The reaction is called :
(a) Reimer - Tiemann reaction
(b) Claisen reaction
(c) Cannizzaro's reaction
(d) Hell - Volhard - Zelinsky reaction

16. Which one of the following compounds will be most readily attacked by an electrophile ?
(a) Chlorobenzene
(b) Benzene
(c) Phenol
(d) Toluene

17. When phenol is treated with excess bromine water. It gives
(a) *m*-Bromophenol
(b) *o*-and *p*-Bromophenols
(c) 2,4-Dibromophenol
(d) 2,4, 6-Tribromophenol.

18. On distillation with Zn dust, phenol gives :
(a) acetophenone
(b) benzoic acid
(c) benzene
(d) benzophenone

19. Phenol is more acidic than alcohol because.
(a) phenol is more stable than water
(b) phenol is aromatic and alcohol is aliphatic
(c) phenoxide ion is resonance stabilised
(d) None of these

20. Phenol is less acidic than :
(a) acetic acid
(b) *p*-methoxyphenol
(c) acetylene
(d) ethanol

21. To distinguish between salicylic acid and phenol, one can use :
(a) $NaHCO_3$ solution
(b) 5% NaOH solution
(c) neutral $FeCl_3$
(d) bromine water

22. What is X in the following reaction ?

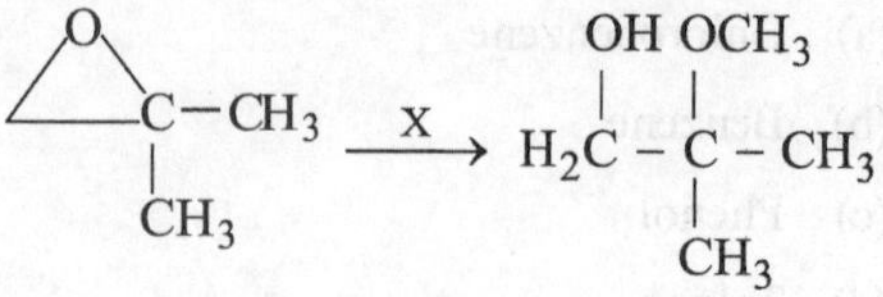

(a) $CH_3OH, H_2SO_4$

(b) $CH_3OH, CH_3O^- \overset{+}{Na}$

(c) $H_2O/H_2SO_4$ followed by $CH_3OH$

(d) $CH_3MgBr$ / ether followed by $H_3O^+$

23. In Williamson's synthesis, ethoxyethane is prepared by

(a) passing ethanol over heated alumina

(b) sodium ethoxide with ethyl bromide

(c) ethyl alcohol with sulphuric acid

(d) ethyl iodide and dry silver oxide

24. The ether that undergoes electrophilic substitution reactions is

(a) $CH_3OC_2H_5$ (b) $C_6H_5OCH_3$

(c) $CH_3OCH_3$ (d) $C_2H_5OC_2H_5$

25. The cleavage of an aryl alkyl ether with cold HI gives :

(a) alkyl iodide and water

(b) aryl iodide and water

(c) alkyl iodide, aryl iodide and water

(d) phenol and alkyl iodide

26. Williamson synthesis of ether is an example of:

(a) Nucleophilic addition

(b) Electrophilic addition

(c) Electrophilic substitution

(d) Nucleophilic substitution

27. In Williamson synthesis of mixed ether having a primary and a tertiary alkyl group if tertiary halide is used, then :

(a) Rate of reaction will be slow due to slow cleavage of carbon-halogen bond.

(b) Alkene will be the main product.

(c) Simple ether will form instead of mixed ether.

(d) Expected mixed ether will be formed.

28. Benzyl alcohol is obtained from benzaldehyde by:

(a) Perkin's reaction

(b) Wurtz reaction

(c) Cannizzaro's reaction

(d) Claisen's reaction

29. The dehydration of 2-methylbutanol with conc. $H_2SO_4$ gives :

(a) 2-Methylbutene as major product

(b) Pentene

(c) 2-Methylbut-2-ene as major product

(d) 2-Methylpent-2-ene

30. Methanol is industrially prepared by

(a) oxidation of $CH_4$ by steam at 900°C

(b) reduction of HCHO using $LiAlH_4$

(c) reaction HCHO with a solution of NaOH

(d) reduction of CO using $H_2$ and $ZnO-Cr_2O_3$.

**ANSWER KEY**

| | | | | | | | | | | | | | | | | | | | |
|---|---|---|---|---|---|---|---|---|---|---|---|---|---|---|---|---|---|---|---|
| 1 | (a) | 4 | (d) | 7 | (b) | 10 | (b) | 13 | (a) | 16 | (c) | 19 | (c) | 22 | (a) | 25 | (d) | 28 | (c) |
| 2 | (a) | 5 | (b) | 8 | (b) | 11 | (d) | 14 | (c) | 17 | (d) | 20 | (a) | 23 | (b) | 26 | (d) | 29 | (c) |
| 3 | (a) | 6 | (a) | 9 | (a) | 12 | (c) | 15 | (a) | 18 | (c) | 21 | (a) | 24 | (b) | 27 | (b) | 30 | (d) |

# 26

# ALDEHYDES, KETONES AND CARBOXYLIC ACIDS

1. 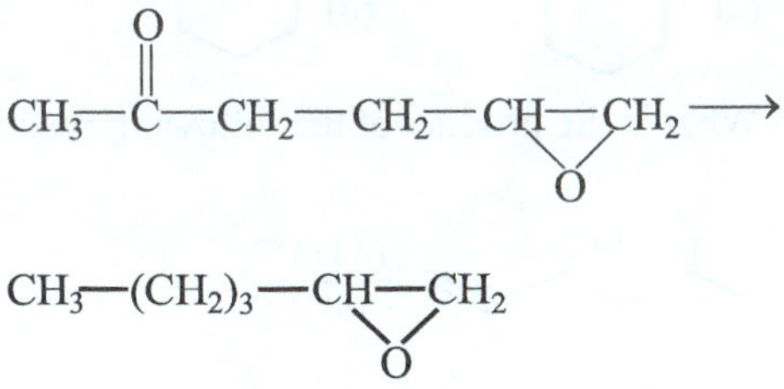

Above conversion can be achived by:

(a) Wolff-Kishner reduction

(b) Clemmensen reduction

(c) HS — $CH_2$— $CH_2$ — SH, following by Raney Ni

(d) None of these

2. $CH_3CHO \xrightarrow[5°C]{10\%\ NaOH} \xrightarrow{\Delta} \xrightarrow[Ni]{H_2} (A)$;

Product (A) of the reaction is:

(a) propanol (b) ethanol

(c) butanol (d) pentanol

3. A compound that gives a positive iodoform test is

(a) 1-pentanol

(b) 2-pentanone

(c) 3-pentanone

(d) pentanal

4. Formaldehyde can be distinguished from acetaldehyde by the use of :

(a) Schiff's reagent

(b) Tollen's reagent

(c) $I_2$/Alkali

(d) Fehling's solution

5. Clemmensen reduction of a ketone is carried out in the presence of :

(a) $LiAlH_4$

(b) Zn-Hg with HCl

(c) Glycol with KOH

(d) $H_2$ with Pt as catalyst

6. *m*-Chlorobenzaldehyde on reaction with conc. KOH at room temperature gives

(a) Potassium *m*-chlorobenzoate and *m*-hydroxybenzaldehyde

(b) *m*-hydroxybenzaldeyde and *m*-chlorobenzyl alcohol

(c) *m*-chlorobenzyl alcohol and *m*-hydroxybenzyl alcohol

(d) Potassium *m*-chlorobenzoate and *m*-chlorobenzyl alcohol

7. Which of the following compound will undergo self aldol condensation in the presence of cold dilute alkali ?

(a) $CH_2 = CH - CHO$

(b) $CH \equiv C - CHO$

(c) $C_6H_5CHO$

(d) $CH_3CH_2CHO$.

8. Which of the following compound will show positive silver mirror test?

(a) HCOOH

(b) $CH_3(CHOH)_3CHO$

(c) $CH_3CO(CHOH)CH_3$

(d) Both (a) and (b)

9. Which of the following is disproportionation reaction?

(a) $2HCHO \xrightarrow{NaOH} CH_3OH + HCOONa$

(b) $2CH_3CHO \xrightarrow{NaOH} CH_3\underset{OH}{\underset{|}{C}H}CH_2CHO$

(c) 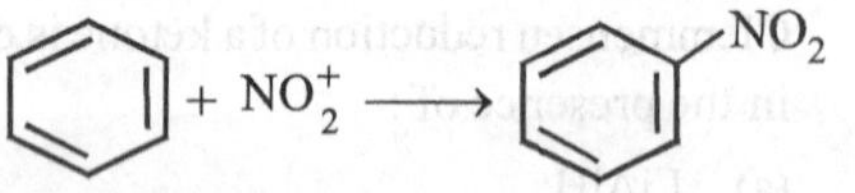

(d) Both (a) & (b)

10. The reactant (X) in the reaction

$(X) \xrightarrow[(CH_3CO)_2O]{CH_3COONa}$ Cinnamic acid, is

(a) 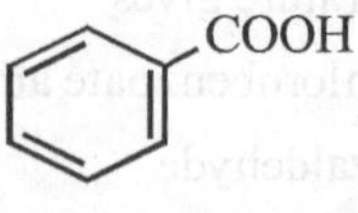 (b) 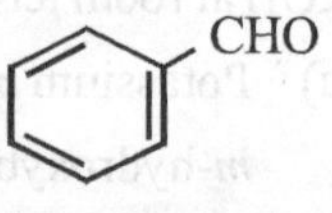

(c) 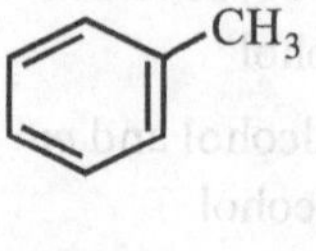 (d) 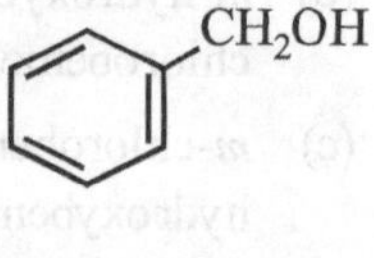

11. Which one of the following reactions will not result in the formation of carbon-carbon bond?

(a) Reimer-Tieman reaction

(b) Friedel Craft's acylation

(c) Wurtz reaction

(d) Cannizzaro reaction

12. 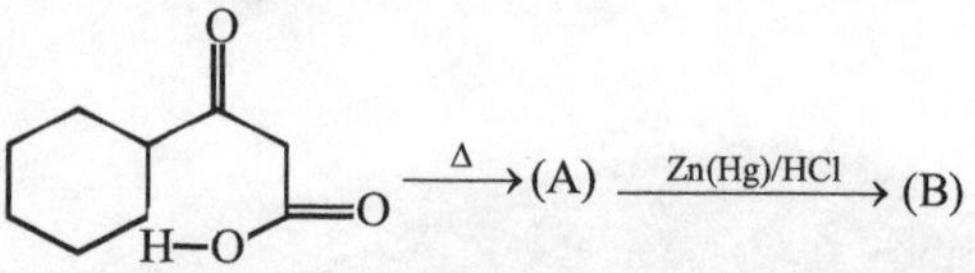

In the above reaction, product (B) is:

(a) 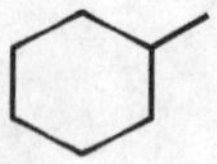 (b) 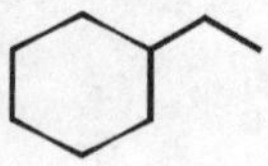

(c) 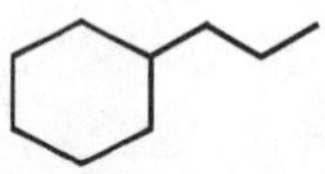 (d) 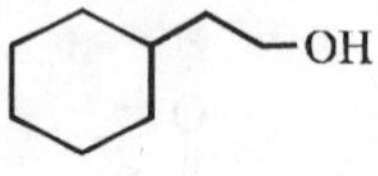

13. What is the product of the following reaction ?

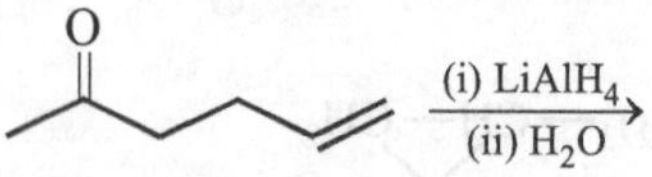

(a) 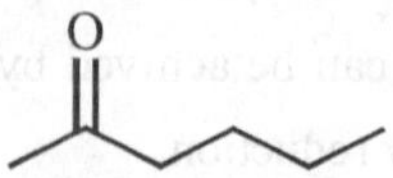

(b) 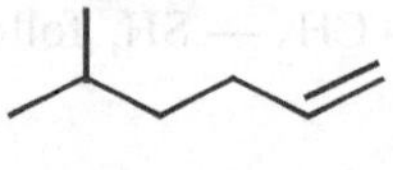

(c) 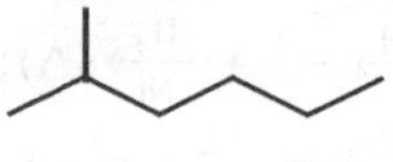

(d) 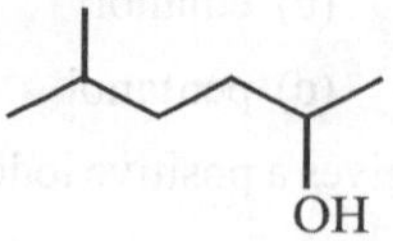

**14.** The major product of the following reaction is :

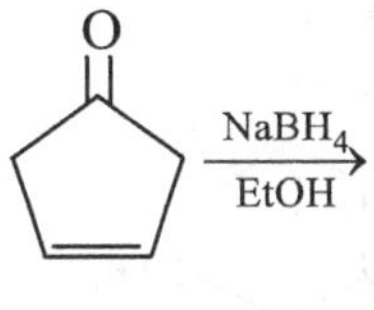

(a) 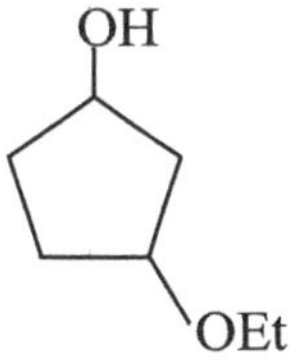 (b) 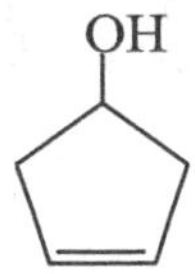

(c) 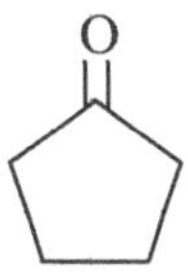 (d) 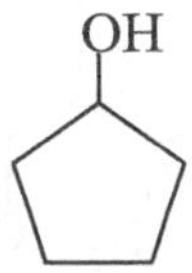

**15.** The correct acidity order of the following is

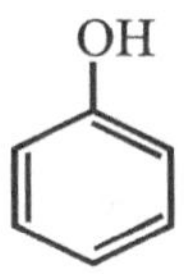 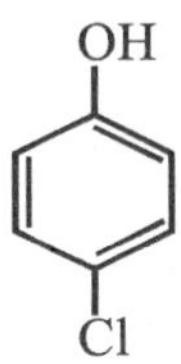 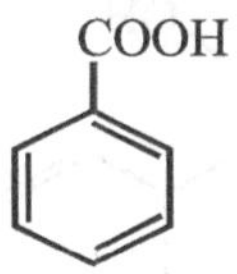 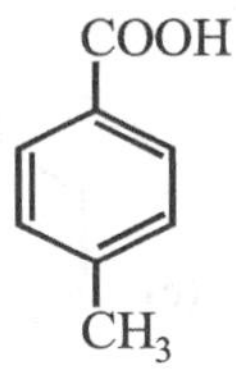

(I) (II) (III) (IV)

(a) (III) > (IV) > (II) > (I)

(b) (IV) > (III) > (I) > (II)

(c) (III) > (II) > (I) > (IV)

(d) (II) > (III) > (IV) > (I)

**16.** 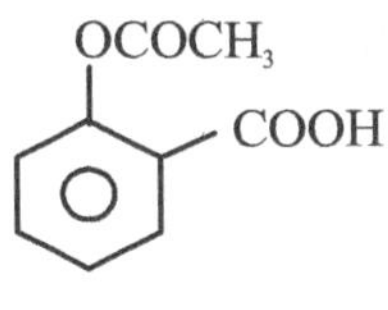 is used as :

(a) Analgesic (b) Insecticide

(c) Antacid (d) Antihistamine

**17.** Benzoyl chloride is prepared from benzoic acid by

(a) $Cl_2$, $hv$ (b) $SO_2Cl_2$

(c) $SOCl_2$ (d) $Cl_2$, $H_2O$

**18.** Formic acid is obtained when

(a) calcium acetate is heated with conc. $H_2SO_4$

(b) calcium formate is heated with calcium acetate

(c) glycerol is heated with oxalic acid at 373 K

(d) acetaldehyde is oxidised with $K_2Cr_2O_7$ and $H_2SO_4$.

**19.** Schotten-Baumann reaction is a reaction of phenols with

(a) benzoyl chloride and sodium hydroxide

(b) acetyl chloride and sodium hydroxide

(c) salicylic acid and conc. $H_2SO_4$

(d) acetyl chloride and conc $H_2SO_4$

**20.** In the Friedel Craft's acylation reaction, the effective electrophile is

(a) $RCOCl^+$ (b) $AlCl_3$

(c) RCOCl (d) $RCO^+$

**21.** $CH_3CH_2COOH \xrightarrow[\text{red P}]{Cl_2} A \xrightarrow{\text{alc.KOH}} B.$

What is $B$?

(a) $CH_3CH_2COCl$ (b) $CH_3CH_2CHO$

(c) $CH_2{=}CHCOOH$ (d) $ClCH_2CH_2COOH$.

**22.** Acetic anhydride reacts with diethyl ether in presence of anhydrous $AlCl_3$ to give :

(a) $CH_3CH_2COOH$

(b) $CH_3CH_2COOC_2H_5$

(c) $CH_3COOCH_3$

(d) $CH_3COOC_2H_5$

23. The major product of the following reaction is:

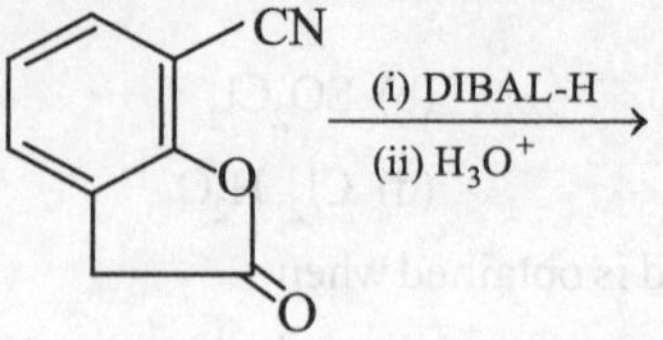

(a) 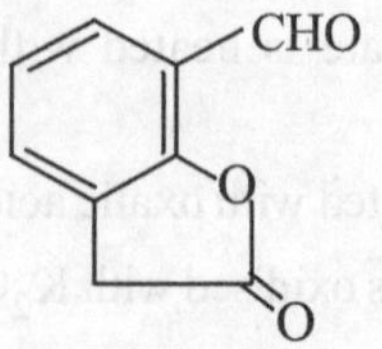

(b) 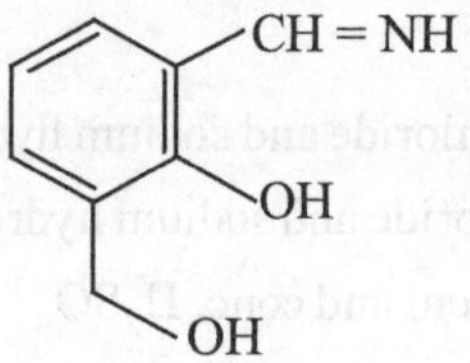

(c) 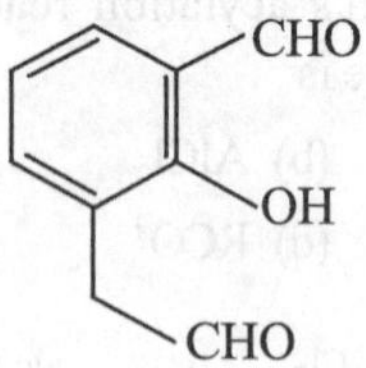

(d) 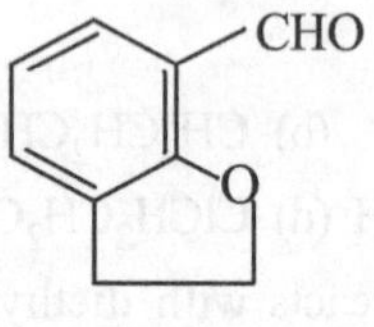

24. The major product obtained in the following reaction is:

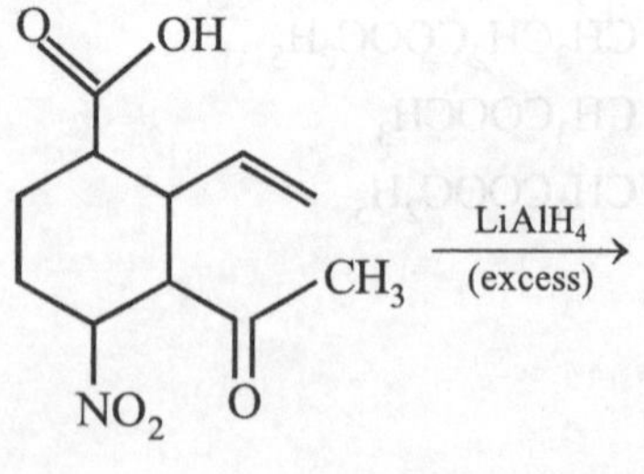

(a) 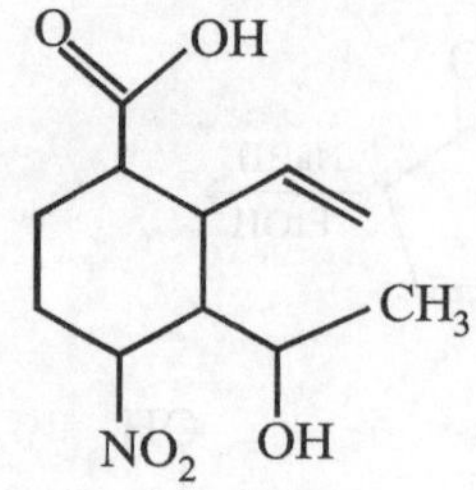

(b) 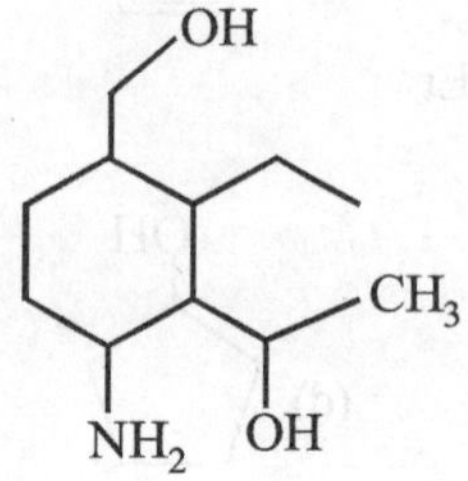

(c) 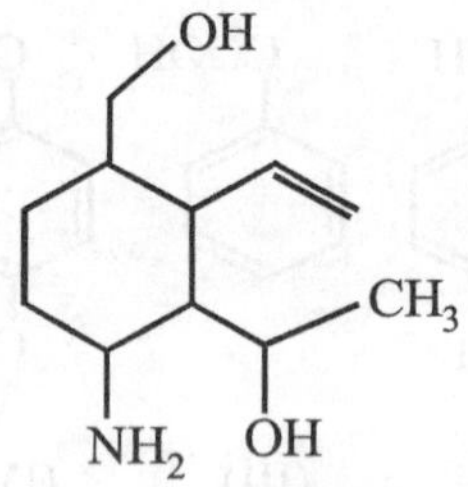

(d) 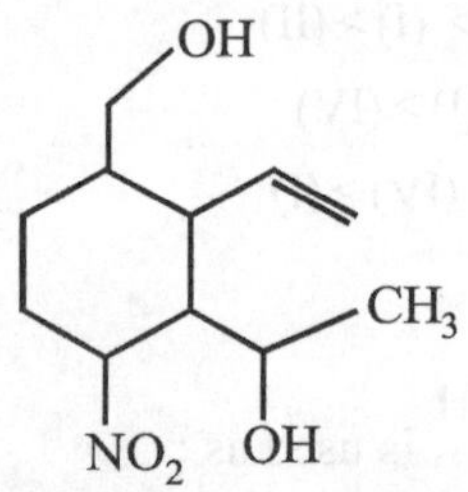

25. The major product of the following reaction is :

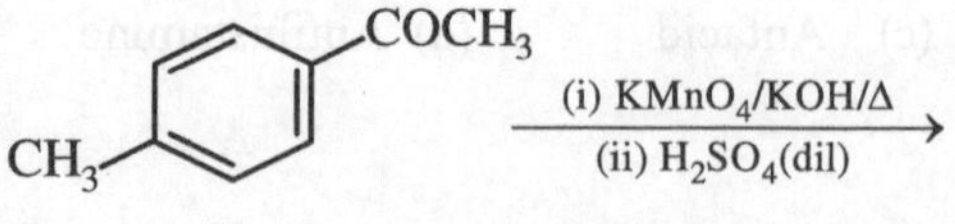

(a) 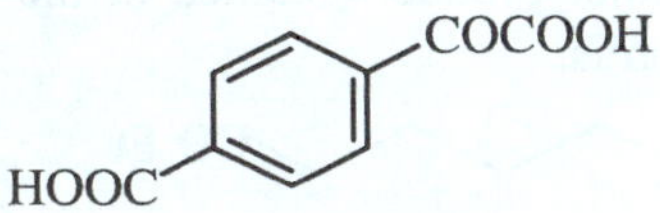

(b) 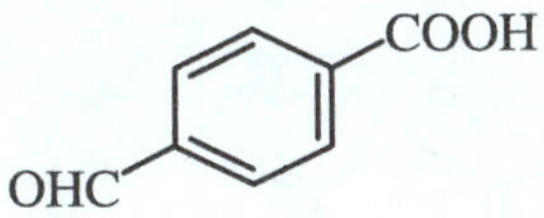

(c) 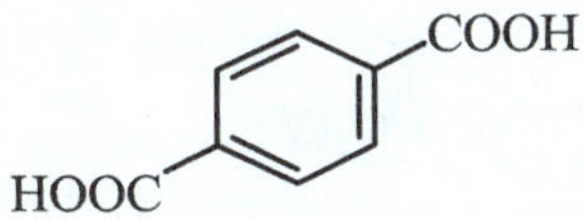

(d) 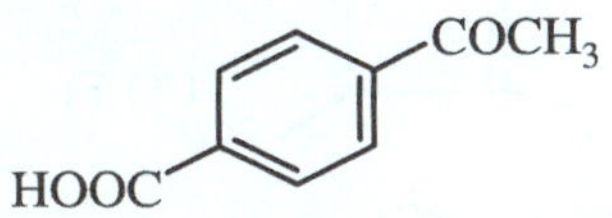

26. Which one of the following compounds will not react with $CH_3MgBr$?
(a) Ethyl acetate
(b) Acetone
(c) Dimethyl ether
(d) Ethanol

27. The compound that undergoes decarboxylation most readily under mild condition is

(a) 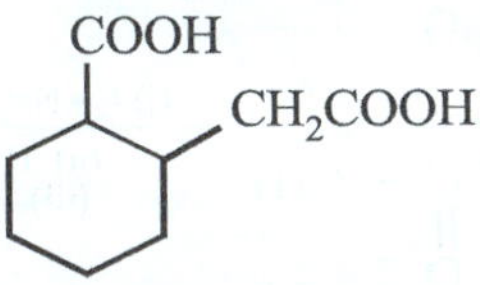

(b) 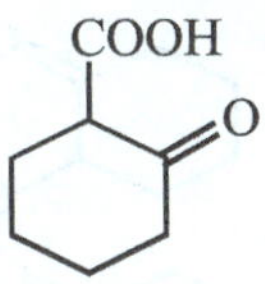

(c) 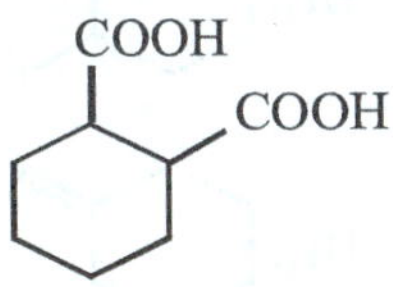

(d) 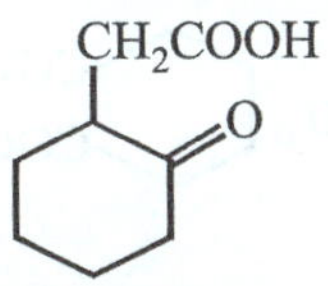

28. Consider the following sequence of reactions.

$$\text{Ketone (A)} \xrightarrow[\text{(ii) } H_2O]{\text{(i) } C_2H_5MgBr}$$

$$\text{(B)} \xrightarrow[-H_2O]{H_2SO_4,\ \text{heat}} \text{(C)} \xrightarrow[\text{(ii) Zn, } H_2O]{\text{(i) } O_3}$$

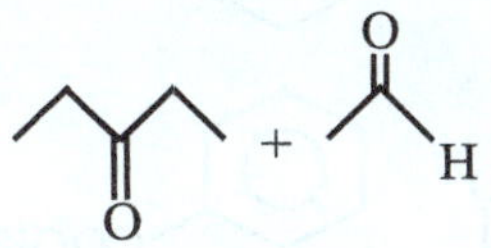

The ketone (A) is:

(a) 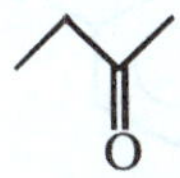
(b) 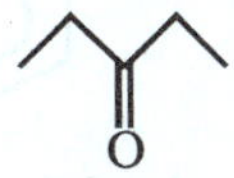
(c) 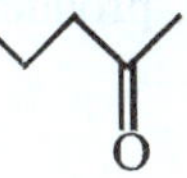
(d) 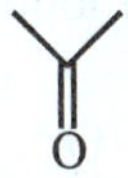

29. 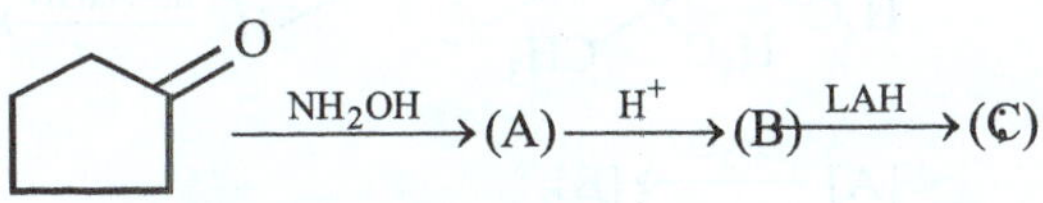

Product (C) of the reaction is:

(a) 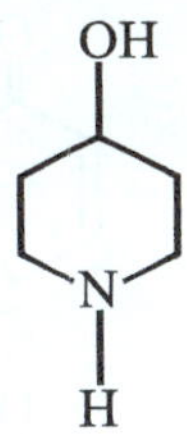
(b) 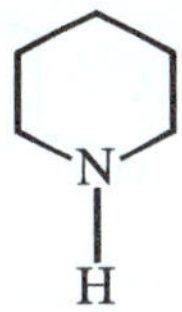
(c) 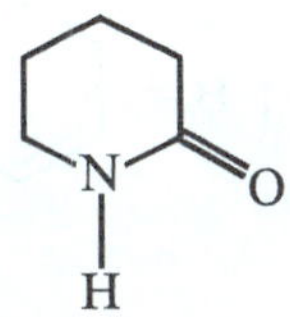
(d) 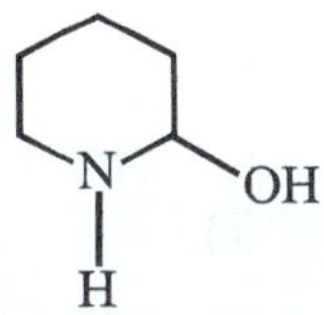

30. 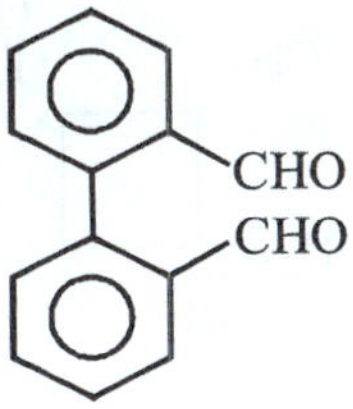

$$\xrightarrow[\Delta]{\text{Conc. KOH}} \text{(A)} \xrightarrow[\Delta]{H^{\oplus}} \underset{\text{Cyclic product}}{\text{(B)}}$$

Structure of (B) is:

(a) 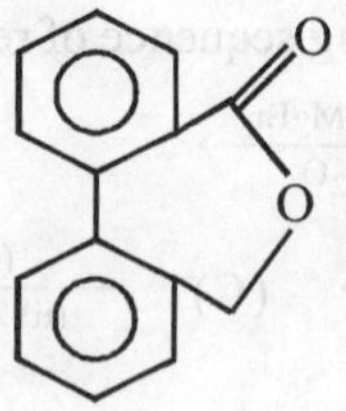 (b) 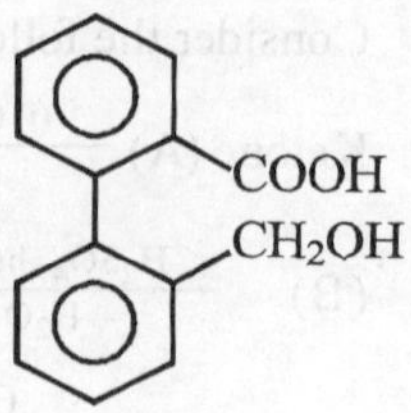

(c) 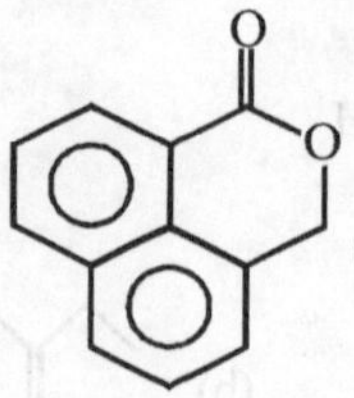 (d) 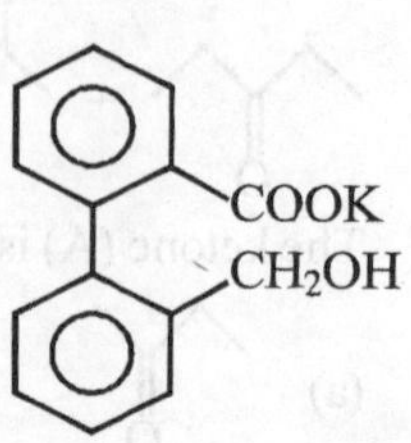

**31.** In the following reactions, products A and B are:

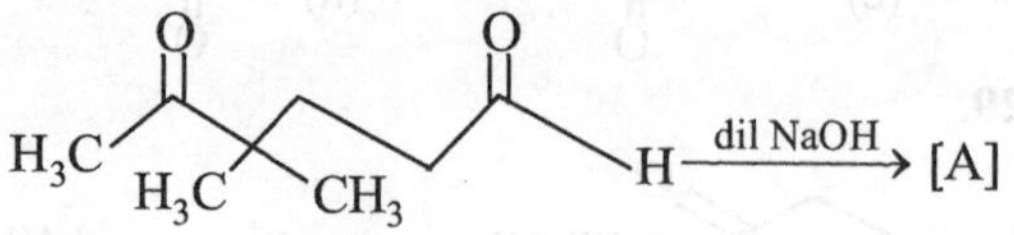

$[A] \xrightarrow{H_3O^+} [B]$

(a)

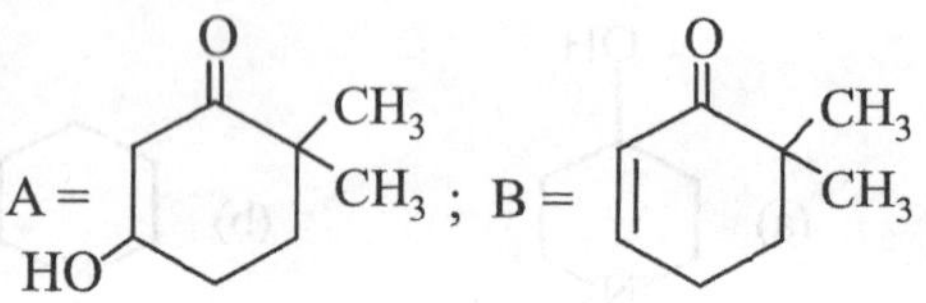

(b)

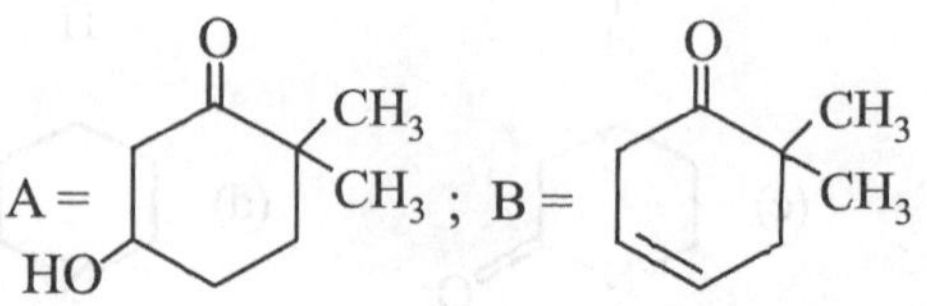

(c)

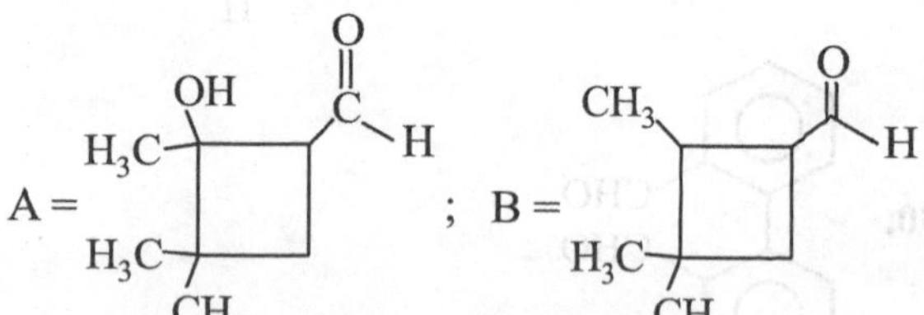

(d)

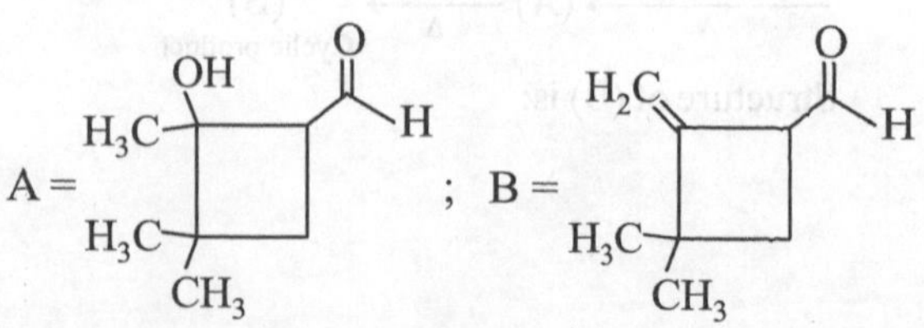

**32.** The major product obtained in the following reaction is:

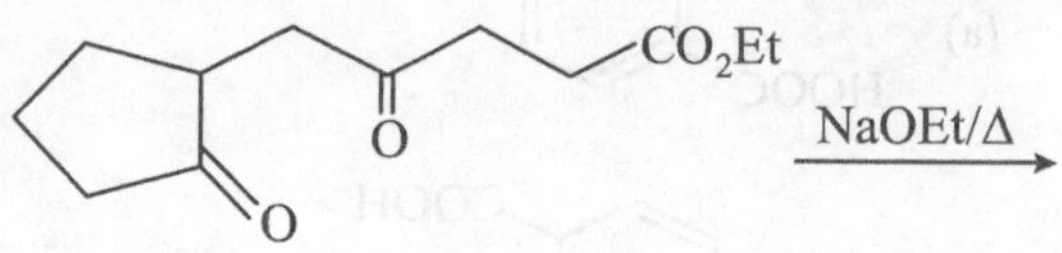

(a) 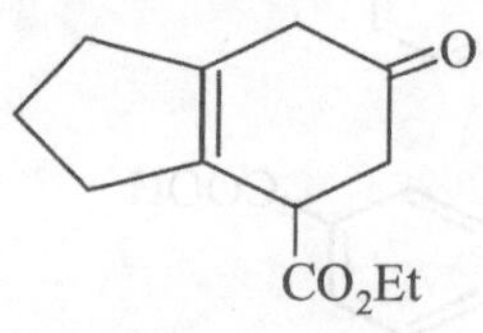

(b) 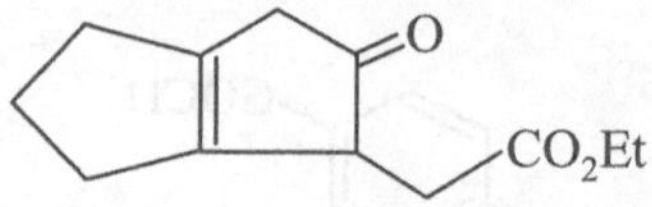

(c) 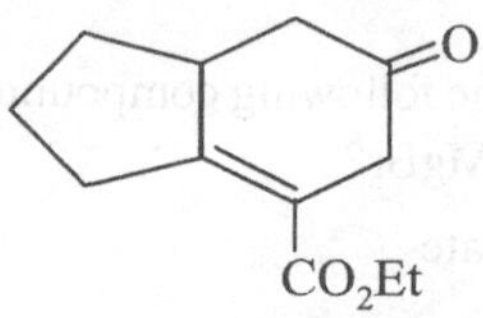

(d) 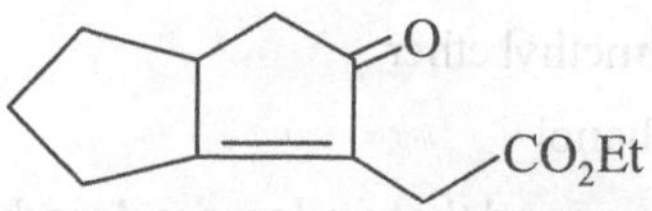

**33.** End product of the following sequence of reactions are:

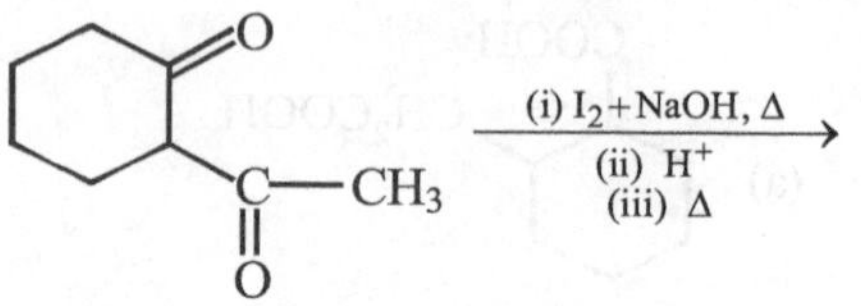

(a) yellow ppt. of $CHI_3$, 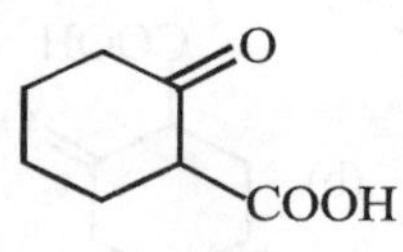

(b) yellow ppt. of $CHI_3$, 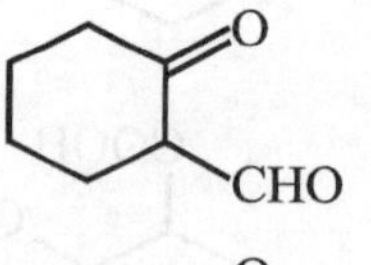

(c) yellow ppt. of $CHI_3$, 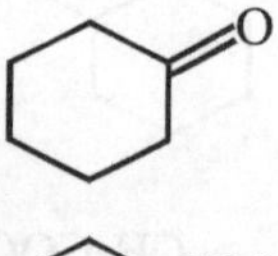

(d) yellow ppt. of $CHI_3$, 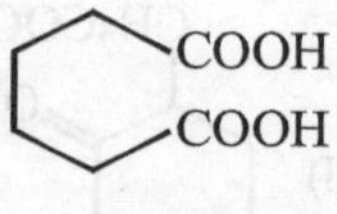

**34.** 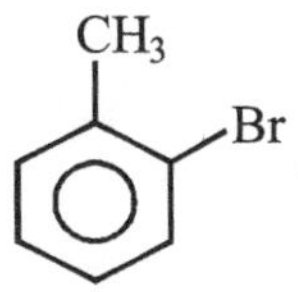 $\xrightarrow[\substack{2.\ H_3O^+ \\ 3.\ KMnO_4/OH^- \\ 4.\ H^+}]{1.\ Mg/Ether}$ A ;

Product A is;

(a) 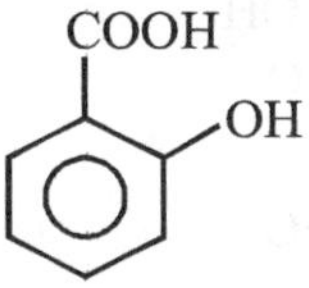 (b) 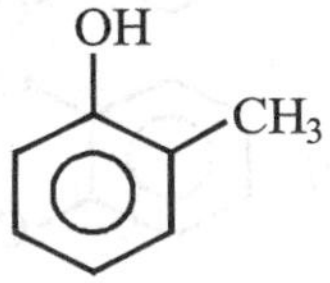

(c) 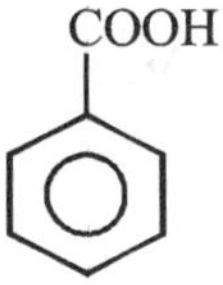 (d) 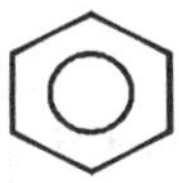

**35.**

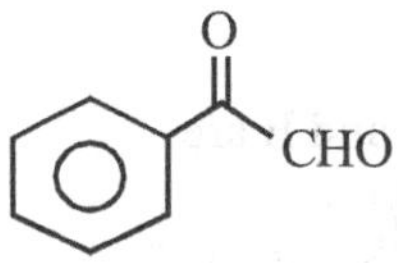 $\xrightarrow{\text{Conc. NaOH}}$ Product should be

(a) 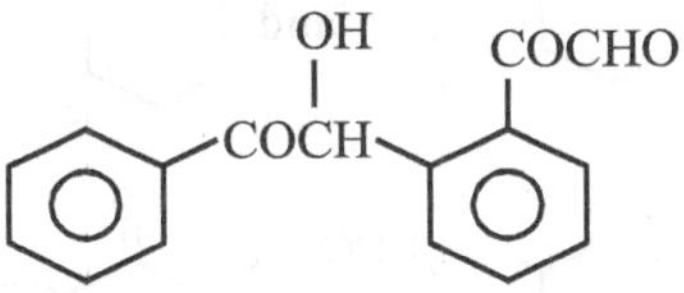

(b) 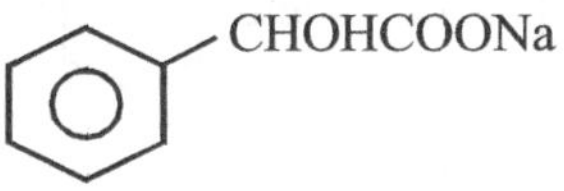

(c)

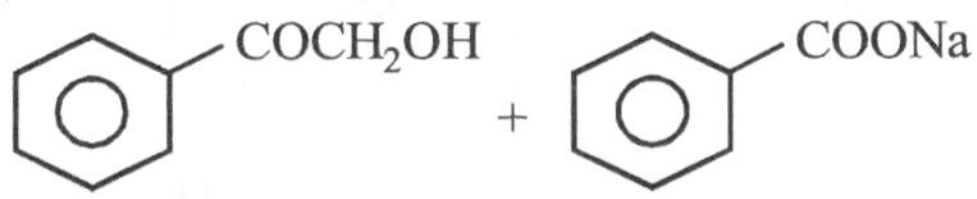

(d) 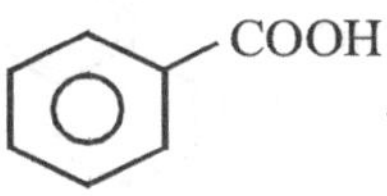

**36.** 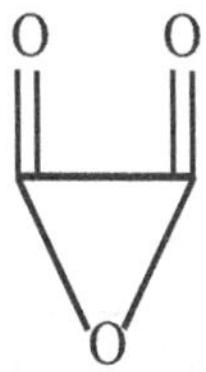

$\xrightarrow[\text{(1 eq.)}]{PhMgBr}$ $\xrightarrow[\text{(1 eq.)}]{CH_3MgBr}$ $\xrightarrow[\text{(1 eq.)}]{H^+/H_2O}$

Product.

The product formed in the reaction is –

(a) 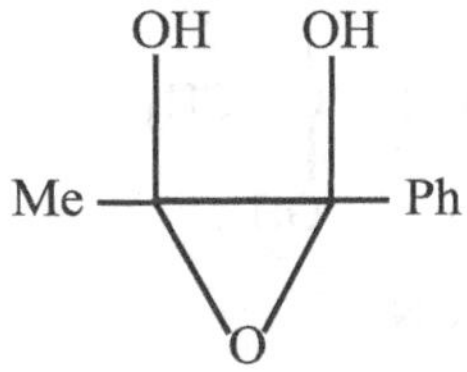

(b) $\mathrm{Me-\overset{\overset{O}{||}}{C}-\overset{\overset{O}{||}}{C}-Ph}$

(c) $\mathrm{Me-\underset{\underset{Ph}{|}}{\overset{\overset{OH}{|}}{C}}-COOH}$

(d) $\mathrm{Ph-\overset{\overset{O}{||}}{C}-\overset{\overset{O}{||}}{C}-O-Me}$

**37.** 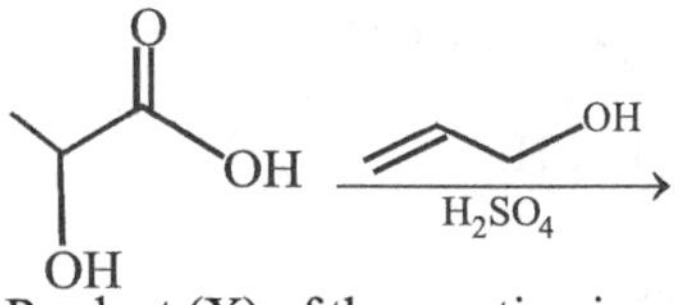 $\xrightarrow[H_2SO_4]{}$ $X + H_2O$

Product (X) of the reaction is–

(a) 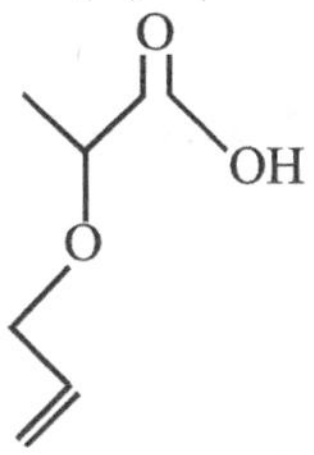 (b) 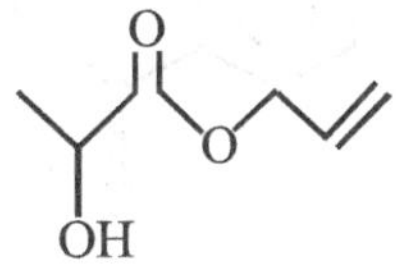

(c) 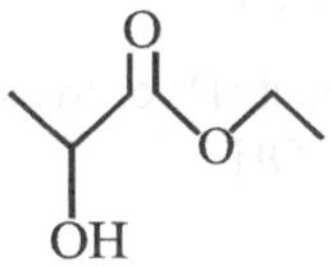 (d) 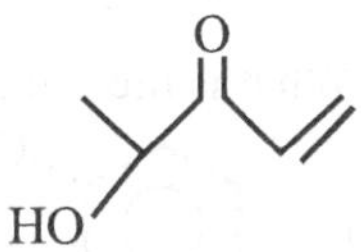

**38.** In a set of reactions, acetic acid yielded a product D.

$$CH_3COOH \xrightarrow{SOCl_2} (A) \xrightarrow[AlCl_3]{Benzene} (B)$$

$$\xrightarrow{HCN} (C) \xrightarrow{HOH} (D)$$

The structure of (D) would be –

(a) 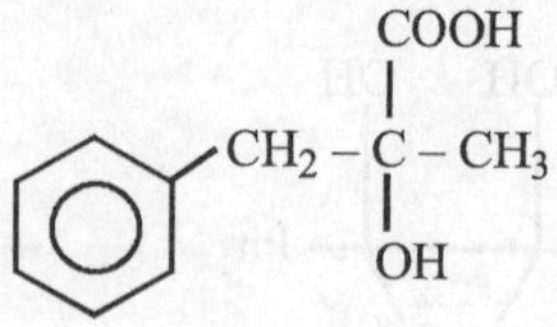

(b) 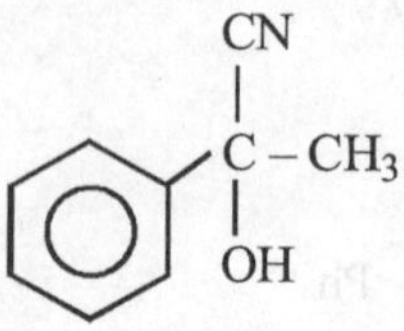

(c) 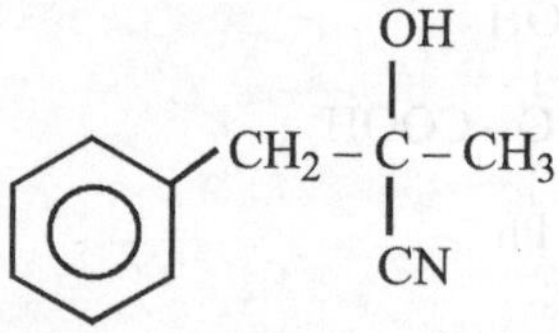

(d) 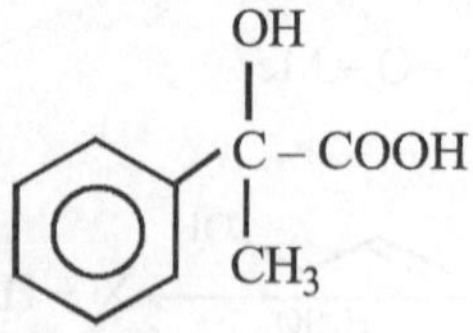

39. 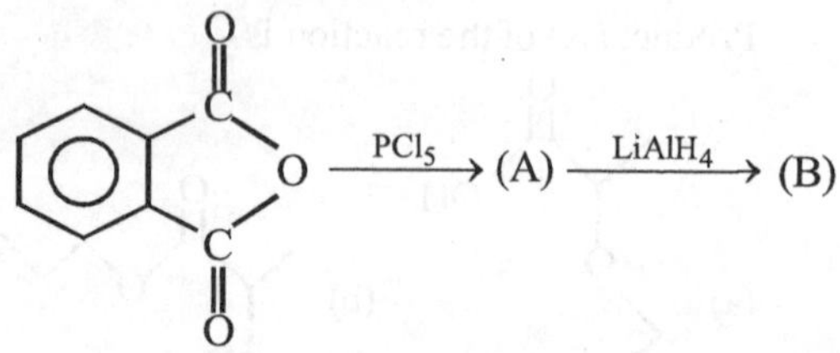

$\xrightarrow{PCC}$ (C) $\xrightarrow[\Delta]{HO^-}$ (D)

What is the final product (D) of the sequence?

(a) 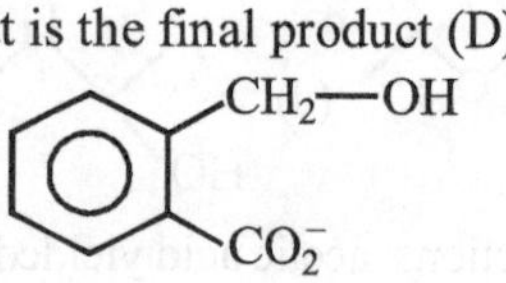

(b) 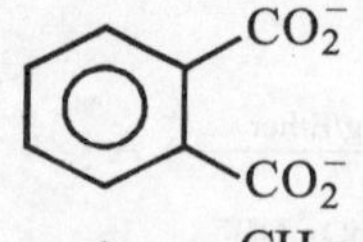

(c) 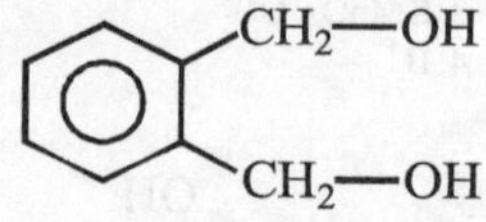

(d) 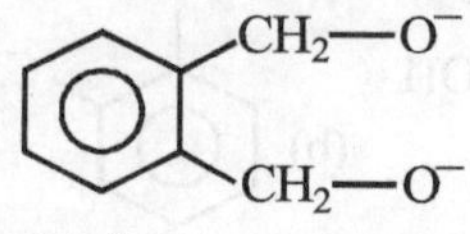

40. 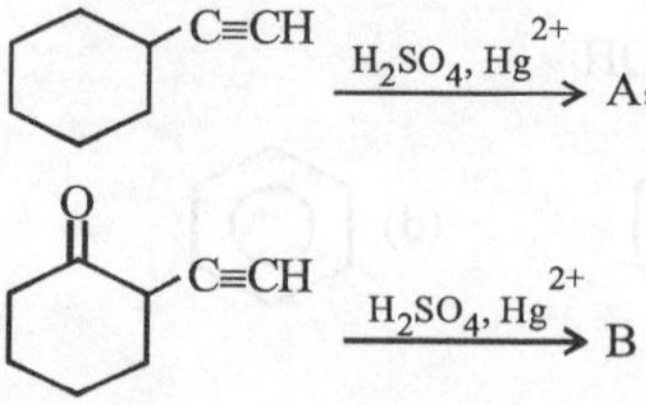

The respective compounds A and B are

(a) 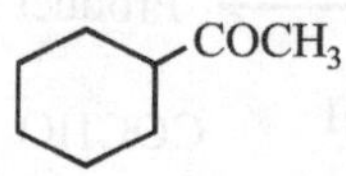 and 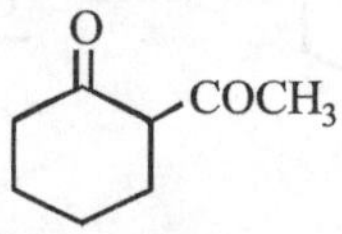

(b) 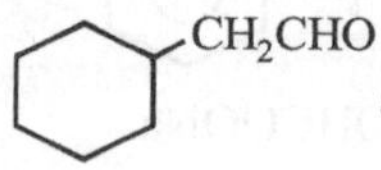 and 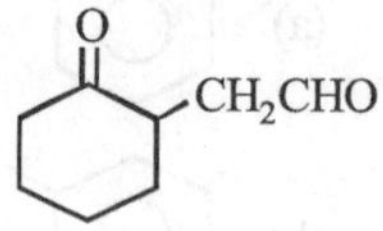

(c) 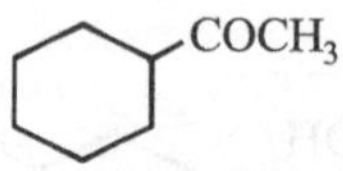 and 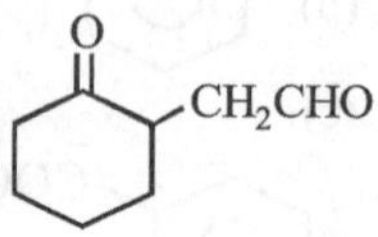

(d) 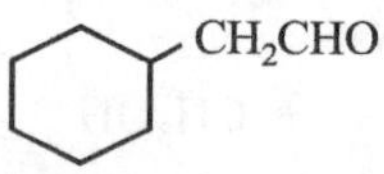 and 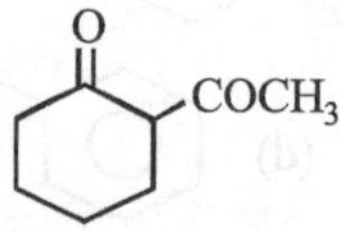

| ANSWER KEY | | | | | | | | | | | | | | | | | | | |
|---|---|---|---|---|---|---|---|---|---|---|---|---|---|---|---|---|---|---|---|
| 1 | (d) | 5 | (b) | 9 | (a) | 13 | (b) | 17 | (c) | 21 | (c) | 25 | (c) | 29 | (b) | 33 | (c) | 37 | (b) |
| 2 | (c) | 6 | (d) | 10 | (b) | 14 | (b) | 18 | (c) | 22 | (d) | 26 | (c) | 30 | (a) | 34 | (c) | 38 | (d) |
| 3 | (b) | 7 | (d) | 11 | (d) | 15 | (a) | 19 | (a) | 23 | (c) | 27 | (b) | 31 | (a) | 35 | (b) | 39 | (a) |
| 4 | (c) | 8 | (d) | 12 | (b) | 16 | (a) | 20 | (d) | 24 | (c) | 28 | (b) | 32 | (d) | 36 | (c) | 40 | (c) |

# 27

# AMINES

1. 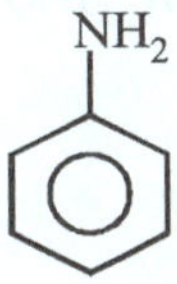 $\xrightarrow[H_2O]{Br_2}$ (A) $\xrightarrow[(ii)\ H_3PO_2]{(i)\ NaNO_2/HCl}$ (B),

Product (B) in this reaction is:

(a) 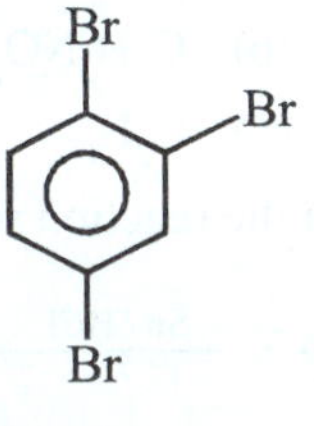 (b) 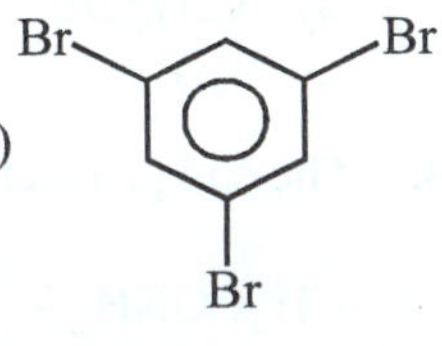

(c) 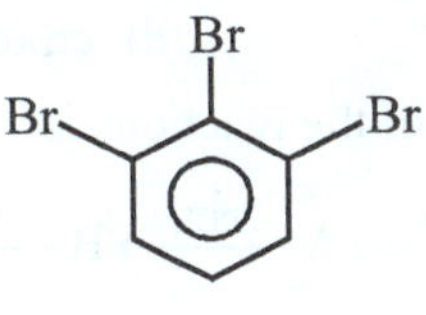 (d) 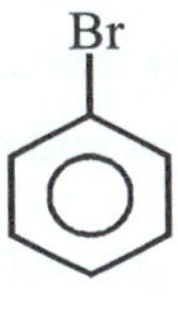

2. For the diazonium ions the order of reactivity towards diazo-coupling with phenol in the presence of dilute NaOH is:

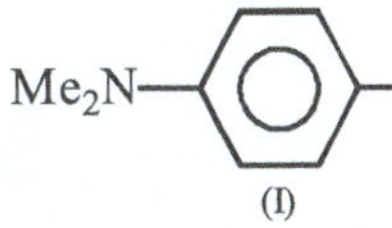
(I)

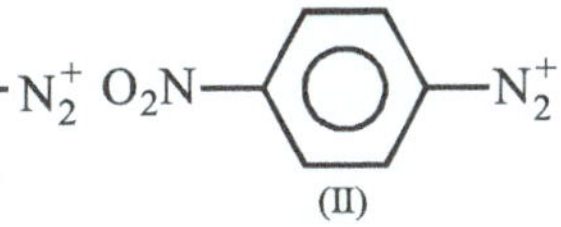
(II)

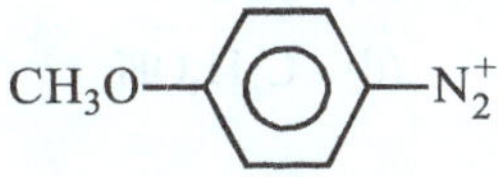
(III)

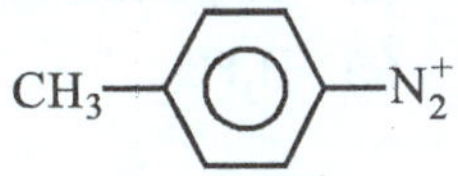
(IV)

(a) I<IV<II<III (b) I<III<IV<II
(c) III<I<II<IV (d) III<I<IV<II

3. Complete reduction of benzene diazonium chloride with Zn/HCl gives:
(a) Aniline (b) Phenylhydrazine
(c) Azobenzene (d) Hydrazobenzene

4. Which of the following reagents will be useful to distinguish between

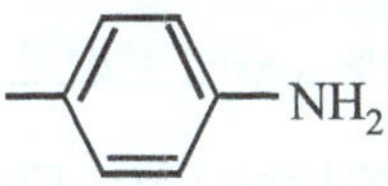 and 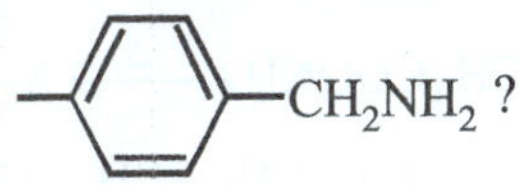 ?

(a) Dilute HCl
(b) $C_6H_5SO_2Cl$ and $OH^-/H_2O$
(c) HONO then β-naphthol
(d) $AgNO_3$ in $H_2O$

**5.** Nitrobenzene is reduced to azoxybenzene using

(a) Sn/HCl (b) $Zn/NH_4Cl$

(c) $As_2O_3/NaOH$ (d) Zn/NaOH

**6.** Which of the following statement is false?

(a) Dimethyl amine as well as trimethyl amine are soluble in water.

(b) Trimethyl amine forms hydrogen bond neither with itself nor with water.

(c) Trimethyl amine can act as hydrogen bond acceptor only, while dimethyl amine can serve as both a hydrogen bond donor and acceptor.

(d) All the three statements are false.

**7.** Which of the following reagents will convert *p*-methylbenzenediazonium chloride into *p*-cresol?

(a) Cu powder (b) $H_2O$

(c) $H_3PO_2$ (d) $C_6H_5OH$

**8.** 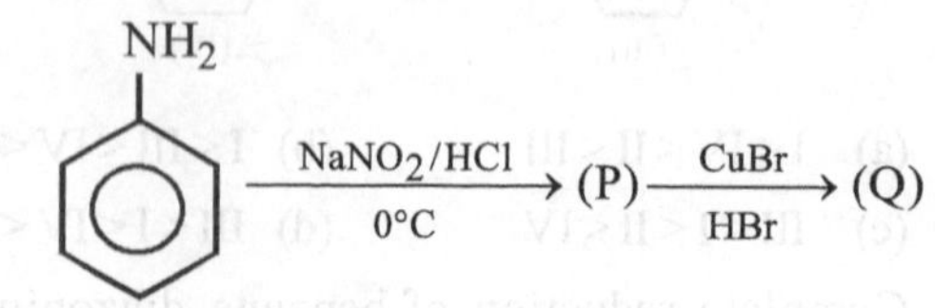


The compound Q is

(a) bromobenzene (b) chlorobenzene

(c) benzyl bromide (d) benzyl chloride

**9.** Identify Z in the following sequence of reactions–

$$CH_3COONH_4 \xrightarrow{\Delta} X \xrightarrow{P_2O_5} Y \xrightarrow{H_2O/H} Z$$

(a) $CH_3-CH_2-CO-NH_2$ (b) $CH_3-CN$

(c) $(CH_3CO)_2O$ (d) $CH_3-COOH$

**10.** The conversion of acetophenone to acetanilide involves :

(a) Beckmann rearrangement

(b) Curtius rearrangement

(c) Lossen rearrangement

(d) Hofmann rearrangement

**11.** An organic amino compound reacts with aqueous nitrous acid at low temperature to produce an oily nitrosoamine. The compound is

(a) $CH_3NH_2$

(b) $CH_3CH_2NH_2$

(c) $CH_3CH_2NHCH_2CH_3$

(d) $(CH_3CH_2)_3N$

**12.** In the following sequence of reactions, the compound C formed would be

$$\underset{\substack{|\\NH_2}}{CH_3-CH-CH_3} \xrightarrow[H_2O]{HNO_2} A \xrightarrow{[O]}$$

$$B \xrightarrow[H^+/H_2O]{CH_3MgI} C$$

(a) 1,1-dimethylethanol

(b) butanol-1

(c) butanol-2

(d) 2-methyl-propanol-1

**13.** Ethylamine reacts with $HNO_2$ giving :

(a) $C_2H_5OH$ (b) $C_2H_5NO_2$

(c) $NH_3$ (d) $C_2H_6$

**14.** The end product (Y) in the reaction sequence

$$CH_3CONH_2 \xrightarrow[\Delta]{P_2O_5} X \xrightarrow{Sn/HCl} Y \text{, is :}$$

(a) ethane nitrile (b) acetic acid

(c) ethanamine (d) chloroethane

**15.** The end product of the reactions is

$$C_2H_5NH_2 \xrightarrow{HNO_2} A \xrightarrow{PCl_5} B \xrightarrow{H.NH_2} C$$

(a) ethyl cyanide (b) ethyl amine

(c) methyl amine (d) acetamide

16. Aniline when treated with conc. $HNO_3$ gives

(a) 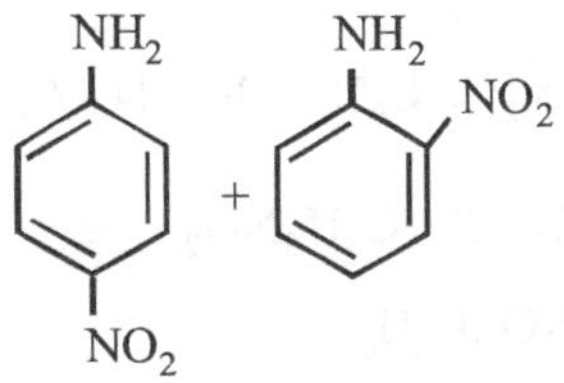

(b) 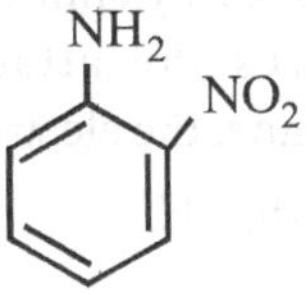

(c) 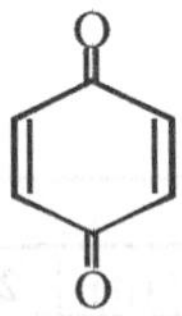
(d) 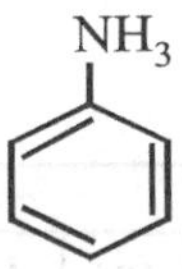

17. Among the following, the strongest base is

(a) $C_6H_5NH_2$ (b) $p-NO_2C_6H_4NH_2$

(c) $m-NO_2C_6H_4NH_2$ (d) $C_6H_5CH_2NH_2$

18. Nitration of aniline also gives *m*-nitroaniline, in strong acidic medium because

(a) in electrophilic substitution reactions, amino group is meta directing

(b) inspite of substituents, nitro group always goes to *m*-position

(c) in strong acidic medium, nitration of aniline is a nucleophilic substitution reaction

(d) in strong acidic medium, aniline is present as anilinium ion

19. The correct order of basicity in amines

(i) $C_2H_5NH_2$ (ii) $CH_3NH_2$

(iii) $(CH_3)_2NH$ (iv) $(CH_3)_3N$

(a) (i) < (iv) < (ii) < (iii)

(b) (iv) < (ii) < (iii) < (i)

(c) (i) < (ii) < (iii) < (iv)

(d) (ii) < (iii) < (iv) < (i)

20. 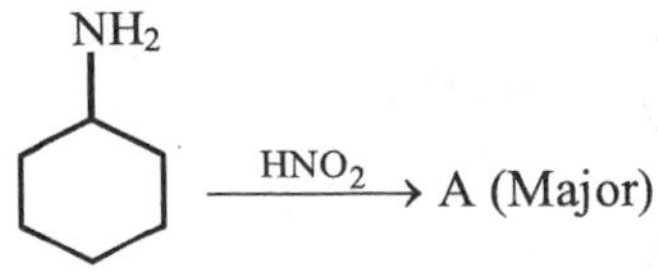

(a) 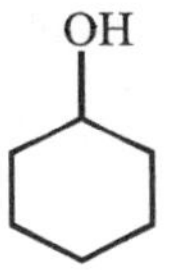
(b) 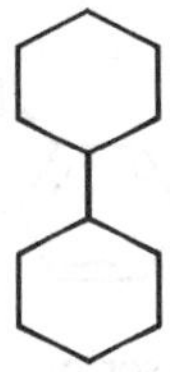

(c) 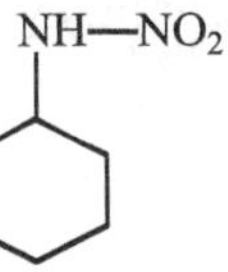
(d) 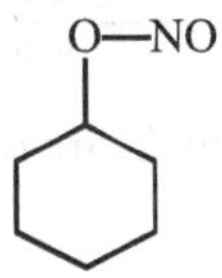

21. Acetanilide on nitration followed by alkaline hydrolysis mainly gives –

(a) *o*-Nitroaniline

(b) *p*-Nitroaniline

(c) *m*-Nitroaniline

(d) 2, 4, 6-Trinitroaniline

22. In the reaction :

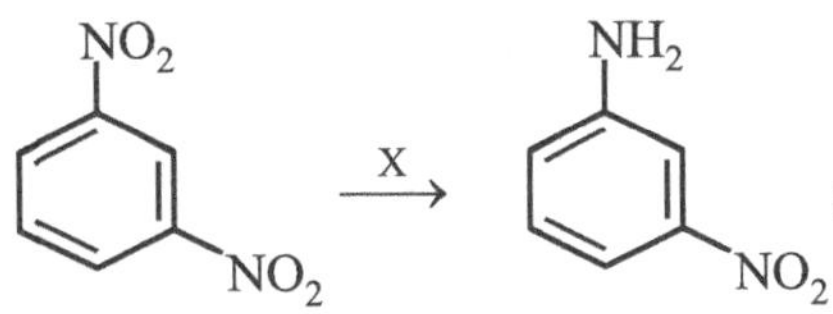

; X is

(a) SiC (b) $H_2SO_4$

(c) $KMnO_4$ (d) $NH_4HS$

23. End product (A) of the following sequence of reactions is :

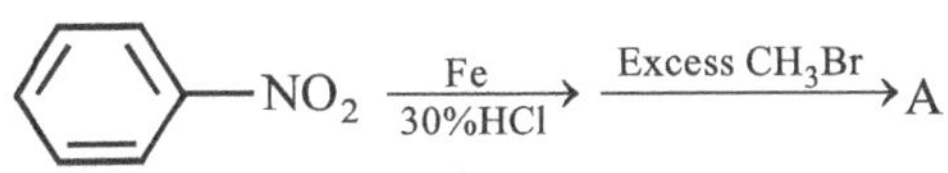

(a) 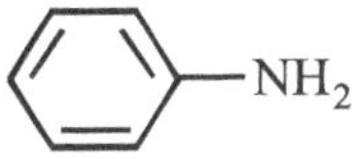

(b) 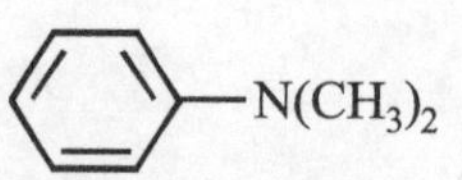


(c) 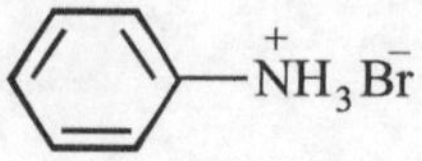


(d) 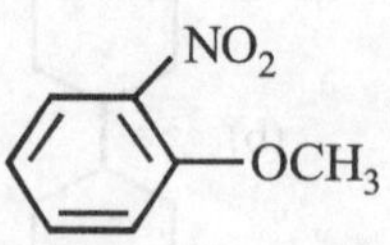


**24.** In the series of reaction

$$C_6H_5NH_2 \xrightarrow[0-5°C]{NaNO_2/HCl} X \xrightarrow[H_2O]{HNO_2} Y + N_2 + HCl,$$

X and Y are respectively

(a) $C_6H_5-N=N-C_6H_5, C_6H_5N_2^+Cl^-$

(b) $C_6H_5N_2^+Cl^-, C_6H_5-N=N-C_6H_5$

(c) $C_6H_5N_2^+Cl^-, C_6H_5NO_2$

(d) $C_6H_5NO_2, C_6H_6$

**25.** Reaction of ethyl amine with alkaline chloroform leads to the formation of carbylamine reaction. This reaction involves the attack of an electrophile on ethyl amine, the electrophile is

(a) $H_3O^+$ (b) $H^+$

(c) $RNH_3^+$ (d) $:CCl_2$

**ANSWER KEY**

| | | | | | | | | | | | | | | | |
|---|---|---|---|---|---|---|---|---|---|---|---|---|---|---|---|
| 1 | (b) | 4 | (c) | 7 | (b) | 10 | (a) | 13 | (a) | 16 | (c) | 19 | (b) | 22 | (d) | 25 | (d) |
| 2 | (b) | 5 | (c) | 8 | (a) | 11 | (c) | 14 | (c) | 17 | (d) | 20 | (a) | 23 | (b) | | |
| 3 | (a) | 6 | (b) | 9 | (d) | 12 | (a) | 15 | (b) | 18 | (d) | 21 | (b) | 24 | (c) | | |

# 28

# BIOMOLECULES

1. Glucose molecule reacts with 'X' number of molecules of phenylhydrazine to yield osazone. The value of 'X' is
   (a) four (b) one
   (c) two (d) three

2. Which of the following will not show mutarotation?
   (a) Maltose (b) Lactose
   (c) Glucose (d) Sucrose

3. Which one of the following is NOT correct?
   (a) D(–) Fructose exists in furanose structure
   (b) D (+) Glucose exists in pyranose structure
   (c) In sucrose the two monosaccharides are held together by peptide linkage
   (d) Maltose is a reducing sugar

4. For $-\overset{\overset{\displaystyle O}{\|}}{C}-\ddot{N}H-$ (peptide bond)

   Which statement is incorrect about peptide bond?
   (a) C — N bond length in proteins is longer than usual bond length of the C — N bond
   (b) Spectroscopic analysis shows planar structure of the $-\underset{\underset{\displaystyle O}{\|}}{C}-NH-$ group
   (c) C — N bond length in proteins is smaller than usual bond length of the C—N bond
   (d) None of the above

5. Denaturation of proteins leads to loss of its biological activity by
   (a) Formation of amino acids
   (b) Loss of primary structure
   (c) Loss of both primary and secondary structures
   (d) Loss of both secondary and tertiary structures

6. In an amino acid, the carboxyl group ionises at $pK_{a_1} = 2.34$ and ammonium ion at $pK_{a_2} = 9.60$. The isoelectric point of the amino acid is at pH
   (a) 5.97 (b) 2.34
   (c) 9.60 (d) 6.97

7. Which amino acid is achiral?
   (a) Alanine (b) Valine
   (c) Proline (d) None of these

8. Which one of the following metals is required as co-factor by all enzymes utilizing ATP in phosphate transfer?
(a) K (b) Ca
(c) Na (d) Mg

9. The reason for double helical structure of DNA is operation of
(a) dipole-dipole interaction
(b) hydrogen bonding
(c) electrostatic attractions
(d) van der Waals' forces

10. Anaemia is caused by the deficiency of vitamin
(a) $B_6$ (b) $B_1$
(c) $B_2$ (d) $B_{12}$

11. The enzyme which hydrolyses triglycerides to fatty acids and glycerol is called
(a) Maltase (b) Lipase
(c) Zymase (d) Pepsin

12. Match the vitamin of column I with deficiency disease given in column II

| Column I | Column II |
|---|---|
| I. Vitamin A | A. Scurvy |
| II. Vitamin $B_{12}$ | B. Sterility |
| III. Vitamin C | C. Xerophthalmia |
| IV. Vitamin E | D. Pernicious anaemia |

(a) I - B, II - D, III - A, IV - C
(b) I - D, II - A, III - C, IV - B
(c) I - C, II - D, III - A, IV - B
(d) I - A, II - D, III - B, IV - C

13. Which one of the following statements is not true?
(a) Lactose contains α-glycosidic linkage between $C_1$ of galactose and $C_4$ of glucose.
(b) Lactose is a reducing sugar and it gives Fehling's test.
(c) Lactose ($C_{11}H_{22}O_{11}$) is a disaccharide and it contains 8 hydroxyl groups.
(d) On acid hydrolysis, lactose gives one molecule of D(+)-glucose and one molecule of D(+)-galactose

14. What are the functional groups present in the structure of maltose?
(a) One ketal and hemiketal
(b) Two acetals
(c) One acetal and one hemiacetal
(d) One acetal and one ketal

15. Two monomers in maltose are:
(a) α-D-glucose and β-D-glucose
(b) α-D-glucose and α-D-galactose
(c) α-D-glucose and α-D-fructose
(d) α-D-glucose and α-D-glucose

16. Which of the given statements is INCORRECT about glycogen ?
(a) It is a straight chain polymer similar to amylose.
(b) Only α-linkages are present in the molecule.
(c) It is present in animal cells.
(d) It is present in some yeast and fungi.

17. Among the following compounds most basic amino acid is:
(a) Asparagine (b) Lysine
(c) Serine (d) Histidine

18. Vitamin $B_6$ is known as
(a) pyridoxine (b) thiamine
(c) tocopherol (d) riboflavin

19. Which one of the following is a non-steroidal hormone?
(a) Estradiol (b) Prostaglandin
(c) Progesterone (d) Estrone

20. Which of the following is correct about H-bonding in nucleotide?
(a) A --- A and T --- T (b) G --- T and A --- C
(c) A --- G and T --- C (d) A --- T and G --- C

**21.** The pair of compounds in which both the compounds give positive test with Tollen's reagent is

(a) glucose and sucrose

(b) fructose and sucrose

(c) acetophenone and hexanal

(d) glucose and fructose

**22.** Which of the following does not reduce Benedict's solution?

(a) Glucose (b) Fructose (c) Sucrose (d) Aldehyde

**23.** The substance that forms the plant cell walls is

(a) cellulose (b) sucrose

(c) vitamins (d) starch

**24.** Among the following organic acids, the acid present in rancid butter is:

(a) Pyruvic acid (b) Lactic acid

(c) Butyric acid (d) Acetic acid

**25.** Pepsin enzyme hydrolyses

(a) proteins to amino acids

(b) fats to fatty acids

(c) glucose to ethyl alcohol

(d) polysaccharides to monosaccharides

**ANSWER KEY**

| | | | | | | | | | | | | | | | | | |
|---|---|---|---|---|---|---|---|---|---|---|---|---|---|---|---|---|---|
| **1** | (d) | **5** | (d) | **9** | (b) | **13** | (a) | **17** | (b) | **21** | (d) | **25** | (a) | | | | |
| **2** | (d) | **6** | (a) | **10** | (d) | **14** | (c) | **18** | (a) | **22** | (c) | | | | | | |
| **3** | (c) | **7** | (d) | **11** | (b) | **15** | (d) | **19** | (b) | **23** | (a) | | | | | | |
| **4** | (a) | **8** | (d) | **12** | (c) | **16** | (a) | **20** | (d) | **24** | (c) | | | | | | |

# 29

# POLYMERS

1. Natural rubber is a polymer of
   (a) butadiene
   (b) isoprene
   (c) 2-methylbutadiene
   (d) hexa-1, 3-diene
2. Which is not an example of copolymer?
   (a) SAN
   (b) ABS
   (c) Saran
   (d) PVC
3. Thermosets are:
   (a) cross-linked polymers
   (b) don't melt or soften on heating
   (c) cross-linking is usually developed at the time of moulding where they harden reversibly
   (d) all of the above
4. Which of the following statements is not correct for fibres?
   (a) Fibres possess high tensile strength and high modulus.
   (b) Fibres impart crystalline nature.
   (c) Characteristic features of fibres are due to strong intermolecular forces like hydrogen bonding.
   (d) All are correct.
5. Which of the following is thermoplastic?
   (a) Bakelite
   (b) Polyethylene
   (c) Terylene
   (d) All of these
6. Perlon is
   (a) Rubber
   (b) Nylon-6
   (c) Terylene
   (d) Orlon

7. Structure of some important polymers are given. Which one represents buna-S?

(a) $\left( CH_2 - \overset{\overset{\Large CH_3}{|}}{C} = CH - CH_2 \right)_n$

(b) $\left( CH_2 - CH = CH - CH_2 - \underset{\underset{\Large C_6H_5}{|}}{CH} - CH_2 \right)_n$

(c) $\left( CH_2 - CH = CH - CH_2 - \underset{\underset{\Large CN}{|}}{CH} - CH_2 \right)_n$

(d) $\left( CH_2 - \overset{\overset{\Large Cl}{|}}{C} = CH - CH_2 \right)_n$

8. Melamine plastic crockery is a codensation polymer of

(a) HCHO and melamine

(b) HCHO and ethylene

(c) melamine and ethylene

(d) None of these

9. Which of the following polymers is synthesized using a free radical polymerization technique ?

(a) Terylene

(b) Melamine polymer

(c) Nylon 6, 6

(d) Teflon

10. Synthetic polymer bakelite can be prepared from following compounds

(a) Styrene and vinyl chloride

(b) Acrylonitrile and vinyl chloride

(c) Adipic acid and ethylene glycol

(d) Phenol and formaldehyde

11. For natural polymers PDI is generally

(a) 0 (b) 1

(c) 100 (d) 1000

12. Caprolactam polymerises to give

(a) terylene

(b) teflon

(c) glyptal

(d) nylon-6

13. The process involving heating of rubber with sulphur is called

(a) galvanisation

(b) vulcanization

(c) bessemerisaion

(d) sulphonation

14. Which of the following polymers do not involve cross linkages?

(a) Melmac

(b) Bakelite

(c) Polythene

(d) Vulcanised rubber

15. Number average molecular mass, $\overline{M}_n$ and weight average molecular mass $(\overline{M}_W)$ of synthetic polymers are related as

(a) $\overline{M}_n = (\overline{M}_W)^{1/2}$ (b) $\overline{M}_n = \overline{M}_W$

(c) $\overline{M}_W > \overline{M}_n$ (d) $\overline{M}_W < \overline{M}_n$

16. Low density polythene is prepared by

(a) Free radical polymerisation

(b) cationic polymerisation

(c) anionic polymerisation

(d) Ziegler-Natta polymerisation

**17.** The polymer used for optical lenses is :

(a) polypropylene

(b) polyvinyl chloride

(c) polythene

(d) polymethyl methacrylate

**18.** The polymer used in making synthetic hair wigs is made up of

(a) $CH_2=CHCl$

(b) $CH_2=CHCOOCH_3$

(c) $C_6H_5CH=CH_2$

(d) $CH_2=CH-CH=CH_2$

**19.** Which of the following is currently used as a tyre cord?

(a) Terylene (b) Polyethylene

(c) Polypropylene d) Nylon - 6

**20.** Which polymer is used for making magnetic recording tapes?

(a) Dacron (b) Acrilan

(c) Glyptal (d) Bakelite

**ANSWER KEY**

| | | | | | | | | | | | | | | | | | | | |
|---|---|---|---|---|---|---|---|---|---|---|---|---|---|---|---|---|---|---|---|
| 1 | (b) | 4 | (d) | 7 | (b) | 10 | (d) | 13 | (b) | 16 | (a) | 19 | (d) | | | | | | |
| 2 | (d) | 5 | (b) | 8 | (a) | 11 | (b) | 14 | (c) | 17 | (d) | 20 | (d) | | | | | | |
| 3 | (d) | 6 | (b) | 9 | (d) | 12 | (d) | 15 | (c) | 18 | (a) | | | | | | | | |

# 30

# CHEMISTRY IN EVERYDAY LIFE

1. An antipyretic is
   (a) quinine (b) paracetamol
   (c) luminal (d) piperazine
2. Salol can be used as
   (a) antiseptic (b) antipyretic
   (c) analgesic (d) None of these
3. Which one of the following is employed as a tranquilizer?
   (a) Naproxen (b) Tetracycline
   (c) Chlorpheninamine (d) Equanil
4. Terfenadine is commonly used as a/an
   (a) tranquilizer (b) antihistamine
   (c) antimicrobial (d) antibiotic
5. Chloramine-T is a/an
   (a) disinfectant (b) antiseptic
   (c) analgesic (d) antipyretic
6. Sulphonamides act as
   (a) Antiseptic (b) Analgesic
   (c) Antimicrobials (d) Antipyretic
7. Which of these is a hypnotic ?
   (a) metaldehyde (b) acetaldehyde
   (c) paraldehyde (d) None of these
8. Barbituric acid and its derivatives are well known
   (a) antipyretics (b) analgesics
   (c) antiseptics (d) traquillizers
9. Sulpha drugs are used for
   (a) precipitating bacteria
   (b) removing bacteria
   (c) decreasing the size of bacteria
   (d) stopping the growth of bacteria
10. Which of the following is not an antiseptic drug?
   (a) Iodoform (b) Dettol
   (c) Gammexane (d) Genation violet
11. Veronal, a barbiturate drug, is used as
   (a) anaesthetic (b) sedative
   (c) antiseptic (d) None of these
12. A drug effective in the treatment of pneumonia, bronchitis, etc, is
   (a) streptomycin (b) chloramphenicol
   (c) penicillin (d) sulphaguanidine
13. The use of chemicals for treatment of diseases is called as
   (a) isothermotherapy (b) angiotherapy
   (c) physiotherapy (d) chemotherapy

**14.** Which of the following acts as an antioxidant in edible oils ?

(a) Vitamin B (b) Vitamin C

(c) Vitamin D (d) Vitamin E

**15.** Which one of the following compounds is an anti-fertility drug?

(a) Aspirin (b) Chloromycetin

(c) Saheli (d) Penicillin

**16.** The formulation of dettol contains

(a) chloroxylenol (b) terpineol

(c) alcohol (d) All of these

**17.** Which of the following is an antidiabetic drug?

(a) Insulin (b) Penicillin

(c) Chloroquine (d) Aspirin

**18.** Which artificial sweetener contains chlorine ?

(a) Sucralose (b) Alitame

(c) Aspartame (d) Saccharin

**19.** Sodium alkyl benzene sulphonate is used as

(a) soap (b) fertilizers

(c) pesticides (d) detergents

**20.** End of detergents have

(a) ester group (b) sodium sulphate

(c) aldehyde (d) amine group

**ANSWER KEY**

| | | | | | | | | | | | | | | | | | | | |
|---|---|---|---|---|---|---|---|---|---|---|---|---|---|---|---|---|---|---|---|
| **1** | (b) | **4** | (b) | **7** | (c) | **10** | (c) | **13** | (d) | **16** | (d) | **19** | (d) | | | | | | |
| **2** | (a) | **5** | (b) | **8** | (d) | **11** | (b) | **14** | (d) | **17** | (a) | **20** | (b) | | | | | | |
| **3** | (d) | **6** | (c) | **9** | (d) | **12** | (c) | **15** | (c) | **18** | (a) | | | | | | | | |

# Mock Test

# NEET Mock Test-1

**1.** Fluorine is more electronegative than either boron or phosphorus. What conclusion can be drawn from the fact that $BF_3$ has no dipole moment but $PF_3$ does ?

(a) $BF_3$ is not spherically symmetrical but $PF_3$ is spherically symmetrical.

(b) $BF_3$ molecule must be linear

(c) The atomic radius of P is larger than that of B

(d) The $BF_3$ molecule must be planar triangular

**2.** At 298 K, equal volumes of $SO_2$, $CH_4$ and $O_2$ are mixed in empty container. The total pressure exerted is 2.1 atm. The partial pressure of $CH_4$ in mixture is :

(a) 0.6 atm. (b) 1.2 atm

(c) 2.4 atm (d) 3.6 atm.

**3.** 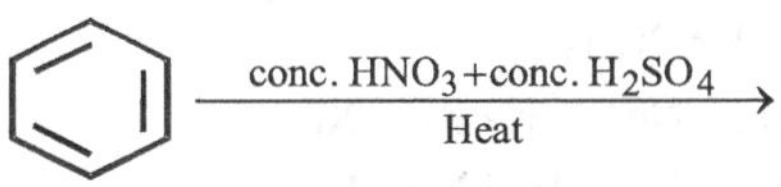

$$X \xrightarrow{Cl_2/FeCl_3} Y$$

The product Y is

(a) *p*-chloronitrobenzene

(b) *m*-chloronitrobenzene

(c) *o*-chloronitrobenzene

(d) *o*-*p*-dichloronitrobenzene

**4.** In the extraction of Cu, the metal is formed in the bessemer converter due to the reaction :

(a) $Cu_2S + 2Cu_2O \longrightarrow 6Cu + SO_2$

(b) $Cu_2S \longrightarrow 2Cu + S$

(c) $Fe + Cu_2O \longrightarrow 2Cu + FeO$

(d) $2Cu_2O \longrightarrow 4Cu + O_2$

**5.** An example of electrophilic substitution reaction is

(a) Chlorination of methane

(b) Conversion of methyl chloride to methyl alcohol

(c) Nitration of benzene

(d) Formation of ethylene from ethyl alcohol.

**6.** Which of the following molecules is most suitable to disperse benzene in water ?

(a) 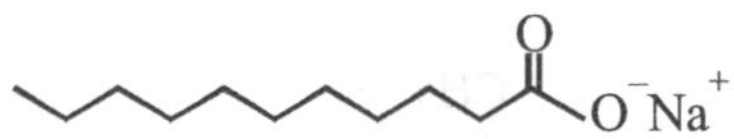

(b) 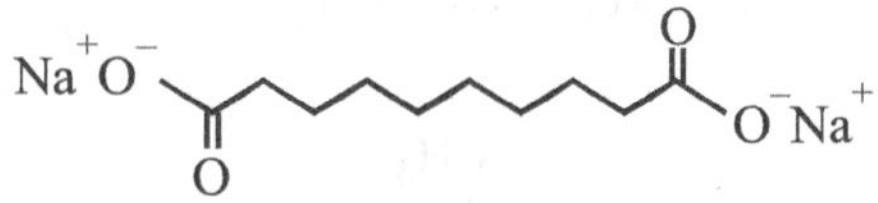

(c) 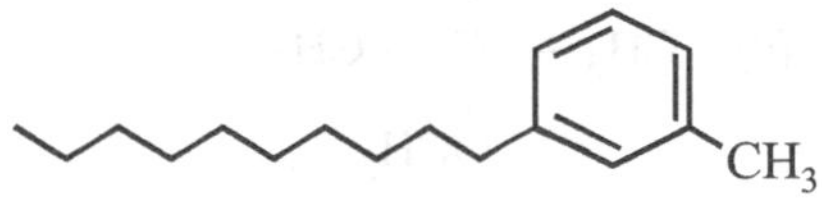

(d) 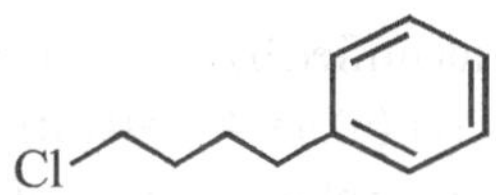

**7.** Ozone hole refers to

(a) Increase in concentration of ozone

(b) Hole in ozone layer

(c) Reduction in thickness of ozone layer in troposphere

(d) Reduction in thickness of ozone layer in stratsophere

**8.** Which of the following does not represent the correct order of the properties indicated

(a) $Ni^{2+} > Cr^{2+} > Fe^{2+} > Mn^{2+}$ (size)

(b) $Sc > Ti > Cr > Mn$ (size)

(c) $Mn^{2+} > Ni^{2+} < Co^{2+} < Fe^{2+}$ (unpaired electron)

(d) $Fe^{2+} > Co^{2+} > Ni^{2+} > Cu^{2+}$ (unpaired electron)

**9.** The major product formed in the following reaction is :

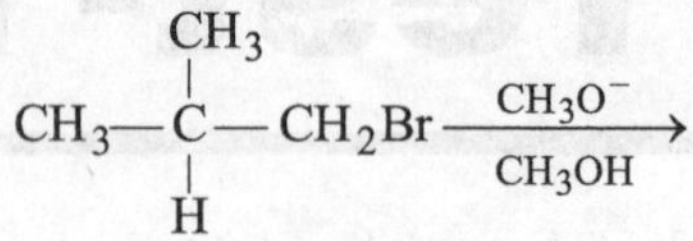

(a) 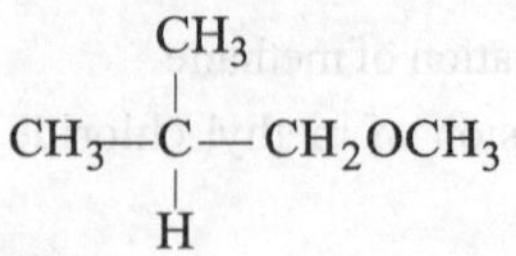

(b) 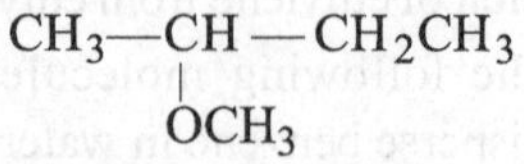

(c) 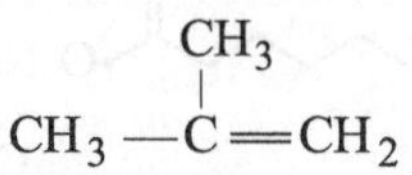

(d) 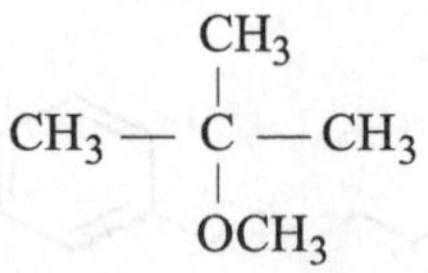

**10.** The electrons, identified by quantum numbers n and l (i) n = 4, l = 1 (ii) n = 4, l = 0 (iii) n = 3, l = 2 (iv) n = 3, l = 1 can be placed in order of increasing energy, from the lowest to highest, as

(a) (iv) < (ii) < (iii) < (i)
(b) (ii) < (iv) < (i) < (iii)
(c) (i) < (iii) < (ii) < (iv)
(d) (iii) < (i) < (iv) < (ii)

**11.** In an adiabatic process which of the following is true?

(a) $q = +w$ (b) $q = 0$
(c) $\Delta E = q$ (d) $P\Delta V = 0$

**12.** In which of the following cases, the stability of two oxidation states is correctly represented

(a) $Ti^{3+} > Ti^{4+}$ (b) $Mn^{2+} > Mn^{3+}$
(c) $Fe^{2+} > Fe^{3+}$ (d) $Cu^{+} > Cu^{2+}$

**13.** Which is not the disproportionation reaction ?

(a) $3H_3PO_2 \longrightarrow 2H_3PO_2 + PH_3$
(b) $HCHO + OH^- \longrightarrow HCOO^- + CH_3OH$
(c) $NH_4NO_3 \longrightarrow N_2O + 2H_2O$
(d) $3Cl_2 + 6OH^- \longrightarrow 5Cl^- + ClO_3^- + 3H_2O$

**14.** The major organic product in the reaction, $CH_3—O—CH(CH_3)_2 + HI \rightarrow$ Product is

(a) $ICH_2OCH(CH_3)_2$
(b) $CH_3O\underset{I}{C}(CH_3)_2$
(c) $CH_3I + (CH_3)_2CHOH$
(d) $CH_3OH + (CH_3)_2CHI$

**15.** For the reaction

$H_2(g) + Br_2(g) \rightleftharpoons 2HBr(g)$, the rate law is rate $= k[H_2][Br_2]^{1/2}$. Which of the following statement is true about this reaction

(a) The reaction is of second order.
(b) Molecularity of the reaction is 3/2
(c) The unit of k is $s^{-1}$
(d) Molecularity of the reaction is 2

**16.** The correct order of solubility in water for He, Ne, Ar, Kr, Xe is

(a) He > Ne > Ar > Kr > Xe
(b) Xe > Kr > Ar > Ne > He
(c) Ne > Ar > Kr > He > Xe
(d) Ar > Ne > He > Kr > Xe

**17.** If uncertainty in position and velocity are equal then uncertainty in momentum will be

(a) $\frac{1}{2}\sqrt{\frac{mh}{\pi}}$ (b) $\frac{1}{2}\sqrt{\frac{h}{\pi m}}$

(c) $\frac{h}{4\pi m}$ (d) $\frac{mh}{4\pi}$

**18.** The correct IUPAC name for

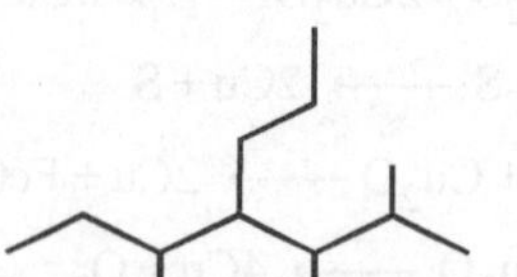

(a) 5-methyl -4-(1'-2'-demethylpropyl) heptane
(b) 3-methyl-4-(1',2'-dimethylpropyl) heptane
(c) 2,3,5-trimethyl-4-propylheptane
(d) 4-propyl-2,3,5-trimethylpeptane

**19.** Which of the following shows iso-structural species?

(a) $NH_4^+$ and $NH_2^-$

(b) $CH_3^-$ and $CH_3^+$

(c) $SO_4^{2-}$, $PO_4^{3-}$ and $[BF_4^-]$

(d) $NH_4^+$ and $NH_3$

**20.** When dihydroxyacetone reacts with $HIO_4$, the product is/are :

(a) HCHO
(b) HCOOH
(c) HCHO and HCOOH
(d) HCHO and $CO_2$

**21.** Hard water when passed through ion exchange resin containing R'COOH groups, becomes free from :

(a) $Cl^-$ (b) $SO_4^{2-}$

(c) $H_3O^+$ (d) $Ca^{2+}$

**22.** A certain compound (X) when treated with copper sulphate solution yields a brown precipitate. On adding hypo solution, the precipitate turns white. The compound is

(a) $K_2CO_3$ (b) KI
(c) KBr (d) $K_3PO_4$

**23.** Consider the following reactions:

(i) $H^+_{(aq)} + OH^-_{(aq)} = H_2O_{(l)}$, $\Delta H = -X_1$ kJ mol$^{-1}$

(ii) $H_{2(g)} + \frac{1}{2}O_{2(g)} = H_2O(l)$, $\Delta H = -X_2$ kJ mol$^{-1}$

(iii) $CO_{2(g)} + H_{2(g)} = CO_{(g)} + H_2O$, $\Delta H = -X_3$ kJ mol$^{-1}$

(iv) $C_2H_{2(g)} + \frac{5}{2}O_{2(g)} = 2CO_2(g) + H_2O(l)'$ $\Delta H = +4X_4$ kJ mol$^{-1}$

Enthalpy of formation of $H_2O_{(l)}$ is

(a) $+X_3$ kJ mol$^{-1}$ (b) $-X_4$ kJ mol$^{-1}$
(c) $+X_1$ kJ mol$^{-1}$ (d) $-X_2$ kJ mol$^{-1}$

**24.** Which of the following possesses a sp-carbon in its structure ?

(a) $CH_2=CCl-CH=CH_2$
(b) $CCl_2=CCl_2$
(c) $CH_2=C=CH_2$
(d) $CH_2=CH-CH=CH_2$.

**25.** A balloon has maximum capacity of 20 L. At one atmospheric pressure 10 L of air is filled in the balloon. It will burst when pressure is (assuming isothermal condition)

(a) $>0.5$ atm (b) $<0.5$ atm
(c) $=0.5$ atm (d) $\geq 0.5$ atm

**26.** Which one of the following complexes will have four different isomers ?

(a) $[Co(en)_2Cl_2]Cl$
(b) $[Co(en)(NH_3)Cl_2]Cl$
(c) $[Co(PPh_3)_2Cl_2]Cl$
(d) $[Co(en)_3]Cl_3$

**27.** Solubility product of a salt AB is $1 \times 10^{-8}$ in a solution in which the concentration of $A^+$ ions is $10^{-3}$ M. The salt will precipitate when the concentration of $B^-$ ions is kept

(a) between $10^{-8}$ M to $10^{-7}$ M
(b) between $10^{-7}$ M to $10^{-8}$ M
(c) $>10^{-5}$ M
(d) $<10^{-8}$ M

**28.** Sucrose in water is dextro-rotatory, $[\alpha]_D = +66.4°$. When boiled with dilute HCl, the solution becomes leavo-rotatory, $[\alpha]_D = -20°$. In this process the sucrose molecule breaks into

(a) L-glucose + D-fructose
(b) L-glucose + L-fructose
(c) D-glucose + D-fructose
(d) D-glucose + L-fructose

**29.** Select correct statement(s).

(a) Cyanamide ion ($CN_2^{2-}$) is isoelectronic with $CO_2$ and has the same linear structure

(b) $Mg_2C_3$ reacts with water to form propyne

(c) $CaC_2$ has NaCl type lattice

(d) All of the above

**30.** For $-\overset{O}{\overset{||}{C}}-\ddot{N}H-$(peptide bond)

Which statement is incorrect about peptide bond?

(a) C — N bond length in proteins is longer than usual bond length of the C — N bond

(b) Spectroscopic analysis shows planar structure of the $-\underset{O}{\underset{||}{C}}-NH-$ group

(c) C — N bond length in proteins is smaller than usual bond length of the C—N bond

(d) None of the above

**31.** Vapour pressure of benzene at 30°C is 121.8 mm. When 15 g of a non volatile solute is dissolved in 250 g of benzene its vapour pressure decreased to 120.2 mm. The molecular weight of the solute (Mo. wt. of solvent = 78)

(a) 356.2 (b) 456.8

(c) 530.1 (d) 656.7

**32.** In nitrogen family, the H-M-H bond angle in the hydrides gradually becomes closer to 90° on going from N to Sb. This shows that gradually

(a) The basic strength of the hydrides increases

(b) Almost pure *p*-orbitals are used for M-H bonding

(c) The bond energies of M-H bonds increase

(d) The bond pairs of electrons become nearer to the central atom

**33.** For reaction $aA \rightarrow xP$, when [A] = 2.2 mM, the rate was found to be 2.4 $mMs^{-}$. On reducing concentration of A to half, the rate changes to 0.6 $mMs^{-1}$. The order of reaction with respect to A is :

(a) 1.5 (b) 2.0

(c) 2.5 (d) 3.0

**34.** The tendency of $BF_3$, $BCl_3$ and $BBr_3$ to behave as Lewis acid decreases in the sequence:

(a) $BCl_3 > BF_3 > BBr_3$

(b) $BBr_3 > BCl_3 > BF_3$

(c) $BBr_3 > BF_3 > BCl_3$

(d) $BF_3 > BCl_3 > BBr_3$

**35.** If 'a' stands for the edge length of the cubic systems : simple cubic, body centred cubic and face centred cubic, then the ratio of radii of the spheres in these systems will be respectively,

(a) $\frac{1}{2}a : \frac{\sqrt{3}}{4}a : \frac{1}{2\sqrt{2}}a$

(b) $\frac{1}{2}a : \sqrt{3}a : \frac{1}{\sqrt{2}}a$

(c) $\frac{1}{2}a : \frac{\sqrt{3}}{2}a : \frac{\sqrt{3}}{2}a$

(d) $1a : \sqrt{3}a : \sqrt{2}a$

**36.** Which of the following is correct order of acidity?

(a) $HCOOH > CH_3COOH > ClCH_2COOH > C_2H_5COOH$

(b) $ClCH_2COOH > HCOOH > CH_3COOH > C_2H_5COOH$

(c) $CH_3COOH > HCOOH > ClCH_2COOH > C_2H_5COOH$

(d) $C_2H_5COOH > CH_3COOH > HCOOH > ClCH_2COOH$

**37.** Penicillin is :

(a) analgesic (b) antipyretic

(c) antimalarial (d) antibiotic

**38.** For the reaction $2NO + Br_2 \longrightarrow 2NOBr$, the following mechanism has been given

$$NO + Br_2 \xrightarrow{\text{fast}} NOBr_2$$

$$NOBr_2 + NO \xrightarrow{\text{slow}} 2NOBr$$

Hence, rate law is

(a) $k'[NO]^2[Br_2]$ (b) $k'[NO][Br_2]$
(c) $k'[NOBr_2][NO]$ (d) $k'[NO][Br_2]^2$

**39.** Which of the following reactions can produce aniline as main product?
(a) $C_6H_5NO_2 + Zn/KOH$
(b) $C_6H_5NO_2 + Zn/NH_4Cl$
(c) $C_6H_5NO_2 + LiAlH_4$
(d) $C_6H_5NO_2 + Zn/HCl$

**40.** Which of the following reactions is used to make a fuel cell?
(a) $Cd(s) + 2Ni(OH)_3(s) \longrightarrow CdO(s) + 2Ni(OH)_2(s) + H_2O(l)$
(b) $Pb(s) + PbO_2(s) + 2H_2SO_4(aq) \longrightarrow 2PbSO_4(s) + 2H_2O(l)$
(c) $2H_2(g) + O_2(g) \longrightarrow 2H_2O(l)$
(d) $2Fe(s) + O_2(g) + 4H^+(aq) \longrightarrow 2Fe^{2+}(aq) + 2H_2O(l)$

**41.** Which does not exist ?
(a) $[SiCl_6]^{2-}$ (b) $[GeF_6]^{2-}$
(c) $[CCl_6]^{2-}$ (d) $[SnCl_6]^{2-}$

**42.** In which case, van't Hoff factor *i* remains unchanged ?
(a) $PtCl_4$ reacts with aq. KCl
(b) aq. $ZnCl_2$ reacts with aq. $NH_3$
(c) aq. $FeCl_3$ reacts with aq. $K_4[Fe(CN)]_6$
(d) $KMnO_4$ reduced to $MnO_2$ in alkaline medium

**43.** The unit of equivalent conductivity is
(a) $S\,cm^{-2}$
(b) ohm $cm^2$ (g - equivalent)
(c) ohm cm
(d) $ohm^{-1}cm^2$ (g equivalent)$^{-1}$

**44.** Perlon is
(a) Terylene (b) Rubber
(c) Nylon – 6 (d) Polyester

**45.** Tertiary nitro compounds do not tautomerise because
(a) there is no double bond
(b) there is no α-hydrogen
(c) oxygen is more electronegative than hydrogen
(d) all of the above

# NEET Mock Test-2

1. IUPAC name of the following compound :

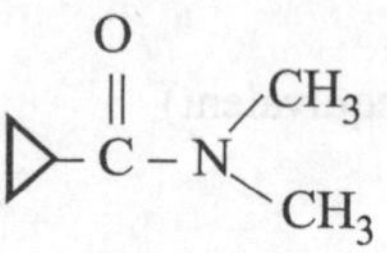

(a) N, N-dimethylcyclopropanecarboxamide
(b) N-methylcyclopropanamide
(c) cyclopropionamide
(d) none of the above

2 The electrical charge on a colloidal particle is observed by:

(a) Ultramicroscope
(b) Scattering
(c) Brownian movement
(d) Electrophoresis

3. A is a lighter phenol and B is an aromatic carboxylic acid. Separation of a mixture of A and B can be carried out easily by using a solution of

(a) Sodium hydroxide (b) Sodium sulphate
(c) calcium chloride (d) Sodium bicarbonate

4. $(Ag + Pb)$ alloy $\xrightarrow[\text{Zinc is added}]{\text{Melt and}}$

$(Ag + Pb + Zn)$ melt $\xrightarrow{\text{Cool}}$ $\xrightarrow[\text{Layer Y}]{\text{Layer X}}$

Select correct statement based on above scheme.

(a) Layer X contains Zn and Ag
(b) Layer Y contains Pb and Ag but amount of silver in this layer is smaller than in layer X
(c) X and Y are immiscible layers
(d) All are correct statements

5. For the reaction : $H_2 + Cl_2 \xrightarrow{\text{sunlight}} 2HCl$ the order of reaction is

(a) 0 (b) 2
(c) 1 (d) 3

6. Which of the following is not correct ?

(a) $3O_2 \underset{\text{disch arge}}{\overset{\text{Silent electric}}{\rightleftharpoons}} 2O_3$; $\Delta H = -284.5$ kJ.
(b) Ozone undergoes addition reaction with unsaturated carbon compounds.
(c) Sodium thiosulphate reacts with $I_2$ to form sodium tetrathionate and sodium iodide.
(d) Ozone oxidises lead sulphide to lead sulphate.

7. (I) $n = 3, l = 2, m_1 = -2$
(II) $n = 3, l = 1, m_1 = 0$
(III) $n = 3, l = 0, m_1 = -1$
(IV) $n = 3, l = 2, m_1 = 0$
(V) $n = 3, l = 3, m_1 = -2$

Of these question state designation which does not describe an allowed state for an electron in an atom ?

(a) I and IV (b) III and V
(c) II and V (d) IV and V

8. Which of the following compounds is a good conductor of electricity in solution state?

(a) covalent (b) molecular solid
(c) metallic solid (d) ionic compounds

9. Which is the most suitable reagent among the following to distinguish compound (3) from rest of the compounds ?

1. $CH_3-C\equiv C-CH_3$
2. $CH_3-CH_2-CH_2-CH_3$
3. $CH_3-CH_2C\equiv CH$
4. $CH_3-CH=CH_2.$

(a) Bromine in carbon tetrachloride
(b) Bromine in acetic acid
(c) Alk $KMnO_4$
(d) Ammonical silver nitrate.

**10.** $N_2+3H_2 \longrightarrow 2NH_3$. In this reaction equivalent weight of $N_2$ is
(a) 4.67 (b) 28
(c) 14 (d) 2.33

**11.** Which of the following is/are the hazardous pollutant(s) present in automobile exhaust gases?
(i) $N_2$ (ii) CO
(iii) $CH_4$ (iv) Oxides of nitrogen
(a) (ii) and (iii) (b) (i) and (ii)
(c) (ii) and (iv) (d) (i) and (iii)

**12.** $Zn^{2+} \rightarrow Zn_{(s)}$ ; $E^0 = -0.76$ V

$Cu^{2+} \rightarrow Cu_{(s)}$ ; $E^0 = -0.34$ V

Which of the following is spontaneous?
(a) $Zn^{2+}+Cu \rightarrow Zn+Cu^{2+}$
(b) $Cu^{2+}+Zn \rightarrow Cu+Zn^{2+}$
(c) $Zn^{2+}+Cu^{2+} \rightarrow Zn+Cu$
(d) None of these

**13.** Cuprous compounds such as CuCl, CuCN and CuSCN are the only salts stable in water due to
(a) high hydration energy of $Cu^+$ ions
(b) their inherent tendency not do disproportionate
(c) diamagnetic nature
(d) insolubility in water

**14.** A compound formed by elements X and Y crystallizes in a cubic structure in which the X atoms are at the corners of a cube and the Y atoms are at the face centres. The formula of the compound is
(a) $XY_3$ (b) $X_3Y$
(c) XY (d) $XY_2$

**15.** An alkene having molecular formula $C_7H_{14}$ was subjected to ozonolysis in the presence of zinc dust. An equimolar amount of the following two compounds was obtained

$(CH_3)(CH_3)C=O$ and $(CH_3)(CH_3CH_2)C=O$

The IUPAC name of the alkene is
(a) 3, 4-dimethyl-3-pentene
(b) 3, 4-dimethyl-2-pentene
(c) 2, 3-dimethyl-3-pentene
(d) 2, 3-dimethyl-2-pentene

**16.** At a particular temperature, the vapour pressures of two liquids A and B are respectively 120 and 180 mm of mercury. If 2 moles of A and 3 moles of B are mixed to form an ideal solution, the vapour pressure of the solution at the same temperature will be (in mm of mercury)
(a) 156 (b) 145
(c) 150 (d) 108

**17.** Which of the following complex ions is expected to absorb visible light?
(a) $[Ti(en)_2(NH_3)_2]^{4+}$
(b) $[Cr(NH_3)_6]^{3+}$
(c) $[Zn(NH_3)_6]^{2+}$
(d) $[Sc(H_2O)_3(NH_3)_3]^{3+}$
(At. no. Zn = 30, Sc = 21, Ti = 22, Cr = 24)

**18.** According to the adsorption theory of catalysis, the speed of the reaction increases because-
(a) Adsorption lowers the activation energy of the reaction
(b) The concentration of reactant molecules at the active centres of the catalyst becomes high due to strong adsorption
(c) In the process of adsorption, the activation energy of the molecules becomes large
(d) Adsorption produces heat which increases the speed of the reaction

**19.** A pressure cooker reduces cooking time for food because

(a) boiling point of water involved in cooking is increased

(b) the higher pressure inside the cooker crushes the food material

(c) cooking involves chemical changes helped by a rise in temperature

(d) heat is more evenly distributed in the cooking space

**20.** Most reactive halide towards $S_N1$ reaction is

(a) *n*-Butyl chloride

(b) *sec*-Butyl chloride

(c) *tert*-Butyl chloride

(d) Allyl chloride

**21.** The absolute configuration of the following :

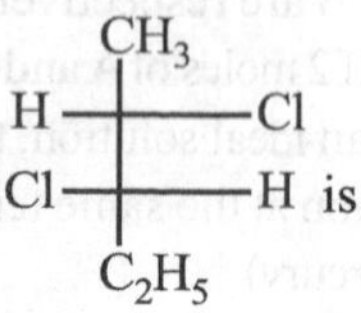

is

(a) 2S, 3R (b) 2S, 3S

(c) 2R, 3S (d) 2R, 3R

**22.** The rate constant $k$, for the reaction

$$N_2O_5(g) \longrightarrow 2NO_2(g) + \frac{1}{2}O_2(g)$$

is $1.3 \times 10^{-2} s^{-1}$. Which equation given below describes the change of $[N_2O_5]$ with time ? $[N_2O_5]_0$ and $[N_2O_5]_t$ corrospond to concentration of $N_2O_5$ initially and at time $t$.

(a) $[N_2O_5]_t = [N_2O_5]_0 + kt$

(b) $[N_2O_5]_0 = [N_2O_5]_t e^{kt}$

(c) $\log [N_2O_5]_t = \log [N_2O_5]_0 + kt$

(d) $\ln \frac{[N_2P_5]_0}{[N_2P_5]_t} = kt$

**23.** Among the following the most stable compound is :

(a) *cis*-1, 2-cyclohexanediol

(b) *trans*-1, 2-cyclohexanediol

(c) *cis*-1,3-cyclohexanediol

(d) *trans*-1, 3-cyclohexanediol

**24.** Which of the following is true?

(a) Coke is found in nature

(b) Producer gas is a mixture of CO & $H_2$

(c) CO is used in the extraction of Ni by Mond's process

(d) $CO_2$ can be prepared by dehydration of formic acid.

**25.** Aniline is reacted with bromine water and the resulting product is treated with an aqueous solution of sodium nitrite in presence of dilute hydrochloric acid. The compound so formed is converted into a tetrafluoroborate which is subsequently heated dry. The final product is

(a) 1,3, 5-tribromobenzene

(b) p-bromofluorobenzene

(c) p-bromoaniline

(d) 2,4, 6-tribromofluorobenzene

**26.** With which one of the following elements silicon should be doped so as to give p-type of semiconductor ?

(a) Germanium (b) Arsenic

(c) Selenium (d) Boron

**27.** 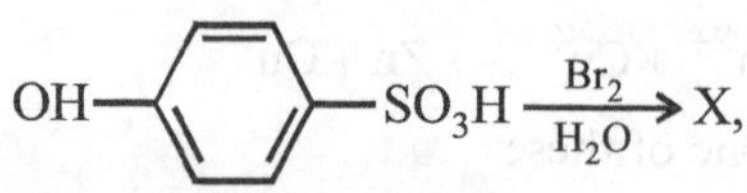

X is identified as

(a) 2, 4, 6-tribromophenol

(b) 2-bromo-4-hydroxylbenzene sulphonic acid

(c) 3, 5-dibromo-4-hydroxybenzene sulphonic acid

(d) 2-bromophenol

28. The appearance of colour in solid alkali metal halides is generally due to
(a) Schottky defect (b) Frenkel defect
(c) Interstitial positions (d) F-centres

29. Which of the following is a basic dye?
(a) Congo red (b) Aniline yellow
(c) Alizarin (d) Indigo

30. Aluminium displaces hydrogen from acids but copper does not. A galvanic cell prepared by combining $Cu/Cu^{2+}$ and $Al/Al^{3+}$ has an e.m.f of 2.0 V at 298°K. If the potential of copper electrode is + 0.34 V, that of aluminium is
(a) +1.66 (b) – 1.66
(c) +2.34 (d) –2.3 V

31. An organic compound X on treatment with pyridinium chlorochromate in dichloromethane gives compound Y. Compound Y reacts with $I_2$ and alkali to form triiodomethane. The compound 'X' is
(a) $C_2H_5OH$ (b) $CH_3CHO$
(c) $CH_3COCH_3$ (d) $CH_3COOH$

32. A sudden large jumps between the values of second and third ionization energies of an element, would be associated with which of the following electronic configuration?
(a) $1s^2, 2s^2, 2p^6, 3s^1$
(b) $1s^2, 2s^2, 2p^6, 3s^1, 3p^1$
(c) $1s^2, 2s^2, 2p^6, 3s^2$
(d) $1s^2, 2s^2, 2p^6, 3s^2, 3p^2$

33. Which of the products is formed when acetone is reacted with barium hydroxide solution?
(a) 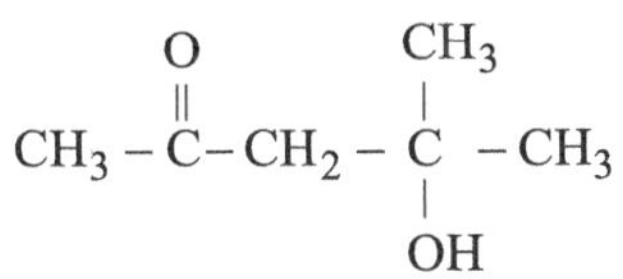
(b) 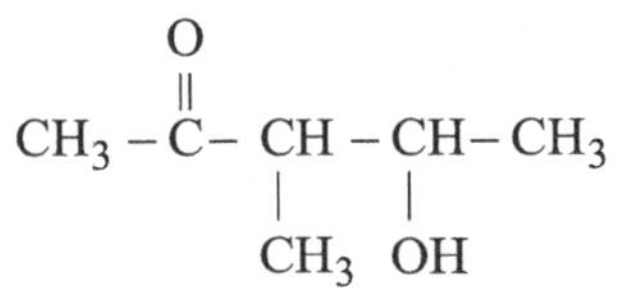
(c) 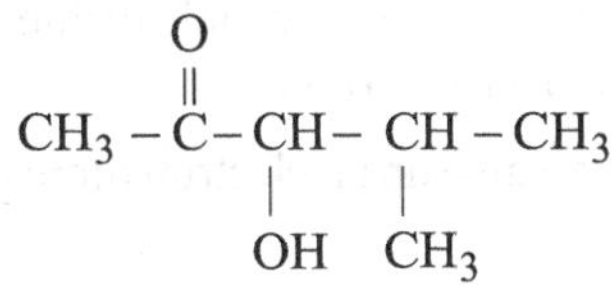
(d) 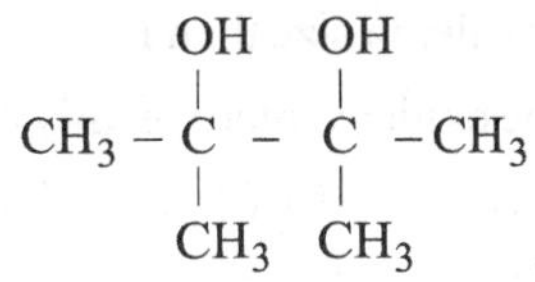

34. For the manufacture of $NH_3$ by the following reaction
$$N_2 + 3H_2 \rightleftharpoons 2NH_3 + 23kcal$$
The favourable conditions are
(a) low temp., high pressure and catalyst
(b) low temp., low pressure and catalyst
(c) high temp., high pressure and catalyst
(d) high temp., low pressure and catalyst

35. Ethanol can be prepared more easily by which reaction ?
(i) $CH_3CH_2Br + H_2O \longrightarrow CH_3CH_2OH$
(ii) $CH_3CH_2Br + Ag_2O$ (in boiling water) $\longrightarrow CH_3CH_2OH$
(a) by (i) reaction
(b) by (ii) reaction
(c) Both reactions proceed at same rate
(d) by none

36. The oxidation states of iodine in $HIO_4$, $H_3IO_5$ and $H_5IO_6$ are respectively
(a) +1, +3, +7 (b) +7, +7, +3
(c) +7, +7, +7 (d) +7, +5, +3

37. Which is correct statement?
(a) Starch is a polymer of α-glucose
(b) In cyclic structure of fructose, there are four carbons and one oxygen atom
(c) Amylose is a component of cellulose
(d) Proteins are composed of only one type of amino acids

**38.** Regarding $F^-$ and $Cl^-$ which of the following statements is/are correct?

(i) $Cl^-$ can give up an electron more easily than $F^-$

(ii) $Cl^-$ is a better reducing agent than $F^-$

(iii) $Cl^-$ is smaller in size than $F^-$

(iv) $F^-$ can be oxidized more readily than $Cl^-$

(a) (i) and (ii) (b) (i), (ii) and (iv)

(c) (iii) and (iv) (d) only (i)

**39.** Among the following, the species having square planar geometry for central atom are

(i) $XeF_4$ (ii) $SF_4$

(iii) $[NiCl_4]^{2-}$ (iv) $[PtCl_4]^{2-}$

(a) (i) and (iv) (b) (i) and (ii)

(c) (ii) and (iii) (d) (iii) and (iv)

**40.** Water glass is :

(a) $Na_2SiO_3$ (b) $Mg_2Si$

(c) $SiCl_4$ (d) $Ca(H_2PO_4)_2$

**41.** Which one of the following statement is *not true*?

(a) In vulcanization the formation of sulphur bridges between different chains make rubber harder and stronger.

(b) Natural rubber has the *trans* -configuration at every double bond

(c) Buna-S is a copolymer of butadiene and styrene

(d) Natural rubber is a 1, 4 - polymer of isoprene

**42.** For a first order reaction, to obtain a positive slope, we need to plot {where [A] is the concentration of reactant A}

(a) $-\log_{10}[A]$ *vs* t (b) $-\log_e[A]$ *vs* t

(c) $\log_{10}[A]$ *vs* log t (d) [A] *vs* t

**43.** Among the following molecules

(i) $XeO_3$ (ii) $XeOF_4$

(iii) $XeF_6$

Those having same number of lone pairs on Xe are

(a) (i) and (ii) only (b) (i) and (iii) only

(c) (ii) and (iii) only (d) (i), (ii) and (iii)

**44.** The de-Broglie wavelength associated with a particle of mass $10^{-6}$ kg moving with a velocity of 10 $ms^{-1}$ is :

(a) $6.63\times10^{-7}$ m (b) $6.63\times10^{-16}$ m

(c) $6.63\times10^{-21}$ m (d) $6.63\times10^{-29}$ m

**45.** Which of the following is not a fat soluble vitamin?

(a) Vitamin B complex

(b) Vitamin D

(c) Vitamin E

(d) Vitamin A

# NEET Mock Test-3

1. If 0.1 M solution of glucose and 0.1 M solution of urea are placed on two sides of the semipermeable membrane to equal heights, then it will be correct to say that
   (a) There will be no net movement across the membrane
   (b) Glucose will flow towards urea solution
   (c) urea will flow towards glucose solution
   (d) water will flow from urea solution to glucose

2. In the Freidel Craft's acylation reaction, the effective electrophile is
   (a) $RCOCl^{\oplus}$  (b) $AlCl_3$
   (c) RCOCl  (d) $RCO^{\oplus}$

3. White lead is
   (a) $Pb_3O_4$
   (b) PbO
   (c) $2PbCO_3.Pb(OH)_2$
   (d) $Pb(CH_3COO)_2.Pb(OH)_2$

4. Specific volume of cylindrical virus particle is $6.02 \times 10^{-2}$ cc/gm. whose radius and length 7 Å & 10 Å respectively. If $N_A = 6.02 \times 10^{23}$, find molecular weight of virus
   (a) $3.08 \times 10^3$ kg/mol
   (b) $3.08 \times 10^4$ kg/mol
   (c) $1.54 \times 10^4$ kg/mol
   (d) 15.4 kg/mol

5. Excess of ethanol and con. $H_2SO_4$ on heating upto 140°C produces
   (a) diethyl ether
   (b) diethyl sulphate
   (c) ethyl hydrogen sulphate
   (d) ethylene

6. Consider the following statements
   I. The radius of an anion is larger than that of the parent atom.
   II. The ionization energy generally increases with increasing atomic number in a period.
   III. The electronegativity of an element is the tendency of an isolated atom to attract an electron.

   Which of the above statements is/are correct?
   (a) I alone  (b) II alone
   (c) I and II  (d) II and III

7. $Cl_2$ changes to $Cl^-$ and $ClO^-$ in cold NaOH. Equivalent weight of $Cl_2$ will be
   (a) M  (b) $\frac{M}{2}$
   (c) $\frac{M}{3}$  (d) $\frac{3M}{3}$

8. Which of the following pentafluoride is not obtained?
   (a) $SbF_5$  (b) $BiF_5$
   (c) $PF_5$  (d) $AsF_5$

9. In the conversion of $Br_2$ to $BrO_3^-$, the oxidation number of Br changes from
   (a) zero to + 5  (b) + 1 to + 5
   (c) zero to − 3  (d) + 2 to + 5

10. Arrange the following phenols in order of their increasing acidity.

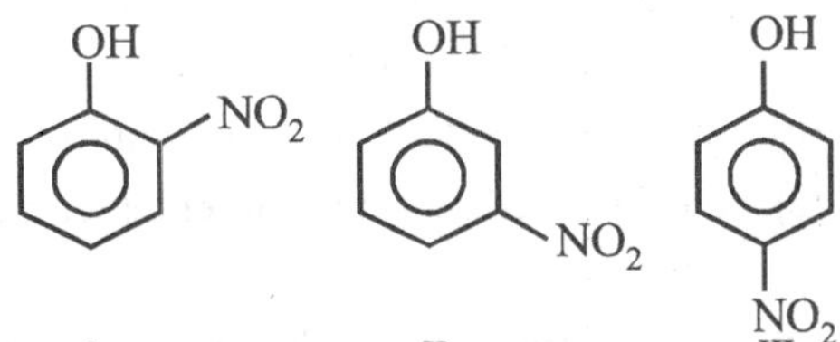

I  II  III

(a) I > III > II (b) I > II > III

(c) III > I > II (d) III > II > I

**11.** The average molecular speed is greatest in which of the following gas samples ?

(a) 1.0 mol of $O_2$ at 560 K

(b) 0.50 mol of Ne at 500 K

(c) 0.20 mol of $CO_2$ at 440 K

(d) 2.0 mol of He at 140 K

**12.** Aniline is an activated system for electrophilic substitution. The compound formed on heating aniline with acetic anhydride is

(a) 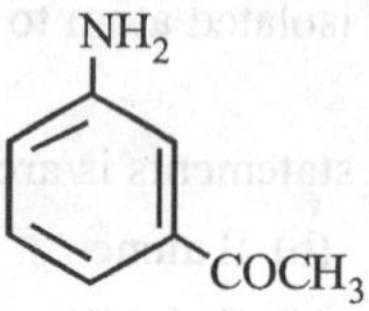


(b) 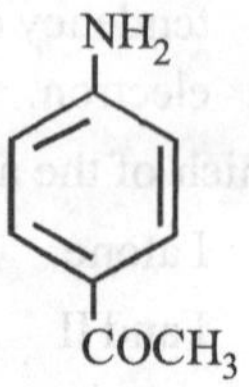


(c) 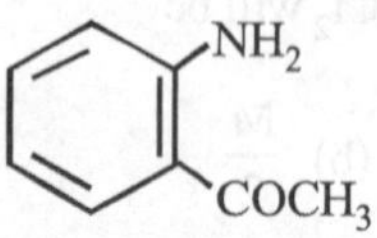


(d) 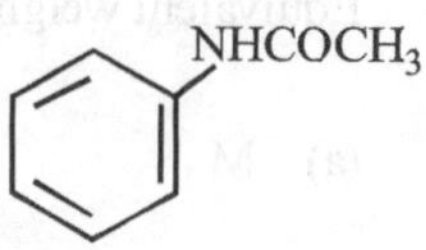


**13.** The formula mass of Mohr's salt is 392. The iron present in it is oxidised by $KMnO_4$ in acid medium. The equivalent mass of Mohr's salt is

(a) 392 (b) 31.6

(c) 278 (d) 156

**14.** Sewage mostly constitutes

(a) Non-biodegradable pollutants

(b) Biodegradable pollutants

(c) Effluents

(d) Air pollutants

**15.** The Langmuir adsorption isotherm is deduced using the assumption

(a) the adsorption sites are equivalent in their ability to adsorb the particles

(b) the heat of adsorption varies with coverage

(c) the adsorbed molecules interact with each other

(d) the adsorption takes place in multilayers.

**16.** Three dimensional molecules with cross links are formed in the case of a

(a) thermoplastic

(b) thermosetting plastic

(c) both (a) and (b)

(d) none of the above

**17.** The volume-temperature graphs of a given mass of an ideal gas at constant pressure are shown below.

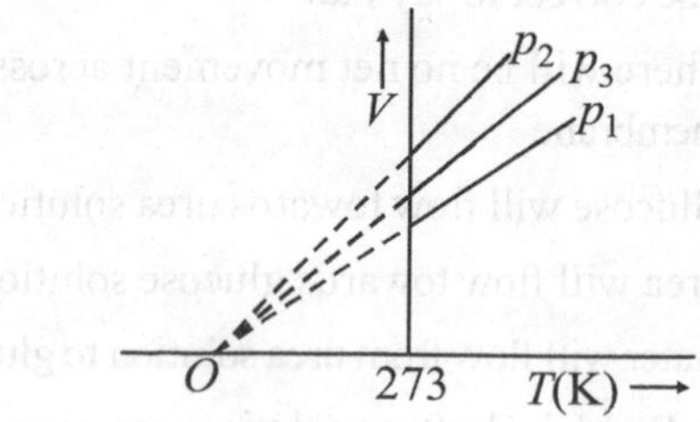


What is the correct order of pressures ?

(a) $p_1 > p_3 > p_2$ (b) $p_1 > p_2 > p_3$

(c) $p_2 > p_3 > p_1$ (d) $p_2 > p_1 > p_3$

**18.** Which of the following is used for making optical instruments?

(a) $SiO_2$ (b) Si

(c) $SiH_4$ (d) SiC

**19.** The correct order of acid strength of oxyacids is:

(a) $HClO > HClO_2 > HClO_3 > HClO_4$

(b) $HClO_2 > HClO_3 > HClO > HClO_4$

(c) $HClO_4 > HClO_3 > HClO_2 > HClO$

(d) $HClO_3 > HClO_4 > HClO > HClO_2$

**20.** 25.3 g of sodium carbonate, $Na_2CO_3$ is dissolved in enough water to make 250 mL of solution. If sodium carbonate dissociates completely, molar concentration of sodium ions, $Na^+$ and carbonate ions, $CO_3^{2-}$ are respectively (Molar mass of $Na_2CO_3 = 106\ g\ mol^{-1}$)

(a) 0.955 M and 1.910 M

(b) 1.910 M and 0.955 M

(c) 1.90 M and 1.910 M

(d) 0.477 M and 0.477 M

21. In which alkyl halide, $S_N2$ mechanism is favoured maximum ?
(a) $CH_3Cl$ (b) $CH_3CH_2Cl$
(c) $(CH_3)_2CHCl$ (d) $(CH_3)_3C-Cl$

22. Equilibrium constant K changes with temperature. At 300 K, equilibrium constant is 25 and at 400 K it is 10. Hence, backward reaction will have energy of activation
(a) equa to that of forward reaction
(b) less than that of forward reaction
(c) greater than that of forward reaction
(d) given values are not sufficient to explain given statement

23. Which of the two ions from the list given below that have the geometry that is explained by the same hybridization of orbitals, $NO_2^-$, $NO_3^-$, $NH_2^-$, $NH_4^+$, $SCN^-$?
(a) $NO_2^-$ and $NO_3^-$ (b) $NH_4^+$ and $NO_3^-$
(c) $SCN^-$ and $NH_2^-$ (d) $NO_2^-$ and $NH_2^-$

24. 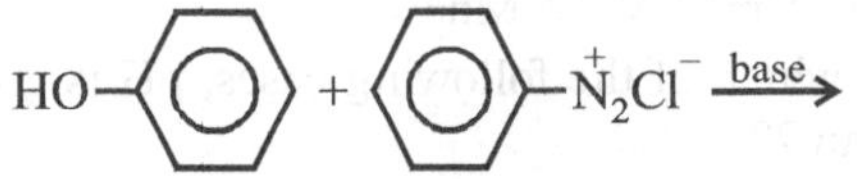

(a) 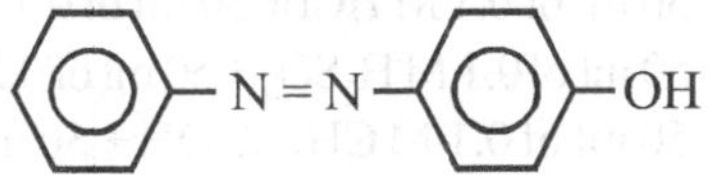

(b) 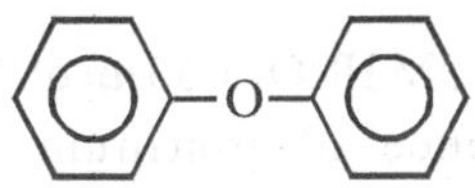

(c) 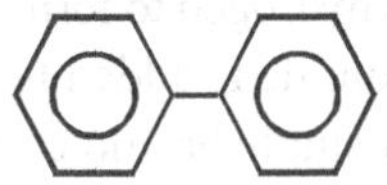

(d) 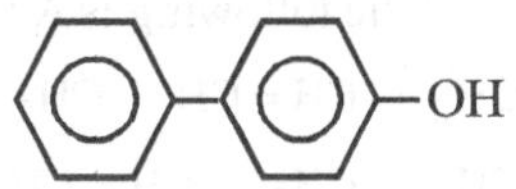

25. White lead is
(a) $Pb_3O_4$
(b) PbO
(c) $2PbCO_3.Pb(OH)_2$
(d) $Pb(CH_3COO)_2.Pb(OH)_2$

26. The commonest method for the extraction of metals from oxide ores involves :
(a) Reduction with carbon and carbon monoxide
(b) Reduction with aluminium
(c) Reduction with hydrogen
(d) Electrolytic method

27. With which one of the following elements silicon should be doped so as to give p-type of semiconductor ?
(a) Germanium (b) Arsenic
(c) Selenium (d) Boron

28. IUPAC name of $[Pt(NH_3)_3(Br)(NO_2)Cl]Cl$ is
(a) Triamminechlorobromonitroplatinum (IV) chloride
(b) Triamminebromonitrochloroplatinum (IV) chloride
(c) Triamminebromochloronitroplatinum (IV) chloride
(d) Triamminenitrochlorobromoplatinum (IV) chloride

29. Van't Hoff factor is:
(a) More than one in case of association
(b) Less than one in case of dissociation
(c) $\dfrac{\text{normal molecular mass}}{\text{observed molecular mass}}$
(d) $\dfrac{\text{observed molecular mass}}{\text{normal molecular mass}}$

30. Which of the following compound will undergo self aldol condensation in the presence of cold dilute alkali ?
(a) $CH_2=CH-CHO$ (b) $CH\equiv C-CHO$
(c) $C_6H_5CHO$ (d) $CH_3CH_2CHO$.

31. When one mole of an ideal gas is compressed to half its initial volume and simultaneously heated to twice in initial temperature, the change in entropy ($\Delta S$) is
(a) $C_V \ln 2$ (b) $C_P \ln 2$
(c) $R \ln 2$ (d) $(C_V - R)\ln 2$

32. If x is amount of adsorbate and m is amount of adsorbent, which of the following relations is not related to adsorption process ?
(a) $x/m = K(p)$ at very low pressure.
(b) $x/m = Kp^{1/n}$ at inter mediate pressure
(c) $\dfrac{x}{m} = K$ at very high pressure
(d) $\dfrac{x}{m} = p$

33. For the reaction of one mole of zinc dust with one mole of sulphuric acid in a bomb calorimeter, $\Delta U$ and w corresponds to
(a) $\Delta U<0, w=0$ (b) $\Delta U<0, w<0$
(c) $\Delta U>0, w=0$ (d) $\Delta U>0, w>0$

**34.** Reactivity of hydrogen atoms attached to different carbon atoms in alkanes has the order
(a) Tertiary > Primary > Secondary
(b) Primary > Secondary > Tertiary
(c) Both (a) and (b)
(d) Tertiary > Secondary > Primary.

**35.** In most cases, for a rise of 10K temperature the rate constant is doubled to tripled. This is due to the reason that
(a) collision frequency increases by a factor of 2 to 3.
(b) fraction of molecules possessing threshold energy increases by a factor of 2 to 3
(c) Activation energy is lowered by a factor of 2 to 3.
(d) none of these

**36.** The restricted rotation about carbon carbon double bond in 2-butene is due to
(a) Overlap of one s- and $sp^2$-hybridized orbitals
(b) Overlap of two $sp^2$- hybridized orbitals
(c) Overlap of one p- and one $sp^2$-hybridized orbitals
(d) Sideways overlap of two p- orbitals.

**37.** Which of the following colligative property can provide molar mass of proteins (or polymers or colloids) with greatest precision ?
(a) Osmotic pressure
(b) Elevation of boiling point
(c) Depression of freezing point
(d) Relative lowering of vapour pressure

**38.** Cyclic hydrocarbon 'A' has all the carbon and hydrogen atoms in a single plane. All the carbon carbon bonds have the same length, less than 1.54 Å, but more than 1.34 Å. The C – C – C bond angle will be
(a) 109°28' (b) 100°
(c) 180° (d) 120°

**39.** The boiling point of three saturated hydrocarbons A, B and C are – 102°C, – 43.4°C and – 0.6°C respectively. The hydrocarbon having the maximum number of carbon atoms in its molecule is
(a) A (b) B
(c) C (d) none of these

**40.** Which of the following electrolyte will have maximum flocculation value for $Fe(OH)_3$ sol?
(a) NaCl (b) $Na_2S$
(c) $(NH_4)_3PO_4$ (d) $K_2SO_4$

**41.** In DNA the complementary bases are
(a) adenine and thymine; guanine and cytosine
(b) uracil and adenine; cytosine and guanine
(c) adenine and guanine; thymine and cytosine
(d) adenine and thymine; guanine and uracil

**42.** What is the correct order of spin only magnetic moment (in BM) of $Mn^{2+}$, $Cr^{2+}$ and $V^{2+}$ ?
(a) $Mn^{2+} > V^{2+} > Cr^{2+}$
(b) $V^{2+} > Cr^{2+} > Mn^{2+}$
(c) $Mn^{2+} > Cr^{2+} > V^{2+}$
(d) $Cr^{2+} > V^{2+} > Mn^{2+}$

**43.** In which of the following cases, pH is greater than 7?
(a) 50 ml of 0.1 M HCl + 50 ml of 0.1 M NaCl
(b) 50 ml of 0.1 M $H_2SO_4$ + 50 ml of 0.2 M NaOH
(c) 50 ml of 0.1 M $CH_3COOH$ + 50 ml of 0.1 M KOH
(d) 50 ml of 0.1 M $HNO_3$ + 50 ml of 0.1 M $NH_3$

**44.** In the presence of platinum catalyst, hydrocarbon A adds hydrogen to form n-hexane. When hydrogen bromide is added to A instead of hydrogen, only a single bromo compound is formed. Which of the following is A?
(a) $CH_3—CH_2—CH=CH—CH_2—CH_3$
(b) $CH_3—CH_2—CH_2—CH=CH—CH_3$
(c) $CH_3—CH=CH—CH_2—CH_2—CH_3$
(d) $CH_2=CH—CH_2—CH_2—CH_2—CH_3$

**45.** $\underset{\text{Benzene}}{C_6H_6} + \underset{\text{Methyl chloride}}{CH_3Cl} \xrightarrow{AlCl_3} \underset{\text{Toluene}}{C_6H_5CH_3} + HCl$

The above reaction is:
(a) Wurtz Fittig reaction
(b) Grignard reaction
(c) Friedel-Craft's reaction
(d) Ullmann reaction

# Hints & Solutions

# HINTS & SOLUTIONS

# 1 Some Basic Concepts of Chemistry

1. (a)

2. (b) Gram molecular weight of CO
$= 12 + 16 = 28$ g
$6.023 \times 10^{23}$ molecules of CO weight 28 g
1 molecule of CO weighs
$$= \frac{28}{6.023 \times 10^{23}} = 4.648 \times 10^{-23} g \approx 4.65 \times 10^{-23} g$$

3. (a) Fe (no. of moles) $= \frac{558.5}{55.85} = 10$ moles $= 10 N_A$ atoms.
No. of moles in 60 g of C $= 60/12 = 5$ moles $= 5 N_A$ atoms.

4. (d) 1 Mole of $Mg_3(PO_4)_2$ contains 8 mole of oxygen atoms
$\therefore$ 8 mole of oxygen atoms $\equiv$ 1 mole of $Mg_3(PO_4)_2$
0.25 mole of oxygen atom
$$\equiv \frac{1}{8} \times 0.25 \text{ mole of } Mg_3(PO_4)_2$$
$$= 3.125 \times 10^{-2} \text{ mole of } Mg_3(PO_4)_2$$

5. (c) 16 g $CH_4$ = 1 mol $= 6.023 \times 10^{23}$ molecules

6. (d) At S.T.P. 22.4 litre of gas contains $6.023 \times 10^{23}$ molecules
$\therefore$ molecules in 8.96 litre of gas
$$= \frac{6.023 \times 10^{23} \times 8.96}{22.4} = 24.092 \times 10^{22}$$

7. (d) 1 molecule of $CO_2$ has one atom of C and two atoms of oxygen.
$\therefore$ 1 mole of $CO_2$ has
$= 6.02 \times 10^{23}$ atoms of C
$= 2 \times 6.02 \times 10^{23}$ atoms of O

8. (b) Total atoms in 1 molecule of $C_{12}H_{22}O_{11}$
$= 12 + 22 + 11 = 45$
$\therefore$ Total atoms in 1 mole of $C_{12}H_{22}O_{11}$
$= 45 \times 6.02 \times 10^{23}$ atoms/mol.

9. (d) 22.4 L of He at STP = 1 mole

10. (a) Let mass of $O_2 = 1$ g
$\therefore$ Mass of $N_2 = 4$g
No. of moles of $O_2 = \frac{1}{32}$
No. of moles of $N_2 = \frac{4}{28}$
Ratio of no. of moles $= \frac{1}{32} : \frac{4}{28} = \frac{1}{32} : \frac{1}{7} = 7 : 32$

11. (b) Moles of $C_{12}H_{22}O_{11} = \frac{25.6}{342.3} = 0.0747$
Number of H-atoms $= 0.0747 \times 22 \times 6.023 \times 10^{23}$
$= 9.91 \times 10^{23}$

12. (a) 5 M $H_2SO_4$ = 10 N $H_2SO_4$,
($\because$ Basicity of $H_2SO_4 = 2$)
$N_1V_1 = N_2V_2$,
$10 \times 1 = N_2 \times 10$ or $N_2 = 1$ N

13. (c) Among all the given options molarity is correct because the term molarity involves volume which increases on increasing temperature.

14. (b) Suppose weight of metallic chloride = 100 g
Then weight of metal = 47.22 g
Weight of chlorine = 100 – 47.22 = 52.78 g

$\therefore$ Equivalent weight of metal $= \frac{47.22}{52.78} \times 35.5$
$= 31.76$

15. (b) Moles of urea present in 100 mL of sol.

$$= \frac{6.02 \times 10^{20}}{6.02 \times 10^{23}}$$

$$\therefore M = \frac{6.02 \times 10^{20} \times 1000}{6.02 \times 10^{23} \times 100} = 0.01M$$

[ $\because$ M = Moles of solute present in 1L of solution]

16. (a) Apply the formula, $d = M\left(\frac{1}{m} + \frac{M_2}{1000}\right)$
where $M$ = molarity, $M_2$ = molecular weight of $CH_3COOH$
$d$ = density, $m$ = molality.

$$\therefore 1.02 = 2.05\left(\frac{1}{m} + \frac{60}{1000}\right)$$

On solving we get, $m = 2.28$ mol/kg.

17. (d) Mass of 1 molecule of water = 18 amu
$= 18 \times 1.66 \times 10^{-24}$ g

Volume of 1 molecule $= \frac{\text{mass}}{\text{density}}$

$= 29.88 \times 10^{-24} = 2.988 \times 10^{-23}$ mL

18. (a) No. of mol $= \frac{\text{Mass}}{\text{Molar mass}}$

$0.0242 = \frac{1.657}{M} \Rightarrow M = 68.47$

$1 + X + 32 = 68.47$
$X = 35.5$

19. (c) Formula of sulphate will be $MSO_4 . 7H_2O$

$$\% \text{ of metal} = \frac{M}{M + 96 + 7 \times 18} \times 100 = 9.87$$

$\Rightarrow M = 24.31$

20. (d) $\overset{+1}{H_3PO_2} \longrightarrow \overset{-3}{PH_3} + \overset{+3}{H_3PO_3}$

$n_1 = |-3-(1)| = |-4| = 4$
$n_2 = |3-(1)| = |2| = 2$

$$\text{n-factor} = \frac{n_1 \times n_2}{n_1 + n_2} = \frac{4 \times 2}{4+2} = \frac{4}{3}$$

$$\text{Eq. mass} = \frac{\text{mol mass}}{\text{n - factor}} = \frac{M \times 3}{4}$$

21. (b) $E_{Element} = 4$, Formula of chloride $M\,Cl_X$
Eq. mass of chloride $= E_{Element} + E_{Chlorine}$

$$\frac{M_{Mass}}{n_f} = E_{Element} + E_{Chlorine}$$

$$\frac{59.25 \times 2}{x} = 4 + 35.5$$

$x = 3$

22. (c) $\underset{28\text{ g}}{C_2H_4} + \underset{96\text{ g}}{3\,O_2} \longrightarrow 2CO_2 + 2H_2O$

$\because$ 28 g of $C_2H_4$ undergo complete combustion by = 96 g of $O_2$
$\therefore$ 2800 g of $C_2H_4$ undergo complete combustion by
= 9600 g or 9.6 kg of $O_2$.

23. (c) 50% of X (Atomic mass 10), 50% of Y (Atomic mass 20). Relative number of atoms of

$X = \frac{50}{10} = 5$

Relative number of atoms of Y $= \frac{50}{20} = 2.5$

$\therefore$ Simple ratio = 2 : 1. Hence simplest formula $X_2Y$

24. (c) Percentage by mass of copper in malachite

$= \frac{2 \times 63.5}{221} = 57.5\%$

25. (c) This is Avogadro's hypothesis.
According to this, equal volume of all gases contain equal no. of molecules under similar condition of temperature and pressure.

# 2 Structure of Atom

1. **(b)** $e/m$ for $He^+ = 1/4$ $e/m$ for $He^{2+} = 2/4$

$e/m$ for $D^+ = 1/2$ $e/m$ for $H^+ = 1/1$

$\therefore$ Value of $e/m$ is highest for $H^+$.

2. **(d)**

(a) $CO_2$ : Atoms $= 1 + 2 = 3$;

Electrons $= 6 + 8 \times 2 = 22\ e^-$

$N_2O$ : Atoms $= 1 + 2 = 3$;

Electrons $= 7 \times 2 + 8 = 22\ e^-$

(b) CaO : Atoms = 2; Electrons $= 20 + 8 = 28\ e^-$

KF : Atoms = 2; Electrons $= 19 + 9 = 28\ e^-$

(c) $OF_2$ : Atoms = 3; Electrons $= 8 + 18 = 26\ e^-$

HClO : Atoms = 3; Electrons $= 1 + 17 + 8 = 26\ e^-$

3. **(b)** Calculating number of electrons

(a).

$$\left.\begin{array}{l} BO_3^{3-} \longrightarrow 5 + 8 \times 3 + 3 = 32 \\ CO_3^{2-} \longrightarrow 6 + 8 \times 3 + 2 = 32 \\ NO_3^{-} \longrightarrow 7 + 8 \times 3 + 1 = 32 \end{array}\right\} \text{iso-electronic species}$$

(b).

$$\left.\begin{array}{l} SO_3^{2-} \longrightarrow 16 + 8 \times 3 + 2 = 42 \\ CO_3^{2-} \longrightarrow 32 \\ NO_3^{-} \longrightarrow 32 \end{array}\right\} \text{non iso-electronic species}$$

(c).

$$\left.\begin{array}{l} CN^{-} \longrightarrow 6 + 7 + 1 = 14 \\ N_2 \longrightarrow 7 \times 2 = 14 \\ C_2^{2-} \longrightarrow 6 \times 2 + 2 = 14 \end{array}\right\} \text{iso-electronic species}$$

(d).

$$\left.\begin{array}{l} PO_4^{3-} \longrightarrow 15 + 8 \times 4 + 3 = 50 \\ SO_4^{2-} \longrightarrow 16 + 8 \times 4 + 2 = 50 \\ ClO_4^{-} \longrightarrow 17 + 8 \times 4 + 1 = 50 \end{array}\right\} \text{iso-electronic species}$$

4. **(d)** This statement is known as uncertainty principle which was given by Heisenberg; it is not a Bohr's postulate.

5. **(b)** P.E. = Work done $= \int_{\infty}^{r} + \frac{Ze^2}{r^2} dr = -\frac{Ze^2}{r}$.

6. **(a)** For hydrogen atom $(n) = 1$ (due to ground state)

Radius of hydrogen atom $(r) = 0.53$ Å.

Atomic number of Li (Z) = 3.

Radius of $Li^{2+}$ ion

$$= r_1 \times \frac{n^2}{Z} = 0.53 \times \frac{(1)^2}{3} = 0.17 \text{ Å}$$

7. **(a)** 2nd excited state will be the 3rd energy level.

$$E_n = -\frac{13.6}{n^2} \text{eV}$$

or $E = -\frac{13.6}{9} \text{eV} = -1.51 \text{ eV}$.

**8.** **(c)** Zeeman effect refers to splitting of lines of an emission spectrum in magnetic field.

**9.** **(d)** $r \propto n^2$

$\therefore \frac{r_1}{r_3} = \frac{(1)^2}{(3)^2}$

$\frac{y}{r_3} = \frac{1}{9}$

$r_3 = 9y$

**10.** **(b)** $r = 0.529 \times \frac{n^2}{Z}$

r = 211.6 pm = 2.11 Å

$\Rightarrow 0.529 \times \frac{n^2}{Z} = 2.11 \text{Å}$

$n = 2$ (Balmer series)

**11.** **(c)** In ${}^{231}_{89}Y$, number of protons and electrons is 89 and number of neutrons = A – Z = 231 – 89 = 142

**12.** **(b)** $r_1$ of H-atom = 0.529 Å

$r_n \text{ (H like atom)} = \frac{n^2}{Z} \times r_1 \text{(H – atom)}$

$r_n \text{ of } Be^{3+} = \frac{n^2}{Z} \times r_1 \text{(H – atom)}$

$\Rightarrow \frac{n^2}{Z} \times 0.529 = 0.529 \Rightarrow n^2 = Z$

$\Rightarrow n^2 = 4 \Rightarrow n = 2$

**13.** **(a)** Total energy $(E_n)$ = K.E + P.E

in first excited state

$$E = \frac{1}{2}mv^2 + \left[-\frac{Ze^2}{r}\right] = +\frac{1}{2}\frac{Ze^2}{r} - \frac{Ze^2}{r}$$

$$-3.4 \ eV = -\frac{1}{2}\frac{Ze^2}{r}$$

$$\therefore \text{K.E} = \frac{1}{2}\frac{Ze^2}{r} = +3.4 \text{ eV}$$

**14.** **(a)** Energy is always absorbed or emitted in whole number or multiples of quantum.

**15.** **(a)** $p_x$ orbital being dumbell shaped, have one nodal plane.

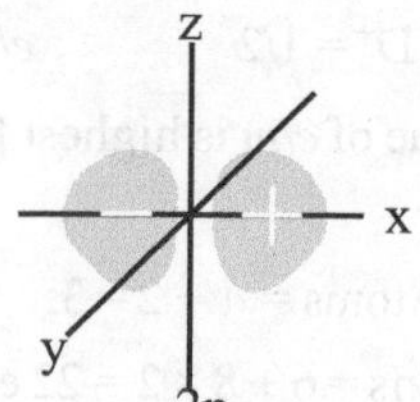


$2p_x$

**16.** **(a)** Number of radial nodes = $(n - l - 1)$

For 3*s*: $n = 3, l = 0$ (Number of radial node = 2)

For 2*p*: $n = 2, l = 1$ (Number of radial node = 0)

**17.** **(d)**

**18.** **(c)** K.E. of emitted electron

$= h\nu - h\nu_0$ (i.e. smaller than $h\nu$).

**19.** **(d)**

(i) Interference and diffraction support the wave nature of electron.

(ii) $E = mc^2$ supports the particle nature of electron.

(iii) $E = h\nu = \frac{hc}{\lambda}$ is de-Broglie equation and it supports both wave nature and particle nature of electron.

**20.** **(a)** The possible quantum numbers for 4*f* electron are

$n = 4, \ell = 3, m = -3, -2 -1, 0, 1, 2, 3$ and $s = \pm\frac{1}{2}$

Of various possiblities only option (a) is possible.

**21. (b)** For $4d$ orbitals, $n = 4$, $l = 2$

$$\begin{bmatrix} \text{For } s \text{ orbital } l = 0 \\ \text{For } p \text{ orbital } l = 1 \\ \text{For } d \text{ orbital } l = 2 \end{bmatrix}$$

$m = -2, -1, 0, +1, +2$

$s = +\frac{1}{2}$ and $-\frac{1}{2}$

Thus choice $b$ having $n = 4$, $l = 2$, $m = 1$ and $s = -\frac{1}{2}$ is correct.

**22. (d)** For $p$ sub-shell, $m = -1, 0, +1$. Therefore, $m = -2$ orbital will not be present in $p$ sub-shell.

**23. (a)** $_{11}Na = 1s^2\, 2s^2 p^6\, 3s^1$ for $3s^1$ $l = 0$.

Hence m = 0.

**24. (a)** m = +2 signifies only one orbital.

**25. (d)** Orbital angular momentum

$= \sqrt{l(l+1)}\frac{h}{2\pi}$; $l = 1$ for $p$-orbital.

# 3 Classification of Elements and Periodicity in Properties

1. (c) F has highest electronegativity, so it is chemically most active non-metal.
2. (c)
3. (d) The electrons are not filled in *d*-subshell monotonically with increase in atomic number among transition elements.
4. (c) $Li^+ (2e^-) = 1s^2$

   $Be^+ (3e^-) = 1s^2 2s^1$

   $B^+ (4e^-) = 1s^2 2s^2$

   $C^+ (5e^-) = 1s^2 2s^2 2p^1$

   Therefore Be < C < B < Li

   Here, $Li^+$ has inert configuration and $B^+$ has fully filled *s*-orbital. Hence these will have high value of second ionisation potential.
5. (d) On moving down in a group atomic radii increases due to successive addition of extra shell hence O < S < Se

   Further As is in group 15 having one less electron in its *p* orbital hence have higher atomic radii than group 16 elements. i.e., O < S < Se < As
6. (c)
7. (c) The correct order of $IE_2$ is Ne > O > F > N
8. (b) Electropositive nature increases down the group and decreases across the period.
9. (b) Due to high stability of half-filled orbitals.
10. (a)

| Species | $Na^+$ | $Mg^{2+}$ | $Al^{3+}$ | $Si^{4+}$ |
|---|---|---|---|---|
| Protons | 11 | 12 | 13 | 14 |
| Electrons | 10 | 10 | 10 | 10 |

   Size of isoelectronic cations decreases with increase in magnitude of nuclear charge

   ∴ Order of decreasing size is

   $Na^+ > Mg^{2+} > Al^{3+} > Si^{4+}$
11. (c) While moving down in a group, effective nuclear attraction decreases due to addition of new orbits. As a result ionisation potential decreases. Hence, the correct order is Li > K > Cs.
12. (c) The element A is $ns^2p^1$ and B is $ns^2p^4$. They can form compound of the type $A_2B_3$
13. (d) Basicity of oxides decreases in a period from left to right. $Na_2O$ is basic oxide, $CO_2$, $SiO_2$ and $SO_2$ are acidic oxides. Alternatively, oxides of metals (e.g., $Na_2O$) are basic, while oxides of non-metals ($SO_2$, $SiO_2$ and $CO_2$) are acidic.
14. (a) CaO is basic as it forms strong base $Ca(OH)_2$ on reaction with water.

   $$CaO + H_2O \longrightarrow Ca(OH)_2$$

   $CO_2$ is acidic as it dissolves in water forming unstable carbonic acid.

   $$H_2O + CO_2 \longrightarrow H_2CO_3$$

   Silica ($SiO_2$) is insoluble in water and acts as a very weak acid.

   $SnO_2$ is amphoteric as it reacts with both acid and base.

   $$SnO_2 + 2H_2SO_4 \longrightarrow Sn(SO_4)_2 + 2H_2O$$

   $$SnO_2 + 2KOH \longrightarrow K_2SnO_3 + H_2O$$
15. (a) Correct order of electron affinity is : Cl > F > S > O

   Electron affinity of 2nd period non-metals is less than that of the respective 3rd period non-metals.
16. (b)

   (a) Correct order → $Ca^{2+} > K^+ > Cl^- > S^{2-}$ (Ionisation energy)

   For isoelectronic species (I.E. $\propto Z_{eff}$)

(b) Correct order → C < N < F < O ($2^{nd}$ I.E.)
Second electron removal from oxygen requires more energy as it acquires stable $2s^22p^3$ configuration after removal of one electron.

(c) Correct order → B > Tl > In > Ga > Al (Electronegativity)
In general, electronegativity increases in boron family from top to bottom due to increase in $Z_{eff}$ on valence shell. However boron has highest E.N. due to its very small size.

(d) Correct order → $Na^+ > Li^+ > Mg^{2+} > Al^{3+} > Be^{2+}$ (Ionic radius)
Ionic radius depends on $Z_{eff}$ and the number of shells.

**17.** **(a)**

**18.** **(a)**

**19.** **(d)** Zero group is also called as buffer group because it is placed between highly electropositive metals (group 1) and highly electronegative non-metals (group 17).

**20.** **(d)** Helium (He) $1s^2$→ Highest ionisation energy due to noble gas in nature.
Fluorine (F) $1s^2\ 2s^22p^3$→ High electronegativity in nature due to small size and –1 oxidation state.
Rubidium (Rb)→ Most electropositive element due to large atomic size.
Lithium (Li) → Strongest reducing agent due to small size and positive oxidation state (+1)

# 4 Chemical Bonding and Molecular Structure

1. **(b)** For compounds containing cations of same charge, lattice energy increases as the size of the cation decreases. Thus, NaF has highest lattice energy. The size of cations is in the order : $Na^+ < K^+ < Rb^+ < Cs^+$

2. **(c)**

3. **(b)** According to Fajan's rule, smaller cation with high charge has greatest covalent character while large cation with smaller charge has greatest ionic character.

4. **(b)** The compounds in which octet of central atom is incomplete are known as electron deficient compounds. Hence $B_2H_6$ is an electron deficient compound.

5. **(a)** For any species to have same bond order we can expect them to have same number of electrons. Calculating the number of electrons in various species.

$$O_2^- (8+8+1=17);\ CN^- (6+7+1=14)$$

$$NO^+ (7+8-1=14);\ CN^+ (6+7-1=12)$$

We find $CN^-$ and $NO^+$ both have 14 electrons so they have same bond order. Correct answer is (a).

6. **(b)** $SF_4$ has permanent dipole moment.

$SF_4$ has $sp^3d$ hybridization and see saw shape (irregular geometry).

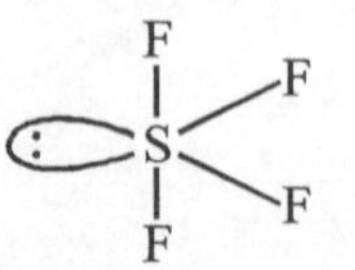


$\mu \neq 0$

Whereas $XeF_4$ shows square planar geometry, $SiF_4$ has tetrahedral shape, and $BF_3$ has trigonal planar shape. All these are symmetric molecules. Hence $\mu = 0$.

7. **(d)**

8. **(d)** In case of anions having same charge, as the size of anion increases, polarisibility of anion also increases.

9. **(d)** Dipole moment cancels each other in $BeF_2$ (F — Be — F) because of linear shape and thus it is non-polar, whereas $H_2O$ is V-shape and is polar.

10. **(c)**

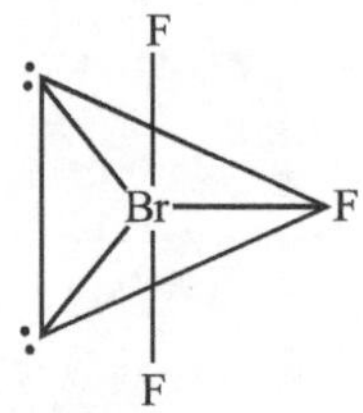


In $BrF_3$, both bond pairs as well as lone pairs of electrons are present. Due to the presence of lone pairs of electrons (*lp*) in the valence shell, the bond angle is contracted and the molecule takes the T-shape. This is due to greater repulsion between two lone pairs or between a lone pair and a bond pair than between the two bond pairs.

11. **(b)** $BH_3$ has $sp^2$ hybridization and hence does not have tetrahedral structure while all others have tetrahedral structures.

12. **(a)** $BF_3$ is $sp^2$ hybridised. So, it is trigonal planar. $NH_3$, and $PCl_3$ have $sp^3$ hybridisation, hence have trigonal pyramidal shape. $IF_3$, has $sp^3d$ hydridisation and has T-shape.

13. (c) The first bond between any two C atoms having multiple bonds is σ and rest are π bonds. Draw detailed structure of compound and find the total bonds in it

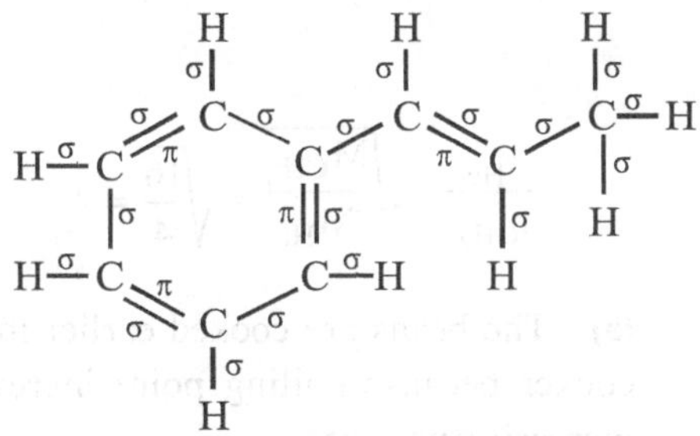

∴ 19 σ bonds and 4π bonds.

14. (a) Both $XeF_2$ and $CO_2$ have a linear structure.
F—Xe—F, O=C=O

15. (a) The structure of $IF_6^-$ is distorted octahedral This is due to presence of a "weak" lone pair.

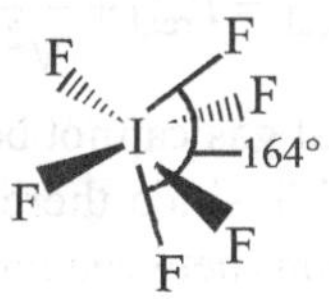

16. (c) $N_2^+ = 7 + 7 - 1 = 13$

Electrons configuration is,

$\sigma 1s^2\ \sigma^* 1s^2\ \sigma 2s^2\ \sigma^* 2s^2\ \pi 2p_x^2$

$= \pi 2p_y^2\ \sigma 2p_z^1$

Bond order =

$$\frac{1}{2}\left(\begin{matrix}\text{No. of } e^-s \text{ in bonding} \\ \text{molecular orbital}\end{matrix} - \begin{matrix}\text{No. of } e^-s \text{ in antibonding} \\ \text{molecular orbital}\end{matrix}\right)$$

$$= \frac{1}{2}(9-4) = \frac{1}{2} \times 5 = 2.5$$

17. (c) Oxygen is paramagnetic due to the presence of two unpaired electrons.

$$O_2 = \sigma 1s^2 \sigma^* 1s^2 \sigma 2s^2 \sigma^* 2s^2$$

$$\sigma 2p_z^2 \pi 2p_x^2 = \pi 2p_y^2\ \pi^* 2p_x^1 = \pi^* 2p_y^1$$

18. (c) $NH_3$ undergoes H-bonding and hence has the highest b.p. Among the remaining hydrides i.e. $PH_3$, $AsH_3$ and $SbH_3$ as we move from $PH_3$ to $BiH_3$, the molecular mass increases. As a result the van der Waal's forces of attraction increases and the boiling point increases regularly from $PH_3$ to $BiH_3$.

19. (c) In ether, there is no H-bonding while alcohols have intermolecular H-bonding.

20. (c) In nitrogen molecule, both the nitrogen atoms have same electronegativity. So it has zero polarity and hence less tendency to break away and form ions.

21. (d) $BCl_3$ has $sp^2$ hybridisation and $NCl_3$ has $sp^3$ hybridisation. There fore, $BCl_3$ is planar whereas $NCl_3$ is pyramidal.

22. (b) The structure of $CaC_2$ is $Ca^{2+}[:C \equiv C:]^{2-}$
i.e, Two π and one σ bonds.

23. (c) The b.p. of *p*-nitrophenol is higher than that of *o*-nitrophenol because in *p*-nitrophenol there is intermolecular H-bonding but in *o*-nitrophenol it is intramolecular H-bonding.

24. (a)

25. (a) $SF_6 \Rightarrow sp^3d^2$
$PF_5 \Rightarrow sp^3d$
$BCl_3 \Rightarrow sp^2$
$C_2H_6 \Rightarrow sp^3$

# 5 States of Matter

1. **(a)** $d \propto P$, Boyle's law, $\left(d = \frac{MP}{RT}\right)$. At sea level pressure is more, hence density of air is more.
2. **(c)**
3. **(d)** $\frac{P_1 v_1}{T_1} = \frac{P_2 v_2}{T_2}$

   Given, $P_1 = 1$ atm, $P_2 = 1$ atm, $V_1 = 5$ L, $V_2 = 10$ L

   $T_1 = 273$K, $T_2 = ?$

   Now, $\frac{1 \times 5}{273} = \frac{1 \times 10}{T_2}$

   $T_2 = 546$ K
4. **(b)** Since, P, V and T are same, here flasks will contain the same number of molecules.
5. **(a)** Dalton's law is applicable for a non-reacting gaseous mixture.

   $SO_2 + Cl_2 \longrightarrow SO_2Cl_2$
6. **(a)** $\frac{r_1}{r_2} = \sqrt{\frac{M_2}{M_1}}$ at constant P and T

   $\frac{r_1}{r_2} = \sqrt{\frac{M_{H_2}}{M_{O_2}}} = \sqrt{\frac{2}{32}}$

   $= \sqrt{\frac{1}{16}} = \frac{1}{4}$
7. **(b)** The real gases show deviation from ideality at low temperature high pressure and low volume. Thus, at very low temperature real gases do not show ideal behaviour.
8. **(b)** Use Grahams' law of diffusion

   $\frac{r_{He}}{r_{CH_4}} = \sqrt{\frac{M_{CH_4}}{M_{He}}} = \sqrt{\frac{16}{4}} = 2$
9. **(a)** The beans are cooked earlier in pressure cooker because boiling point increases with increasing pressure.
10. **(b)** $K.E. = \frac{1}{2}mv^2$
11. **(b)** $K.E_{avg} = \frac{3}{2}k_B T$
12. **(d)** $P_{ideal} = P_{real} + \frac{n^2 a}{V^2}$
13. **(d)** Ideal gas cannot be liquefied at any value of P and T since there are no intermolecular interactions between molecules.
14. **(b)** Apply $\frac{U_1}{U_2} = \sqrt{\frac{T_1 M_2}{T_2 M_1}}$

   $\frac{U_{SO_2}}{U_{O_2}} = \sqrt{\frac{T_{SO_2} \times 32}{64 \times 303}} = \sqrt{\frac{T_{SO_2}}{606}} \Rightarrow T_{SO_2} = 606$K

   (since $U_{SO_2} = U_{O_2}$)
15. **(a)** Root mean square speed, average speed, and the most probable speed have following relationship $^u$rms > uav > kmp. Thus option (a) is correct.
16. **(a)** $u_{rms} = \sqrt{\frac{3RT}{M}}$ or $u_{rms} \propto \sqrt{T}$

   $\frac{u_{rms}}{u'_{rms}} = \sqrt{\frac{T}{T'}}$

Given $u'_{rms} = 2\,u_{rms}$

$$\frac{1}{2} = \sqrt{\frac{T}{T'}} \quad \text{or} \quad \frac{1}{4} = \frac{T}{T'}$$

$\therefore$ $T' = 4T$

$\therefore$ When rms velocity is doubled, the temperature increases four times.

17. **(c)** Here volume is constant. Again the mass of $H_2$ is fixed so the number of moles of the gas do not change. As temperature increases the pressure also increases. The rate of collision among the gas molecules and their energy also increases.

18. **(b)** No work is required to tear apart the molecules due to the absence of attractive forces in an ideal gas.

19. **(d)** $Z > 1$ real gas shows positive deviation from ideal behaviour and are difficult to compress.

    $Z < 1$ real gas shows negative deviation from ideal behaviour.

20. **(c)** At low pressure and high temperature terms a and b are negligible hence PV= nRT.

21. **(a)** Since for $H_2$ and He,

    $$PV > nRT \text{ and } Z = \frac{PV}{nRT}.$$

    Hence Z is more than 1

22. **(c)** van der Waal's equation,

    $$\left(P + \frac{a}{V^2}\right)(V - b) = RT;$$

    Here $\left(P + \frac{a}{V^2}\right)$ represents the intermolecular forces.

23. **(b)**

24. **(d)**

25. **(a)**

# 6 Thermodynamics

1. **(b)** $C_P - C_V = nR = 2R$
2. **(b)** $\Delta H = \Delta U + \Delta n_g RT$

$$\Rightarrow 82.8 = \Delta U + \frac{1 \times 8.314 \times 298}{1000}$$

$$\Rightarrow \Delta U = 80.32 \text{ kJ}$$

3. **(a)** $\Delta E = \Delta Q + W$

For adiabatic expansion, $\Delta Q = 0$

$\Rightarrow \Delta E = +W$

In expansion, work is done by the system on the surroundings, hence W is negative, accordingly $\Delta E$ is negative *i.e.,* decrease in internal energy.

4. **(b)** $\Delta n_g = 2 - 4 = -2$, $\Delta H = \Delta E - 2RT$.
5. **(d)** As $\Delta H = \Delta E + \Delta n_g RT$

if $n_p < n_r$; $\Delta n_g = n_p - n_r = -ve$

Hence $\Delta H < \Delta E$

6. **(c)** During isothermal expansion of ideal gas, $\Delta T = 0$, Now $H = E + PV$

$\because \Delta H = \Delta E + \Delta(PV)$

$\therefore \Delta H = \Delta E + \Delta(nRT)$;

Thus if $\Delta T = 0.$, $\Delta H = \Delta E = 0$

This means enthalpy remains unaffected.

7. **(b)** As volume is constant hence work done in this process is zero therefore heat supplied is equal to change in internal energy.
8. **(a)** $q = +10$ kJ, $w = -4$ kJ

$\because \Delta E = q + w$

$= 10 - 4 = 6$ kJ

So, energy increases by 6 kJ

9. **(b)** $\Delta_r H = (\Delta_f H)_P - (\Delta_f H)_R$

Heat of formation of $F_2$ is zero.

$\Delta_r H = -113 + 3 \times (-269) + 46.2 = -873.8$ kJ

10. **(c)** $SO_2 + \frac{1}{2}O_2 \longrightarrow SO_3$

$$\Delta H = \Delta H_f^\circ (SO_3) - \Delta H_f^\circ (SO_2)$$

$$= -98.2 + 298.2 = 200 \text{ kJ/mole}$$

11. **(c)** Standard heat of formation of a substance is a amount of heat evolved or absorbed when one mole of substance is formed from its elements in their standard states. Since standard state of carbon and hydrogen are graphite and gaseous $H_2$ respectively. Hence standard heat of formation of methane is given by

$$C_{(graphite)} + 2H_2\,(g) \longrightarrow CH_4\,(g)$$

12. **(d)** 13.7 kcal = 57 kJ = $5.7 \times 10^4$ J.
13. **(b)**

$$S\,(s) + 3F_2\,(g) \rightarrow SF_6\,(g),\ \Delta H = -1100 \text{ kJ mol}^{-1}$$

Hence,

$$\Delta H_f(S\,(g)) + 6\Delta H_f(F\,(g)) - 6\Delta H_{S-F} = -1100$$

or $275 + 6 \times 80 - 6\Delta H_{S-F} = -1100$

$$\Rightarrow H_{S-F} = 309.16$$

14. **(b)** According to 3rd law of thermodynamics. At absolute zero temperature entropy of perfectly crystalline substance is taken to be zero.
15. **(b)**

16. (d) Entropy of a gas is greater than liquid and solid because gaseous particles are quite apart from each other and are in random motion.

17. (d) In the process of synthesis of ammonia from $N_2$ and $H_2$, number of moles decrease which implies that the change in entropy will be negative

$$N_2(g) + 3H_2(g) \longrightarrow 2NH_3(g)$$

18. (d) Since the process is at equilibrium $\Delta G = 0$ for $\Delta G = 0$, they should be $\Delta H > 0, \Delta S > 0$.

19. (a) The relation between free energy change and equilibrium constant is given by Nernst equation

$$E = E^\circ - \frac{RT}{nF}\ln Q$$

At equilibrium, $E = 0$ and $Q = K$

$$\therefore E^\circ = \frac{RT}{nF}\ln K \quad ...(i)$$

Again, $\Delta G^\circ = -nE^\circ F$

$$E^\circ = \frac{-\Delta G^\circ}{nF}$$

By substituting value of E° in equation (i), we get

$$\frac{-\Delta G^\circ}{nF} = \frac{RT}{nF}\ln K \; ; \; \Delta G^\circ = -RT\ln K$$

20. (a) If $\Delta G_{system} = 0$, the system has attained equilibrium is right choice.

In alternative (d) is most confusing as when $\Delta G > 0$, the process may be spontaneous when it is coupled with a reaction which has $\Delta G < 0$ and total $\Delta G$ is negative, so right answer is (a).

21. (d)

$\Delta H = \Delta U + \Delta n_g RT$ ; $\Delta n_g = 1$ in (d); $\Delta n_g = 0$ in other cases.

22. (c) $\Delta H = 200 \text{ J mol}^{-1}$

$\Delta S = 40 \text{ JK}^{-1} \text{ mol}^{-1}$

For spontaneous reaction,

$\Delta G < 0$

$$\Delta H - T\Delta S < 0; \Delta H < T\Delta S; \frac{\Delta H}{\Delta S} < T$$

$5 < T$

So, minimum temperature is 5 K

23. (d)

24. (b) At Melting Point $\Delta S_{fus} = \frac{\Delta H_{fus}}{T}$

$$\Rightarrow T = \frac{\Delta H}{\Delta S} = \frac{9.95 \times 1000}{35.7} = 278.7 \text{ K}$$

25. (b) For the reaction

$2\,ZnS \rightarrow 2\,Zn + S_2$ ; $\Delta G_1^\circ = 293$ kJ ...(i)

$2\,Zn + O_2 \rightarrow 2\,ZnO$ ; $\Delta G_2^\circ = -480$ kJ ...(ii)

$S_2 + 2\,O_2 \rightarrow 2\,SO_2$ ; $\Delta G_3^\circ = -544$ kJ ...(iii)

$\Delta G^\circ$ for the reaction

$$2\,ZnS + 3\,O_2 \rightarrow 2\,ZnO + 2\,SO_2$$

can be obtained by adding eqs. (i), (ii) and (iii)

$\Rightarrow \Delta G^\circ = 293 - 480 - 544 = -731$ kJ

# 7 Equilibrium

1. **(b)** $K_p = K_c (RT)^{\Delta n_g}$

$\therefore K_p = K_c$ only when $\Delta n_g = 0$

For reaction, $N_2(g) + O_2(g) \rightleftharpoons 2NO(g)$

$\Delta n_{(g)} = 2 - 2 = 0$

$\therefore K_p = K_c (RT)^0$ or $K_p = K_c$

2. **(a)**

| | $2HI(g)$ | $\rightleftharpoons$ | $H_2(g)$ | $+ I_2(g)$ |
|---|---|---|---|---|
| $t = 0$ | c M | | 0 | 0 |
| $t_{eq.}$ | $(c - c\alpha)$ | | $\frac{\alpha c}{2}$ | $\frac{\alpha c}{2}$ |

Given : $\alpha = 0.5$

So $$K_{eq} = \frac{[H_2][I_2]}{[HI]^2} = \frac{\frac{c\alpha}{2} \cdot \frac{c\alpha}{2}}{c^2(1-\alpha)^2} = \frac{c^2\alpha^2}{4c^2(1-\alpha)^2}$$

$$= \frac{\alpha^2}{4(1-\alpha)^2} = \frac{0.5 \times 0.5}{4(1-0.5)^2} = 0.25$$

3. **(d)**

| | $CH_3COOH$ | $+ C_2H_5OH \rightarrow$ | $CH_3COOC_2H_5$ | $+ H_2O$ |
|---|---|---|---|---|
| At start | 1 mole | 1 mole | 0 | 0 |
| At eqm. | $1 - \frac{2}{3}$ | $1 - \frac{2}{3}$ | $\frac{2}{3}$ | $\frac{2}{3}$ |

$$K_{eq} = \frac{\frac{2}{3} \times \frac{2}{3}}{\frac{1}{3} \times \frac{1}{3}} = \frac{2 \times 2}{3 \times 3} \times 3 \times 3 = 4$$

4. **(c)** $N_2 + 3H_2 \rightleftharpoons 2NH_3$

$\therefore K = [NH_3]^2 / [N_2][H_2]^3$ .... (i)

$$\frac{1}{2}N_2 + \frac{3}{2}H_2 \rightleftharpoons NH_3$$

$\therefore K' = [NH_3]/[N_2]^{1/2}[H_2]^{3/2}$ .... (ii)

Dividing equation (i) by equation (ii),

we get $K' = \sqrt{K}$

5. **(c)** Addition of inert gas at constant volume has no effect on equilibrium.

6. **(a)** With the increases of temperature, K value decreases, so the forward reaction decreases with increase of temperature. This implies that reaction will proceed in forward direction with decrease of temperature, i.e., heat is liberated and hence forward reaction is exothermic.

7. **(a)** As the temperature is increased, solubility of solid in liquid increases and hence equilibrium shifts to the right and hence the amount of solid decreases.

8. **(a)** Reactions in which number of moles of gaseous reactants and gaseous products is equal (i.e. $\Delta n = 0$) are not affected by change in pressure **(Le-Chatelier principle)**

$H_2(g) + I_2(g) \rightleftharpoons 2HI(g)$

9. **(d)** For reaction to proceed from right to left $Q > K_c$, i.e the reaction will be fast in backward direction i.e $r_b > r_f$.

10. **(b)** Le-Chatelier principle is not applicable to solid-solid equilibrium.

11. **(b)** Because $NH_3$ after losing a proton ($H^+$) gives $NH_2^-$.

$$NH_3 + H_2O \rightleftharpoons NH_2^- + H_3O^+$$

(Conjugate acid-base pair differ only by a proton)

12. **(a)** $NH_3 + H_2O \rightleftharpoons NH_4^+ + OH^-$

$$K_b = \frac{[NH_4^+][OH^-]}{[NH_3]} = \frac{x \times x}{0.1}$$

or $1.8\times10^{-5} = \frac{x^2}{0.1}$

$x^2 = 1.8 \times 10^{-6}$

$x = 1.35 \times 10^{-3}$

Thus at equilibrium, $[OH^-] = 1.35 \times 10^{-3}$

$pOH = -\log(1.35 \times 10^{-3}) = 2.87$

$\therefore$ pH $= 14.00 - 2.87 = 11.13$

13. (c) $AlCl_3$ is a Lewis acid as it can accept a lone pair of electrons.

14. (a) We know, $pH = -\log[H^+]$

$[H^+] = N.\alpha$ [α is degree of ionisation]

$= N.1$ [HCl is completely ionised]

$= 0.0001 = 1 \times 10^{-4}$

$\therefore pH = -\log[1 \times 10^{-4}] = 4$

15. (a) The neutral water has $[OH^-] = 1 \times 10^{-7}$ M

By adding $10^{-8}$ M NaOH, a concentration of $OH^-$ has increased in solution.

Thus, total $[OH^-] = 10^{-8} + 10^{-7}$

$= 10^{-8} + 10 \times 10^{-8} = 11 \times 10^{-8}$

$pOH = -\log 11 \times 10^{-8} = 6.9586$

$pH = 14 - 6.9586 = 7.04$

16. (b) pH of $1 \times 10^{-8}$ M HCl is below 7.

$$H_2PO_4^- + H_2O \rightleftharpoons HPO_4^{2} + H_3O^+$$

conjugate base of $H_2PO_4^-$ is $HPO_4^{2-}$

K (Autoprotolysis constant of water i.e. ionic product of water) increases with temperature.

For half neutralisation of a weak acid by a weak base,

$$pH = pK_a + \log\frac{[Salt]}{[Acid]}$$

[Salt] = [Acid], $\therefore pH = pK_a$

17. (b) $\frac{\alpha_1}{\alpha_2} = \sqrt{\frac{K_{a_1}}{K_{a_2}}} = \sqrt{\frac{3.14\times10^{-4}}{1.96\times10^{-5}}} = 4:1$

18. (a) $K_a = c\alpha^2 = 0.1\times\left(\frac{1.34}{100}\right)^2$

$= 1.79 \times 10^{-5} \approx 1.8 \times 10^{-5}$

19. (d) $A_2B_3 \rightleftharpoons \underset{2S}{2A^{3+}} + \underset{3S}{3B^{2-}}$

$K_{sp} = (2S)^2(3S)^3 = 108\,S^5 = 108\times(10^{-4})^5$

$= 108 \times 10^{-20} = 1.08 \times 10^{-18}$

20. (d) Aspirin is a weak acid. Due to common ion effect, it is unionised in acid medium but completely ionised in alkaline medium.

21. (c) Solubility of weak electrolyte decreases in solvent having common ion. So solubility of AgI in NaI solution is less than in pure water because of common ion effect.

22. (b) Let solubility of $BaCl_2 = x$ mol/L

$$BaCl_2 \rightleftharpoons Ba^{2+} + 2Cl^-$$

No. of moles $x$    $x$    $2x$

$K_{sp} = [Ba^{2+}][Cl^-]^2 = (x) \times (2x)^2 = 4x^3$

$\therefore 4 \times 10^{-9} = 4x^3$

or, $x = \sqrt[3]{\frac{4\times10^{-9}}{4}} = 1\times10^{-3}$

23. (c) Due to common ion effect, addition of $NH_4Cl$ in group (III) suppresses the ionisation of $NH_4OH$ with the result concentration of $OH^-$ decreases.

24. (b) $HClO_4$ is a strong acid

$HNO_2$ is a weak acid.

$NH_2^-$ is a very good proton acceptor and thus, it is a base.

$H_2SO_4$ is a strong acid hence its conjugate base $(HSO_4^-)$ will be a weak base.

25. (a) $N_2(g) + O_2(g) \rightleftharpoons 2NO(g) + Heat$

No. of moles of reactants = No. of moles of products.

The reaction in which number of moles of reactants are equal to number of moles of products are not affected by change in pressure (Le-Chatelier's principle).

# 8 Redox Reactions

1. (a) Intermolecular redox reaction and redox reactions are same.
2. (a) O.N. of Mn in $MnO_4^-$ is +7 and in $Mn^{2+}$ it is +2. The difference is of 5 electrons.
3. (d) $2I^- \rightarrow I_2$ is oxidation (loss of electrons) ; Cr (+6) changes to Cr (+3) by gain of electrons. Hence Cr is reduced.
4. (a) In this reaction, $H_2S$ is oxidised because the oxidation state of 'Sulphur' changes from –2 to 0.
5. (b) $SO_2$ bleaches by reduction, while chlorine bleaches colour of flowers by oxidation.
6. (a) In this reaction oxidation occurs.
7. (a) If an electronegative element is in its lowest possible oxidation state in a compound or in free state. It can act as a powerful reducing agent. e.g. $I^-$
8. (d) Oxidizing agent itself, undergoes reduction during a redox reaction

$$\overset{+3}{HAsO_2} + \overset{+2}{Sn} \longrightarrow \overset{0}{As} + \overset{+4}{Sn} + H_2O$$

Hence, here $HAsO_2$ is acting as an oxidizing agent.

9. (a) Fluorine has highest E° value and more reactive than $MnO_2$.
10. (b)
11. (d) $\overset{0}{Fe}\overset{0}{CO_5}$ Oxidation state of Fe = 0
12. (d) Let the oxidation no. of N in $HNO_3 = x$

$\therefore \quad 1 + x + [3 \times (-2)] = 0$

$\therefore \quad x = +5$

13. (a) Let $x$ = oxidation no. of Cr in $K_2Cr_2O_7$.

$\therefore (2 \times 1) + (2 \times x) + 7(-2) = 0$

or $2 + 2x - 14 = 0$ or $x = +6$.

14. (c) $K[Co(CO)_4]$

Let O.N. of Co be $x$ then

$$\underset{\text{for K}}{1 \times (+1)} + \underset{\text{for Co}}{x} + 4 \times (0) = 0$$

$\therefore$ O.N. of Co is = –1

15. (a) $K_4[Fe(CN)_6]$

Let O.N. of Fe be $x$ then $4 \times (+1) + 1 \times (x) + 6 \times (-1) = 0$

$\therefore \; x = +2$

16. (b) O.N. of iodine in $I_3^-$ is –1/3
17. (d) It is a disproportionation reaction, and hence, $Br_2$ is both reduced and oxidised.
18. (d)

$$8KMnO_4 + 3NH_3 \longrightarrow 8MnO_2 + 3KNO_3 + 5KOH + 2H_2O$$

19. (d) In disproportionation reaction, one element of a compound will simultaneously get reduced and oxidised. In $ClO_4^-$, oxidation number of Cl is + 7 and it can not increase it further. So, $ClO_4^-$ will not get oxidised and so will not undergo disporportionation reaction.
20. (a)

$$\left(Cr_2O_7^{2-} + 14H^+ + 6e^- \longrightarrow 2Cr^{3+} + 7H_2O\right)\frac{1}{3}$$

$$Sn^{2+} - 2e^- \longrightarrow Sn^{4+}$$

On adding,

$$\frac{1}{3}Cr_2O_7^{2-} + \frac{14}{3}H^+ + Sn^{2+} \longrightarrow \frac{2}{3}Cr^{3+} + \frac{7}{3}H_2O + Sn^{4+}$$

# 9 Hydrogen

1. (d)
2. (a) N and B belong to p-block and since the electronegativity difference between these elements and H is very less, they form covalent hydrides.
3. (a) In ionic hydrides, oxidation state of H is – 1, whereas in covalent hydrides, HF, its oxidation state is +1.
4. (c)
5. (a) $Mg + \text{dil. } HNO_3 \rightarrow Mg(NO_3)_2 + H_2$

   (Mg and Mn give $H_2$ with dil $HNO_3$)
6. (c) Hydrogen behaves as a metal at very high pressure.
7. (b)
8. (c)
9. (a)
10. (d)
11. (d)
12. (b) Heavy water is $D_2O$ hence
    number of electrons $= 2 + 8 = 10$
    number of protons $= 10$
    Atomic mass of $D_2O = 4 + 16 = 20$
    hence number of neutron
    $=$ Atomic mass – number of protons
    $= 20 - 10 = 10$
13. (a) Polarity of bond depends on difference in electronegativity of the two concerned atoms. $H_2O$ is more polar than $H_2S$ because oxygen (in O–H) is more electronegative than sulphur (in S–H).
14. (a) Calgon process is used to remove permanent hardness of water
15. (c) Potash alum is used for purifying water.
16. (a) The triple point of any substance is that temperature and pressure at which the material can exist in all three phases (solid, liquid and gas) in equilibrium specifically the triple point of water is 273. 16K at 611.2 Pa.
17. (d)
18. (d) Although $H_2O_2$ is a better polar solvent than $H_2O$. However it cannot be used as such because of the strong auto-oxidation ability.
19. (a) Glycerol, phosphoric acid or acetanilide is added to $H_2O_2$ to retard its decomposition.
20. (c)

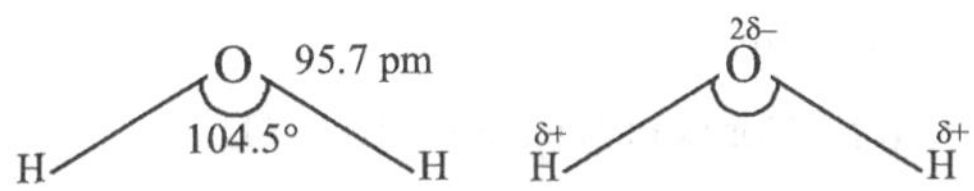


(i) (ii)

# 10 The s-Block Elements

1. **(a)** Only Li reacts with $N_2$ to form stable nitride

$$6Li + N_2 \rightarrow 2Li_3N$$

2. **(a)** $4KO_2 + 2CO_2 \rightarrow 2K_2CO_3 + 3O_2$

3. **(d)**

4. **(a)** It is due to more ionic character of $Cs_2CO_3$.

5. **(a)**

6. **(c)** Ionic radii of alkali metals in water follows the order $Li^+ < Na^+ < K^+ < Rb^+ < Cs^+$

Thus in aqueous solution due to the smallest ionic radius $Li^+$ has the lowest mobility and hence the correct order of ionic mobility is

$$Li^+ < Na^+ < K^+ < Rb^+$$

7. **(c)** With the same anion, smaller the size of the cation, higher is the lattice energy. The correct order of size of cations is –

$$Na^+ < K^+ < Rb^+ < Cs^+$$

Hence, the lattice energy of NaF will be maximum. i.e., NaF.

8. **(c)** Borax is $Na_2B_4O_7 . 10\,H_2O$.

9. **(a)** NaOH is a strong alkali. It combines with acidic and amphoteric oxides to form salts. Since CaO is a basic oxide hence does not react with NaOH.

10. **(c)** Mixture of $K_2CO_3$ and $Na_2\,CO_3$ is called fusion mixture.

11. **(c)**

12. **(d)** (i) $Na_2CO_3.10H_2O \longrightarrow$ Solvay process

(ii) $Mg(HCO_3)_2 \longrightarrow$ Temporary hardness

(iii) $NaOH \longrightarrow$ Castner-Kellener process

(iv) $Ca_3Al_2O_6 \longrightarrow$ Portland cement

13. **(c)** Be is transparent to X-rays so it is used in making X-ray tube windows.

14. **(a)**

15. **(c)** Mg reacts both with $O_2$ and $N_2$ present in air to form MgO and $Mg_3N_2$

$$2Mg + O_2 \rightarrow 2MgO$$

$$3Mg + N_2 \rightarrow Mg_3\,N_2$$

16. **(a)** $Al_4C_3 + 12H_2O \longrightarrow 4Al\,(OH)_3 + 3CH_4$

17. **(d)** Stability of ionic compounds decreases with decrease in lattice enthalpy. Thus stability of alkaline earth metal hydroxides decreases with decrease in lattice enthalpy as the size of alkali earth metal cations increases down the group.

18. **(c)** MgO, $Mg^{2+}$ ion is smallest in size and double the charge in comparison to $Li^+$ and $Na^+$ ions.

19. **(b)** Colemanite is a mineral having composition as $Ca_2B_6O_{11}.5H_2O$

20. **(a)**

# 11 The p-Block Elements (Group 13 and Group 14)

1. **(b)**
2. **(b)**
3. **(b)**
4. **(c)** $Al_2O_3$ is electrolyte, $Na_3AlF_6$ is used to decrease the melting point of $Al_2O_3$ and to increase the conductivity.
5. **(b)** Thermite is a mixture of $Fe_2O_3 + Al$.
6. **(a)** van Arkel method is used for refining of Ti, Zr and V, and not for Al.
7. **(b)** Down the group basic character of oxides increases.
   $B_2O_3$ - Acidic
   $Al_2O_3$ - Amphoteric
   $Ga_2O_3$ - Amphoteric
   $In_2O_3$ - Basic
   $Tl_2O_3$ - Basic
8. **(b)** Cryolite, $Na_3AlF_6$ is added
   (1) To decrease the melting temperature.
   (2) To increase the electrical conductivity of solution.
9. **(b)**
10. **(d)**
11. **(c)**
12. **(b)** Two dimensional sheet structures are formed when three oxygen atoms of each $[SiO_4]^{4-}$ tetrahedral are shared.
13. **(b)** $2Pb + 2H_2O + O_2 \rightarrow 2Pb(OH)_2$
14. **(b)** Due to the small size of carbon atom effective, lateral overlapping between $2p$ and $2p$ occurs.
15. **(a)** The stability of +2 O.S. follows the order:

    $Pb^{2+} > Sn^{2+} > Ge^{2+}$

    Hence order of reducing power is:

    $Ge > Sn > Pb$
16. **(c)** Glass is a super cooled liquid.
17. **(a)** Red lead is $Pb_3O_4$. It is a mixed oxide of Pb (II) and Pb (IV). It acts as a powerful oxidising agent.
18. **(a)** A buff coloured crystalline state of PbO is known as litharge.
19. **(c)** Graphite is composed of flat two-dimensional sheets of carbon atoms. Each sheet is a hexagonal network of C atoms. The 3 electrons of C form three $\sigma$ bonds and 4th electron is a $\pi$ $e^-$ and is delocalized over the whole sheet and is thus mobile. Conduction of electricity is due to these delocalized electrons within each layer. Conduction does not occur from one sheet to another.
20. **(d)** Tin is oxidised to metastannic acid when it is treated with nitric acid.

$$Sn + 4HNO_3 \longrightarrow \underset{\text{Meta stannic acid}}{H_2SnO_3} + 4NO_2 + H_2O$$

21. **(c)** White lead is $2PbCO_3.Pb(OH)_2$ also known as basic lead carbonate.
22. **(d)** Catenation power of the elements decreases as we move down in the group. Therefore, Pb does not show catenation behaviour.
23. **(d)**
24. **(d)** $4Al + 3O_2 \longrightarrow 2Al_2O_3,\ \Delta H = -ve$
25. **(a)** $B_2O_3 + 3C + 3Cl_2 \rightarrow 2BCl_3 + 3CO$

# 12 Organic Chemistry – Some Basic Principles and Techniques

1. **(c)** The cyclic portion contains more C-atoms than acyclic portion. Hence it is derivative of cyclopentane.
2. **(d)**

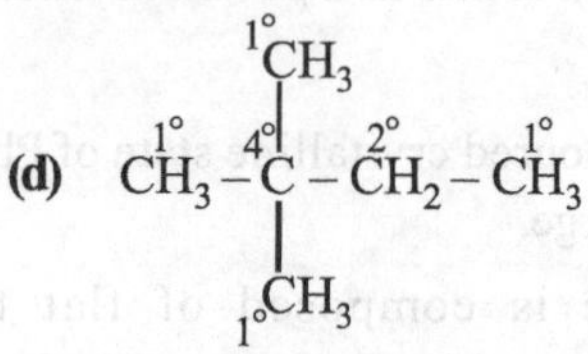

3. **(d)** Maleic acid and fumaric acids are geometrical isomers.

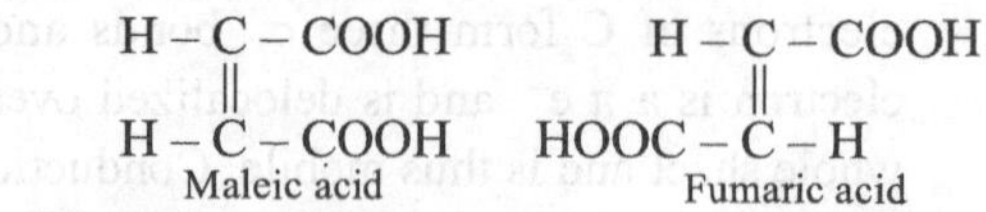


4. **(b)**

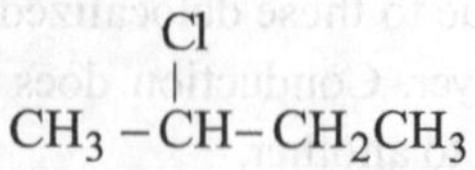

contains asymmetric C - atom.

5. **(d)** They are metamers.
6. **(c)** Diastereomers since they have different melting points, boiling points, solubilities etc.
7. **(d)** Tautomerism is exhibited by the oscillation of hydrogen atom between two polyvalent atoms present in the molecule. As (d) has α-hydrogen atom therefore it shows tautomerism whereas other structures do not.

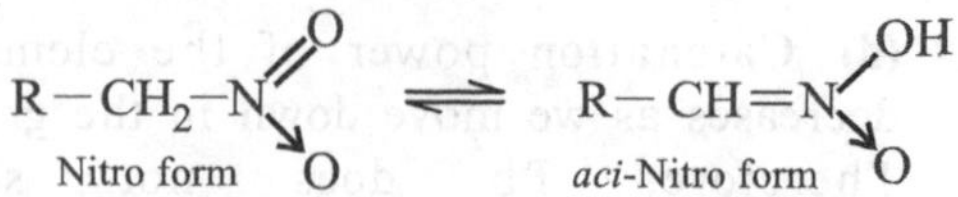


8. **(a)**

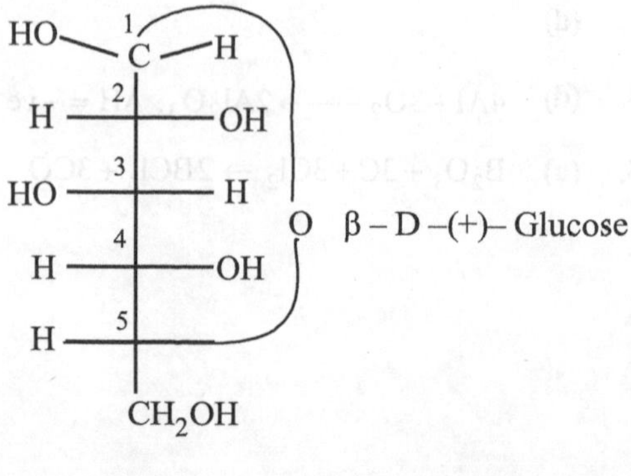


Carbon atoms from $C_1$ to $C_5$ are chiral while $C_6$ is not chiral because it has two hydrogen atoms.

9. **(b)** Optical and geometrical isomerism pair up to exhibit stereoisomerism. This is because the isomers differ only in their orientation in space.
10. **(b)** No. of optical isomers $= 2^n$ (where $n$ = no. of chiral atoms)

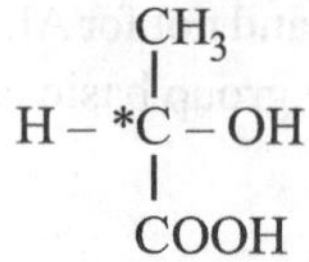

Lactic acid

∴ No. of optical isomers of lactic acid $= (2)^1 = 2$

11. **(d)** Keto-enol tautomerism is shown by carbonyl compounds having α-hydrogen atom.
12. **(d)** A and B are enantiomers.
13. **(b)** In diphenylmethane, monochlorination at following positions (1, 2, 3, 4) will produce structural isomers

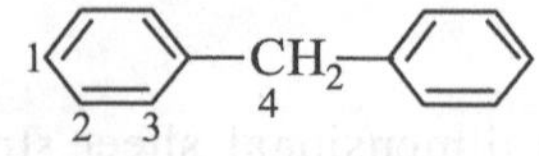

14. **(a)** In 1, 2-dichlorobenzene the two dipoles are at 60° (i.e. unsymmetric). Thus possesses dipole moment.
15. **(b)**

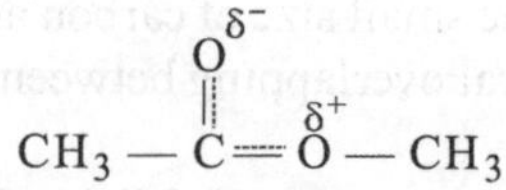

The correct relation is b > a because bond 'a' has partial double bond characters due to resonance.

16. **(c)** Phenol is less acidic than $H_2CO_3$ so reaction does not favours in forward direction.

17. (d) Stability of alkene $\propto$ no. of '$\alpha$' H-atoms or more hyper conjugation.

18. (b) It is free radical addition.

19. (b)

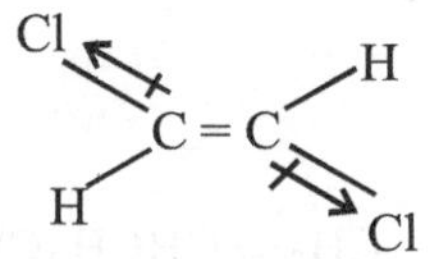

has zero dipole moment.

20. (b)

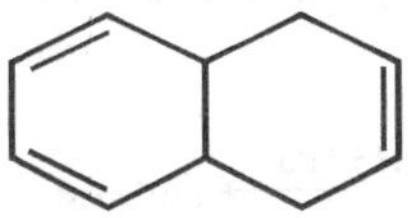

Non-aromatic (unconjugated $6\pi$ electrons)

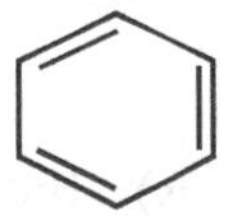

Aromatic (conjugated $6\pi$ electrons)

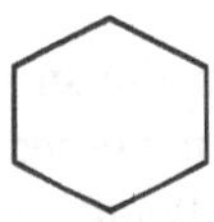

Alicyclic

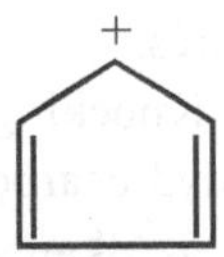

Antiaromatic (conjugated $4\pi$ electrons)

21. (d) Aliphatic halides react by $S_N2$ mechanism.

22. (a) Among the three given hybrid orbitals, *sp* hybrid orbital is most electronegative. Contribution of *s* in *sp* hybrid orbital is maximum so this orbital is closer to nucleus. Naturally it will have greater tendency to pull electron towards it. Hence it becomes more electronegative and $sp^3$ becomes least electronegative.

23. (b) The order of stability of free radicals

$$(C_6H_5)_3\dot{C} > (C_6H_5)_2\dot{C}H > (CH_3)_3\dot{C} > (CH_3)_2\dot{C}H$$

The stabilisation of the first two is due to resonance and last two is due to inductive effect.

24. (d)

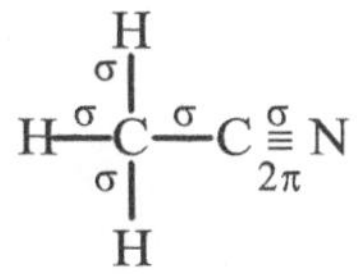

25. (b) Methyl carbanion is $sp^3$ hybridised, with three bond pairs and one lone pair, same is the case with $NH_3$.

26. (b) Sodium cyanide ($Na + C + N \rightarrow NaCN$).

27. (c) $CH_3 - \overset{\overset{O}{||}}{C} - H$

$$\xrightarrow[\text{(Tollen's reagent)}]{Ag_2O} CH_3 - \overset{\overset{O}{||}}{C} - OH$$

$$Ph - \overset{\overset{O}{||}}{C} - CH_3 \xrightarrow[\text{(Tollen's reagent)}]{Ag_2O} \text{No}$$

reaction.

28. (d) The Beilstein test is a simple qualitative chemical test for halides.

29. (c) Formaldehyde cannot produce iodoform, since only those compounds which contain either $CH_3 - \underset{\underset{OH}{|}}{CH} -$ group or $CH_3 - \underset{\underset{O}{||}}{C} -$ group on reaction with potassium iodide and sodium hypochlorite yield iodoform.

30. (b) Hydrazine ($NH_2NH_2$) does not contain carbon and hence on fusion with Na metal, it cannot form NaCN; consequently hydrazine does not show Lassaigne's test for nitrogen.

# 13 Hydrocarbons

1. (b) $2CH_3CH_2Cl \xrightarrow[\text{Dry ether}]{Na} CH_3CH_2CH_2CH_3$

Open chain alkane having even number of carbons and symmetrical can be achieved by Wurtz reaction.

2. (b) For isomeric alkanes, the one having longest straight chain has highest b.p. because of larger surface area.

3. (d) The order of substitution in alkanes is

$$3° > 2° > 1°$$

Thus the bromination of 2-methylbutane mainly gives 2-bromo - 2 - methylbutane

$$\underset{\text{2-Methylbutane}}{CH_3-CH_2-\overset{\overset{CH_3}{|}}{C}H-CH_3} \xrightarrow{Br_2}$$

$$\underset{\substack{\text{1-Bromo-2 methylbutane}\\\text{(minor)}}}{CH_3-CH_2-\overset{\overset{CH_3}{|}}{C}H-CH_2Br} + \underset{\substack{\text{2-Bromo-2-methylbutane}\\\text{(major)}}}{CH_3-CH_2-\overset{\overset{CH_3}{|}}{\underset{\underset{Br}{|}}{C}}-CH_3}$$

4. (d) Half chair is less stable due to angle strain.

5. (a) Addition of HBr to alkenes is an electrophilic addition reaction. The reaction proceeds via formation of carbocation. Since 3° carbocation is most stable, hence the reactant which involves formation of 3° carbocation will react most easily with HBr.

$$\underset{\text{(a)}}{(CH_3)_2C=CH_2} \xrightarrow{H^+} \underset{\text{3° Carbocation}}{(CH_3)_2\overset{+}{C}-CH_3}$$

6. (c) Anti-Markovnikoff's addition of HBr is observed only with unsymmetrical alkenes, *a*, *b*, and *d*.

$$\underset{\text{(a)}}{CH_3CH=CH_2} \qquad \underset{\text{(b)}}{CH_2=CHCH_2CH_3}$$

$$\underset{\text{(c)}}{CH_3CH=CHCH_3} \qquad \underset{\text{(d)}}{CH_3CH=CHCH_2CH_3}$$

7. (c) Butene - 1 $\xrightarrow{H_2/Pd}$ Butane

8. (d) The $\pi$-bonds of double bond are easily attacked by electrophiles as compared to $\pi$ bonds of triple bond because $sp^2$ orbitals of double bond are less electronegative than *sp* of alkynes.

9. (c) Knocking depends upon the structure of the hydrocarbon and follows the order

*n*-Alkanes > branched alkanes > straight chain alkenes > branched alkenes > arenes

10. (a) Only alkenes and alkynes (compounds having C = C or C ≡ C) decolourise alkaline $KMnO_4$ solution. Only (a) is alkene, other three are alkanes.

11. (d)

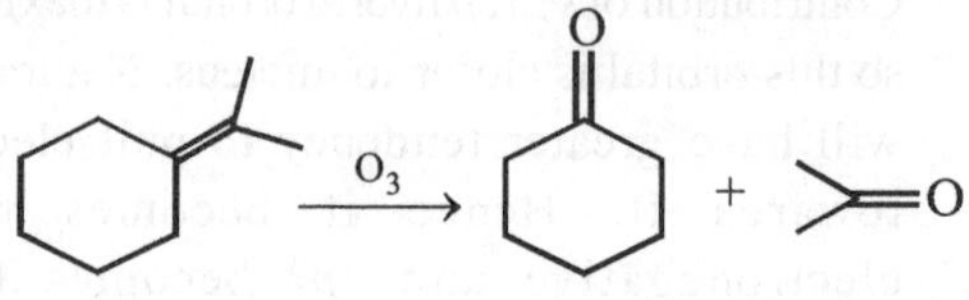

12. (a)

13. (d) $R-CH_2-CCl_2-R$

$$\xrightarrow{\text{alc.KOH}} R-CH=C(Cl)-R$$

$$\xrightarrow{NaNH_2} R-C\equiv C-R$$

14. (a) Acetylene reacts with the other three:

15. (a) Terminal alkynes give a white precipitate on reaction with ammonical silver nitrate solution.

**16.** **(c)**

$$CaC_2 \xrightarrow{H_2O} \underset{\text{Acetylene (A)}}{HC \equiv CH} \xrightarrow[Hg^{+2}]{Dil.H_2SO_4} \underset{\text{Acetaldehyde (B)}}{CH_3CHO} \xrightarrow[H_2]{Ni} \underset{(C)}{C_2H_5OH}$$

**17.** **(b)** 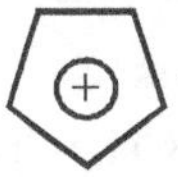 $4\pi e$ (Anti-aromatic)

**18.** **(b)** $I - \ddot{Cl}: \xrightarrow{AlCl_3} I^+AlCl_4^- \xrightarrow{Ph.H} Ph - I$

**19.** **(c)** The Friedal-Crafts alkylation reaction will give propyl phenyl ketone which further on Clemmensen reduction will give butyl benzene

$$C_6H_6 + CH_3CH_2CH_2COCl \xrightarrow{AlCl_3} C_6H_5COCH_2CH_2CH_3 \xrightarrow{Zn\text{-}Hg/HCl} \underset{\text{Butyl benzene}}{C_6H_5CH_2CH_2CH_2CH_3}$$

**20.** **(d)**

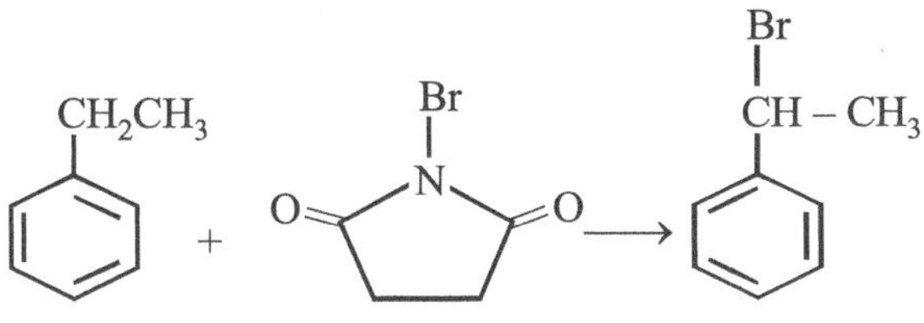

N – Bromosuccinimide

**21.** **(d)** **22.** **(a)**

**23.** **(b)** $HNO_3$ accepts a proton from $H_2SO_4$.

**24.** **(d)**

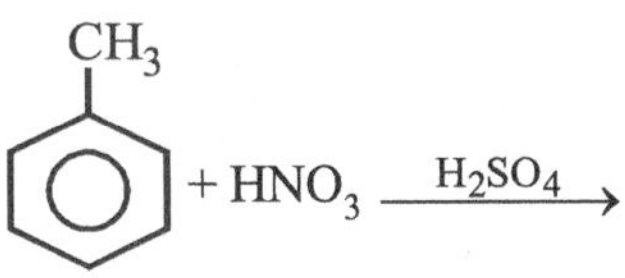

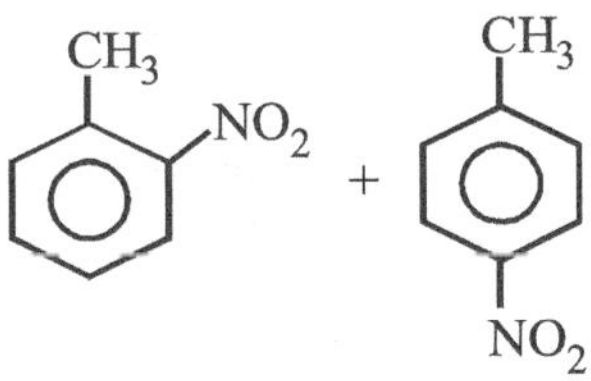

*o*-Nitrotoluene *p*-Nitrotoluene

Under vigorous conditions, toluene produces TNT or trinitrotoluene.

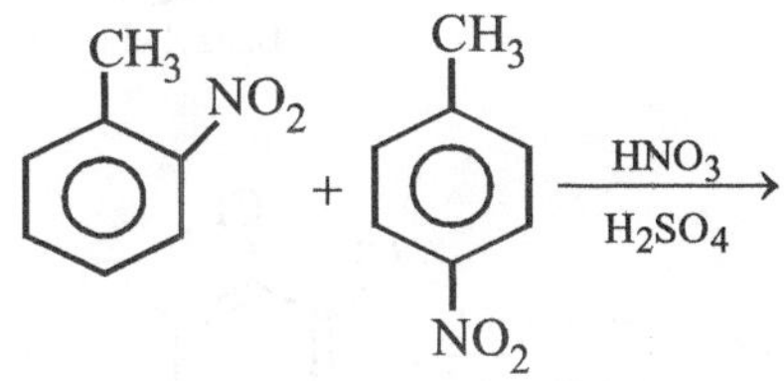

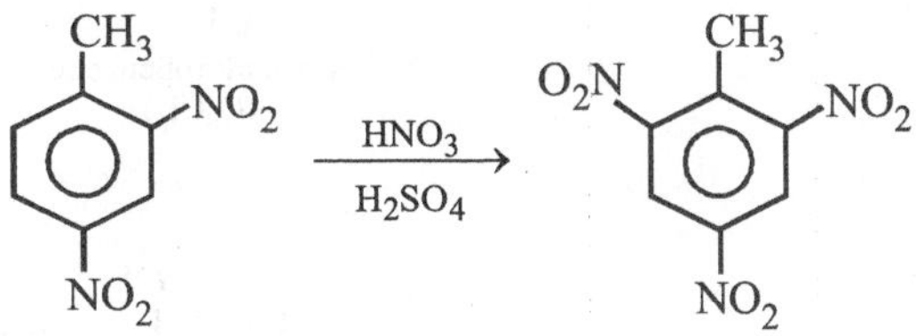

(TNT or 2,4,6 –Trinitrotoluene)

**25.** **(a)** Resonance energy is the difference in observed and calculated heat of hydrogenation of benzene, higher is its value, more is its stability. So, resonance energy represents stability of benzene.

**26.** **(a)**

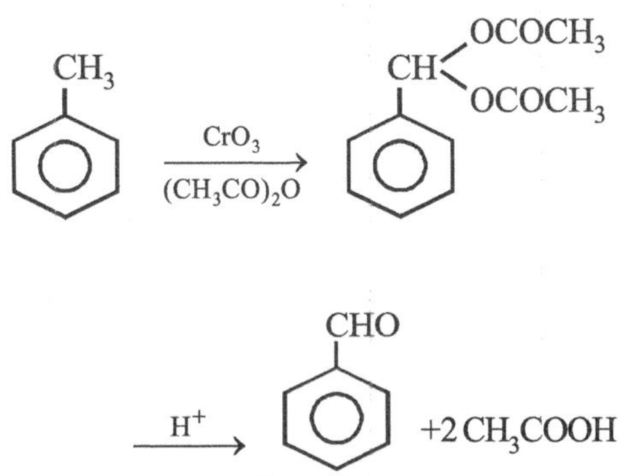

Benzaldehyde

**27.** **(c)**

**28.** **(b)**

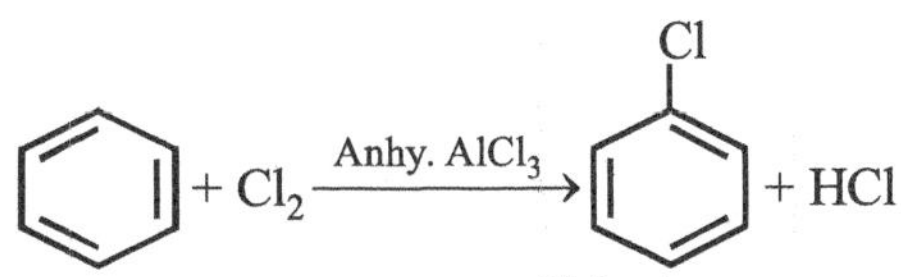

Chlorobenzene

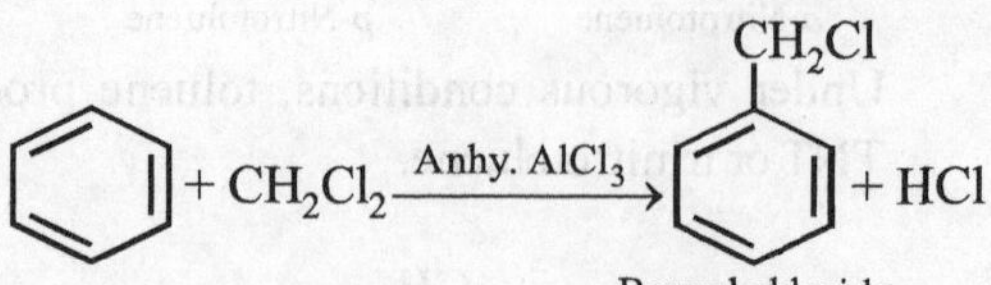

Benzyl chloride

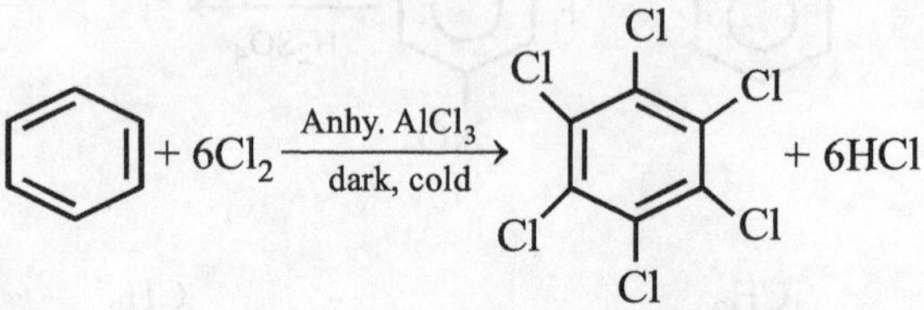

Hexachlorobenzene
($C_6Cl_6$)

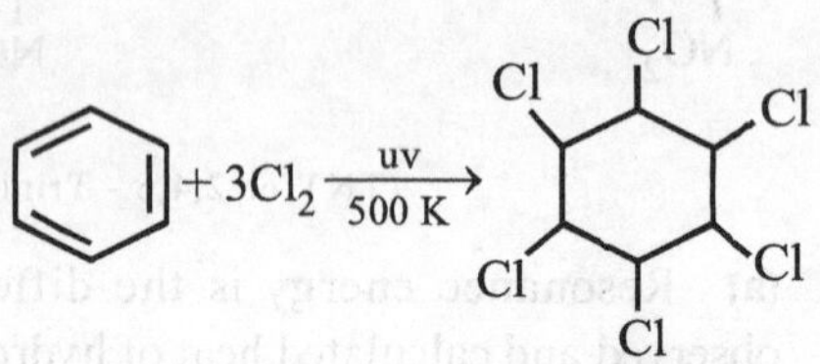

Benzene hexachloride.
(BHC)

**29.** **(c)**

$$CH_3-\underset{\underset{Cl}{|}}{CH}-CH_3+CH_3C\equiv C^-Na^+\xrightarrow[\text{Base}]{}$$

$$\underset{\text{Propene}}{CH_3-CH=CH_2} + \underset{\text{Propyne}}{CH_3C\equiv CH} + NaCl$$

**30.** **(d)** Order of acidic strength is

$$CH\equiv CH > CH_3-C\equiv CH > CH_2=CH_2$$

# 14 Environmental Chemistry

1. (b)
2. (b)
3. (d)
4. (c)
5. (d) P.A.N is produced by photochemical smog.
6. (c) $SO_2$ and $NO_2$ are responsible for the discoloured and lustureless nature of marble.
7. (d) Green house gases are those gases that absorbs and emits radiation within the thermal IR range. These are $CO_2$, $CH_4$ $N_2O$ and $O_3$.
8. (b) High concentration of $SO_2$ leads to stiffness of flower buds.
9. (c)
10. (d)
11. (a)
12. (b)
13. (b) Green chemistry may be defined as the programme of developing new chemical products and chemical processes or making improvements in the already existing compounds and processes so as to make them less harmful to human health and environment. This means the same as to reduce the use and production of hazardous chemicals.
14. (a)
15. (a)
16. (d)
17. (d)
18. (a) Excessive concentration of nitrate in drinking water is harmful and can cause methemoglobinemia (blue baby syndrome).
19. (d)
20. (b) Ethanal is commerically prepared by one step oxidation of ethene in the presence of ionic catalyst in aqueous medium with a yield of 90%.

$$CH_2=CH_2+O_2 \xrightarrow[\text{Pb(II)|Cu(II) (in water)}]{\text{Catalyst}} CH_3CHO$$

# 15 The Solid State

1. (d) Crystals show good cleavage because their constituent particles are arranged in planes.

2. (c) Tetrahedral & octahedral holes are present in *hcp* & *ccp*.

3. (b) Triclinic-unsymmetrical

$\alpha \neq \beta \neq \gamma \neq 90°, a \neq b \neq c$

Cubic-symmetrical

$\alpha = \beta = \gamma = 90°, a = b = c$

4. (b) In ZnS structure, sulphide ions occupy all *fcc* lattice points while $Zn^{2+}$ ions are present in alternate tetrahedral voids.

5. (d) Effective number of 'A' atoms

$$= \left(8 \times \frac{1}{8}\right) + \left(4 \times \frac{1}{2}\right) = 3$$

Effective number of 'B' atoms $= \left(12 \times \frac{1}{4}\right) + 1$

$= 4$

$\therefore$ Formula of the solid $= A_3B_4$.

6. (b) For orthorhombic system, $\alpha = \beta = \gamma = 90°$

7. (b) C.N. of A = x (B)

C.N. of B = y (A)

Formula $A_yB_x$

8. (c)

9. (b) Since C.No. is 6, it is octahedral and

$$\frac{r^+}{r^-} = 0.414 - 0.73.$$

10. (b) 14 kinds of Bravais lattices (space lattices) are possible in a crystal.

11. (d) Simple cubic; $a = 2r$, $r = \frac{a}{2}$

12. (d) Body diagonal (*d*) of a cubic crystal of edge length (a) is given by, $d = a\sqrt{3}$

putting $a = 400$ pm, we get

$d = \sqrt{3} \times 400 \text{ pm} = 692.8 \text{ pm} \approx 693 \text{ pm}.$

13. (b)

$$d = \frac{ZM}{N_A a^3} \Rightarrow 6.25 = \frac{Z \times 120}{6.02 \times 10^{23} \times \left(4 \times 10^{-8}\right)^3}$$

Z= 2 (No. of effective atoms per unit cell)

Therefore, the crystal lattice should be *bcc* type

14. (b)

$$d = \frac{Z \times M}{N_A \times a^3} = \frac{2 \times 100}{6.023 \times 10^{23} \times (400 \times 10^{-10})^3}$$

$$= 5.188 \text{ g/cm}^3$$

15. (c) For *bcc* structure $d = \frac{\sqrt{3}\,a}{2}$

where $d$ = distance between two atoms

$a$ = edge length

$$1.73 = \frac{\sqrt{3}}{2} a$$

$$a = \frac{2 \times 1.73}{\sqrt{3}} = 2\text{Å} = 200\text{pm}$$

16. (b) Distance between $K^+$ and $F^-$

$= \frac{1}{2} \times$ length of the edge

17. (b)

18. **(d)** Ferrimagnetism is observed when the magentic moments of the domains in the substance are aligned in parallel and antiparallel directions in unequal numbers.

19. **(c)** Two $Ag^+$ ions will be replaced by one $Cd^{2+}$, so there is one vacancy for each $Cd^{2+}$ added.

20. **(c)** Electrical conductivity of semiconductors lies in the range $10^{-8} - 10^2 \text{ ohm}^{-1} \text{ cm}^{-1}$.

21. **(d)** In KCl, co-ordination number of cation and anion is 6 and 6 respectively. KCl is highly ionic so Schottky defect is common.

    **Note :** Schottky defect is common in compounds having high coordination number while Frenkel defect is common in compounds with low coordination number.

22. **(b)** When equal number of cations ($Na^+$) and anions ($Cl^-$) are missing from their regular lattice positions, we have Schottky defect.

23. **(b)** For *bcc*, $r = \frac{\sqrt{3}}{4}a$

    Edge length not covered by atom = $a - 2r$

    $$= a - 2 \times \frac{\sqrt{3}}{4}a = a\left[\frac{2-\sqrt{3}}{2}\right]$$

    $\therefore$ % of fraction not covered

    $$= \frac{a\left[\frac{2-\sqrt{3}}{2}\right]}{a} \times 100 = 0.134 \times 100 = 13.4\%$$

24. **(d)** Here, $A_2B_3$ can be written as $A_4B_6$.

    Thus, hcp has six atom so 'B' forms hcp lattice and 'A' is present in void.

    total tetrahedral void = 12

    $\therefore$ Fraction of tetrahedral voids occupied by

    $$A = 4/12 = \frac{1}{3}$$

25. **(c)** $C_6H_6$ is diamagnetic (i – 5)

    $CrO_2$ is ferromagnetic (ii – 3)

    MnO is antiferromagnetic (iii – 1)

    $Fe_3O_4$ is ferrimagnetic (iv – 2)

    $Fe^{3+}$ is paramagnetic with 5 unpaired electron (v – 4)

# 16 Solutions

1. (d) According to Henry's law

$$\frac{P_1}{P_2}=\frac{S_1}{S_2}$$

$$\frac{500}{750}=\frac{0.01}{S_2}$$

$$\therefore S_2=\frac{750\times 0.01}{500}=0.015\ g/L$$

2. (b) Density = 1.17 g/cc (Given)

As $d=\frac{\text{Mass}}{\text{Volume}}$

Volume = 1cc $\quad\therefore$ Mass = $d$ = 1.17g

$$\text{Molarity}=\frac{\text{No. of moles}}{\text{Volume in litre}}=\frac{1.17\times 1000}{36.5\times 1}$$

$$=\frac{1170}{36.5}=32.05\text{M}$$

3. (b) Both molality and mole fraction are not related to the volume of solution, thus they are both independent of temperature.

4. (b) When A – B interaction is weaker than A – A and B – B interaction, then mixture of A and B show positive deviation.

5. (c) $P_{Total}=P_A^\circ x_A+P_B^\circ x_B$

$=P_A^\circ x_A+P_B^\circ(1-x_A)$

$=P_B^\circ-(P_B^\circ-P_A^\circ)x_A$ ...(i)

Given, $P=254-119x_A$ ...(ii)

Comparing, (i) and (ii), we get

$P_B^\circ=254,\ P_A^\circ=254-119=135$

6. (b) Positive deviations are shown by such solutions in which solvent-solvent and solute-solute interactions are stronger than the solute-solvent interactions. In such solution, the interactions among molecules becomes weaker. Therefore their escaping tendency increases which results in the increase in their partial vapour pressures.

In pure methanol there exists intermolecular H–bonding.

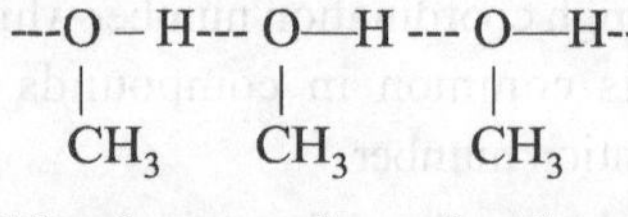

On adding benzene, its molecules come between ethanol molecules thereby breaking H-bonds which weaken intermolecular forces. This results in increase in vapour pressure.

7. (b) Moles of glucose $=\frac{18}{180}=0.1$

Moles of water $=\frac{178.2}{18}=9.9$

Total moles = 0.1 + 9.9 = 10

$P_{H_2O}$ = Mole fraction × Total pressure

$$=\frac{9.9}{10}\times 760$$

$$=752.4\text{ Torr}$$

8. (b) $K_2HgI_4 \rightleftharpoons 2K^+ + [HgI_4]^{2-};\ n=3$

$\because\ \alpha=\frac{i-1}{n-1};\ 0.4=\frac{i-1}{3-1}$

$i=1.8$

9. (d) Colligative property ∝ moles of non-volatile solute.

10. (a)

| | $XY_2$ | $\rightleftharpoons$ | $X^{2+}$ | + | $2Y^-$ |
|---|---|---|---|---|---|
| Initially | 1 | | 0 | | 0 |
| at equilibrium | $1-\alpha$ | | $\alpha$ | | $2\alpha$ |

Total no. of moles $= 1-\alpha+\alpha+2\alpha = 1+2\alpha$

$$i = \frac{\text{Normal molar mass}}{\text{Observed molar mass}};\ \frac{1+2\alpha}{1} = \frac{164}{65.6}$$

$\therefore \quad \alpha = 0.75; \% \alpha = 75\%$

11. **(d)** According to the question we can write
$\Delta T_b = K_b m$ ; $K_b(1) = 2$ ; $K_b = 2\ \text{Km}^{-1}$
$\Delta T_f = K_f m$ ; $K_f(2) = 2$ ; $K_f = 1\ \text{Km}^{-1}$
$\therefore K_f = 0.5\, K_b$
$\therefore K_b = 2K_f$

12. **(c)** $\Delta T_f = K_f m = \dfrac{K_f \times w \times 1000}{\text{m} \times W}$

$$= 5.12 \times \frac{1}{250} \times \frac{1000}{51.2} = 0.4\text{K}$$

13. **(c)** $\Delta T_b = K_b \times m$
Elevation in boiling point is a colligative property, which depends upon the no. of particles (concentration of solution). Thus greater the number of particles, greater is the elevation in boiling point and hence greater will be its boiling point.

$$Na_2SO_4 \rightleftharpoons 2Na^+ + SO_4^{2-}$$

Since $Na_2SO_4$ has maximum number of particles (c) hence it will exhibit maximum boiling point.

14. **(a)** (i) $i = \dfrac{\text{No. of particles after ionisation}}{\text{No. of particles before ionisation}}$

(ii) $\Delta T_b = i \times K_b \times m$

$$CuCl_2 \longrightarrow Cu^{2+} + 2Cl^-$$

| | $CuCl_2$ | $Cu^{2+}$ | $2Cl^-$ |
|---|---|---|---|
| | 1 | 0 | 0 |
| | $(1-\alpha)$ | $\alpha$ | $\alpha$ |

$$i = \frac{1+2\alpha}{1},\ i = 1+2\alpha$$

Assuming 100% ionization
So, $i = 1+2 = 3$
$\Delta T_b = 3 \times 0.52 \times 0.1 = 0.156 \approx 0.16$

$$\left[m = \frac{13.44}{134.4} = 0.1\right]$$

15. **(b)** $\pi = \dfrac{nRT}{V}$ or $T = \dfrac{\pi V}{nR}$

10% (w/v) aqueous solution of glucose means 10 g glucose is present in 100 mL of $H_2O$

$$= \frac{14 \times 100 \times 10^{-3} \times 180}{0.082 \times 10} = 307.3\ \text{K}$$

16. **(d)** Osmotic pressure is directly proportional to the number of particles in the solution. KCl will dissociate completely in the solution, while $CH_3COOH$ and sucrose are weak electrolyte. Hence correct order will be :
KCl > $CH_3COOH$ > Sucrose

17. **(a)** Van't Hoff factor ($i$)

$$= \frac{\text{No. of particles after association or dissociation}}{\text{No. of particles before association or dissociation}}$$

For $\quad MX_2 \rightleftharpoons M^+ + 2X^-$

| | $MX_2$ | $M^+$ | $2X^-$ |
|---|---|---|---|
| $t = 0$ | 1 | 0 | 0 |
| at eq. | $1-\alpha$ | $\alpha$ | $2\alpha$ |

Total no. of particles $= 1-\alpha+\alpha+2\alpha = 1+2\alpha$

$$\therefore i = \frac{1+2\alpha}{1} = 2.$$

$\therefore \alpha = 0.50$ or 50%.

18. **(d)** $\Delta T_b = K_b \times$ Molality
$\Delta T_f = K_f \times$ Molality

$$\therefore \frac{\Delta T_b}{\Delta T_f} = \frac{K_b}{K_f} \Rightarrow \Delta T_b = \frac{\Delta T_f \times K_b}{K_f} = \frac{0.186 \times 0.512}{1.86}$$

$= 0.0512$

19. **(d)** $\dfrac{P^\circ - P}{P^\circ} = \dfrac{n_2}{n_1+n_2}$

$$\frac{640-600}{640} = \frac{2.5/m}{39/78}$$

$$m = \frac{640 \times 78 \times 2.5}{39 \times 40} = 80$$

20. **(c)** $N_1V_1 + N_2V_2 = NV$
$4x + 10(1-x) = 6 \times 1; -6x = -4 ; x = 0.67$
Thus 0.67 litre of 4N HCl
$1-x = 1-0.67 = 0.33$ litre of 10 N HCl

**21. (d)**

$$2NaHCO_3 + H_2C_2O_4 \longrightarrow Na_2C_2O_4 + 2CO_2 + 2H_2O$$

Moles of $CO_2$ evolved $= \frac{0.25}{25 \times 10^3} = 10^{-5}$

$\therefore$ moles of $NaHCO_3 = 10^{-5}$

$\therefore$ mass of $NaHCO_3 = 84 \times 10^{-5}$ g $= 0.84 \times 10^{-3}$ g $= 0.84$ mg

$\therefore$ % by weight $= \frac{0.84}{10} \times 100 = 8.4\%$

**22. (d)** $P_M^o = 450$ mmHg, $P_N^o = 700$ mmHg

$P_M = P_N^o x_M = y_M P_T$

$P_M^o = \frac{y_M}{x_M}(P_T)$

Similarly, $P_N^o = \frac{y_N}{x_N}(P_T)$

Given, $P_M^o < P_N^o$

$\frac{y_M}{x_M} < \frac{y_N}{x_N}$

$\frac{y_M}{y_N} < \frac{x_M}{x_N}$

**23. (c)** $x_A' = \frac{P_A}{P_{total}} = \frac{P_A^\circ x_A}{P_{total}} \Rightarrow \frac{x_A'}{x_A} = \frac{P_A^\circ}{P_{total}} < 1$

(since the liquid

$A$ is less volatile, $P_A^\circ < P_{total}$)

**24. (b)** $P_{total} = P_A^\circ x_A + P_B^\circ x_B$

$550 = P_A^\circ \times \frac{1}{4} + P_B^\circ \times \frac{3}{4}$

$P_A^\circ + 3P_B^\circ = 550 \times 4$ ...(i)

In second case

$P_{total} = P_A^\circ \times \frac{1}{5} + P_B^\circ \times \frac{4}{5}$

$P_A^\circ + 4P_B^\circ = 560 \times 5$ ...(ii)

Subtract (i) from (ii)

$\therefore P_B^\circ = 560 \times 5 - 550 \times 4 = 600$

$\because P_A^\circ = 400$

**25. (b)** $\Delta H_1 = \Delta H_2$, because similar attractive forces between solvent molecules in pure state and solution must be overcome for vaporisation. Due to increase in randomness during mixing of solute and solvent, $S_{solution} > S_{solvent}$.

Hence $(S_{vapour} - S_{solvent}) > (S_{vapour} - S_{solution})$.

**26. (b)** One molal solution means one mole of solute is present in 1 kg (1000 g) solvent

i.e., mole of solute = 1

Mole of solvent $(H_2O) = \frac{1000\,g}{18\,g} = \frac{1000}{18}$

Mole fraction of solute $= \frac{1}{\left(1 + \frac{1000}{18}\right)} = \frac{18}{1008}$

$= 0.018.$

**27. (b)**

$$K_3\left[Fe(CN)_6\right] \rightleftharpoons 3K^+ + \left[Fe(CN)_6\right]^{3-}$$

| | $K_3[Fe(CN)_6]$ | $3K^+$ | $[Fe(CN)_6]^{3-}$ |
|---|---|---|---|
| At t = 0 | 1 | 0 | 0 |
| After ionisation | (1 – α) | 3 α | α |

$i = 1 + 3\alpha$

Since, $i = \frac{M_{normal}}{M_{abnormal}}$;

$\therefore \frac{1+3\alpha}{1} = \frac{M_{normal}}{M_{abnormal}}$

$\therefore M_{abnormal} = M_{normal}(1 + 3\alpha)^{-1}$

**28.** **(a)** $(\Delta T_f)_x = (\Delta T_f)_y$

$$k_f.m_x = k_f.m_y$$

$$\frac{4 \times 1000}{A \times 96} = \frac{12 \times 1000}{m_y \times 88}$$

$$m = 3.27\ A$$

$$m \simeq 3\ A$$

**29.** **(a)** van't Hoff equation is

$\pi V = inRT$

For depression in freezing point.

$\Delta T_f = i \times K_f \times m$

For elevation in boiling point.

$\Delta T_b = i \times K_b \times m$

For lowering of vapour pressure,

$$\frac{P^{\circ}_{\text{solvent}} - P_{\text{solution}}}{P^{\circ}_{\text{solvent}}} = i\left(\frac{n}{N+n}\right).$$

**30.** **(a)** The vapour pressure of a solution of glucose in water can be calculated using the relation

$$\frac{P^{\circ} - P}{P^{\circ}} = \frac{\text{Moles of glucose in solution}}{\text{Moles of water in solution}}$$

or $\frac{17.5 - P}{17.5} = \frac{18/180}{178.2/18}$ $[\because P^{\circ} = 17.5]$

or $17.5 - P = \frac{17.5 \times 18 \times 18}{180 \times 178.2}$

$P = 17.323$ mm Hg.

# 17 Electrochemistry

1. **(a)** $E^0 = \frac{0.0591}{2}\log K_{eq}; \log K_{eq} = \frac{2\times 0.22}{0.0591}$

$\log K_{eq} = 7.44$ or $K_{eq} \approx 2.8\times 10^7$

2. **(d)** Oxidation potential of Co is more than Ag, hence cell reaction will be

$Co + 2Ag^+ \longrightarrow Co^{2+} + 2Ag$

$E_{cell} = E^0_{cell} - \frac{RT}{nF}\ln\frac{[Co^{2+}]}{[Ag^+]^2}$, the lesser the value of the factor $\frac{[Co^{2+}]}{[Ag^+]^2}$ greater will be value of $E_{cell}$.

3. **(d)** Here Ni is anode and Au is cathode

Given $E^0_{Ni^{2+}/Ni} = -0.25V$

and $E^0_{Au^{3+}/Au} = +1.5V$

$E^0_{cell} = E^0_C - E^0_A$

$= 1.5-(-0.25) = 1.5+0.25 = 1.75\ V$

$Ni(s) \longrightarrow Ni^{2+}(aq) + 2e^-$ ... (i) × 3

$Au^{3+}(aq) + 3e^- \longrightarrow Au(s)$ ... (ii) × 2

$3Ni(s) + 2Au^{3+} \longrightarrow 3Ni^{2+}(aq) + 2Au(s)$

$n = 6$

$E_{cell} = E^0_{cell} - \frac{0.059}{n}\log\frac{[Ni^{+2}]^3}{[Au^{+3}]^2}$

$E_{cell} = 1.75 - \frac{0.059}{6}\log\frac{(1)^3}{(1)^2} = 1.75\ V$

4. **(b)** Maximum work done $= W_{max}$ $\because 1V = 1JC^{-1}$

$= -nFE^0_{cell} = -2\times 96500\times 1.10$

$= -212.30$ kJ

5. **(b)** (i) $A^{3+} + e^- \longrightarrow A^{2+}, \Delta G_1 = -1\,F\,y_2$

(ii) $A^{2+} + 2e^- \longrightarrow A, \Delta G_2 = -2F(-y_1) = 2Fy_1$

Add, (i) and (ii) we get

$A^{3+} + 3e^- \longrightarrow A; \Delta G_3 = -3FE^0$

$\Delta G_3 = \Delta G_1 + \Delta G_2$

$-3FE^0 = -Fy_2 + 2Fy_1$

$-3FE^0 = -F(y_2 - 2y_1)$

$E^\circ = \frac{y_2 - 2y_1}{3}$

6. **(b)** Equivalent conductivity of $BaCl_2$

$\Lambda^\infty_m(BaCl_2) = \lambda^\infty_m(Ba^{2+}) + 2\lambda^\infty_m(Cl^-)$

$= 127 + 2\times 76 = 279\ ohm^{-1}\ cm^2\ eq^{-1}$.

7. **(d)** Green vitriol ($FeSO_4.7H_2O$), potash alum ($K_2SO_4.\ Al_2(SO_4)_3.24H_2O$) and chile salt petre ($NaNO_3$) are electrolytes. Hence their solutions will be conducting whereas ethyl alcohol is a non-electrolyte i.e., does not produce ions in solution, hence will be non-conducting.

8. **(a)** $\Lambda_{eq} = \kappa\times\frac{1000}{N} = \frac{1}{R}\times\frac{l}{A}\times\frac{1000}{N}$

$= \frac{1}{R}\times \text{cell constant}\times\frac{1000}{N}$

$= \frac{1}{220}\times 0.88\times\frac{1000}{0.01}$

$= 400\ mho\ cm^2\ g\ eq^{-1}$

9. (c) $W = ZIt = \frac{\text{Eq.wt. of subs.}}{96,500} \times I \times t$

$\frac{W}{E} = \frac{I \times t}{96500}; \frac{0.195}{195} \times 4 = \frac{5 \times 60 \times 60 \times I}{96,500}$,

$I = 21.44\,mA$

10. (b)

$\text{No. of moles} = \frac{\text{Given mass}}{\text{Molar mass}} = \frac{0.25}{92.9} = 0.00269$

$\overset{+5}{Nb} + 5e^- \longrightarrow Nb$

Each $Nb^{5+}$ would require $5e^-$

0.00269 Mole of $Nb^{5+}$ require

$= 0.00269 \times 5 = 0.0134$ mole of $e^-$

1 Faraday = 1 mole of electrons

0.0134 mole of electrons

$= 0.0134F = 1.34 \times 10^{-2}F$

11. (c) $Ag^+ + e^- \longrightarrow Ag$

1 F is required for 1 mole. So 3 F will produce 3 mole

$Ca^{2+} + 2e^- \longrightarrow Ca$

2F is required for 1 mole. So 3 F will produce

$\frac{1}{2} \times 3 = \frac{3}{2}$ mole.

$Al^{+3} + 3e^- \longrightarrow Al$

3F is required for 1 mole. So 3F will produce 1 mole.

Molar ratio $3 : \frac{3}{2} : 1 = 6 : 3 : 2$

12. (a) $M^{n+} + ne^- \longrightarrow M$

$\text{Mole of metal deposited} = \frac{2.977}{106.4} = 0.028 \text{ mole}$

1 mole of M deposited by n Faraday

$= n \times 96500\,C$.

0.028 mole of metal deposited by charge

$= n \times 96500 \times 0.028$

$\therefore n \times 96500 \times 0.028 = 10800\,C$

$\therefore n - 4$

13. (b) Given: current (I) = 0.5 amp;

Time (t) = 100 minutes × 60 = 6000 sec

Equivalent weight of silver (E) = 108.

According to Faraday's first law of electrolysis

$w = \frac{E \times I \times t}{96500} = \frac{108 \times 0.5 \times 6000}{96500} = 3.3575\,g$

14. (d)

$C_6H_5NO_2 + 6H^+ + 6e^- \longrightarrow C_6H_5NH_2 + 2H_2O$

$E_{C_6H_5NO_2}(\text{eq.wt}) = \frac{123}{6} = 20.5$

$\text{Number of coulombs required} = \frac{W \times 96500}{\text{Eq. wt}}$

$= \frac{12.3 \times 96500}{20.5}$

$= 57900\,C$

15. (a) Cathodic protection is best method to prevent iron from rusting. In this method iron is made cathode by application of external current. Saline water is highly conducting and hence accelerates the formation of rust.

16. (b) During charging, the lead storage battery behaves like an electrolytic cell. So, at anode the reaction is

$PbSO_4 + 2H_2O \longrightarrow PbO_2 + SO_4^{2-} + 4H^+ + 2e^-$

17. (a) An oxidising agent with a higher reduction potential will oxidise only reducing agent with a lower reduction potential.

18. (d) $E = E^0 - \frac{0.0591}{1} \log \frac{[Fe^{3+}]}{[Ag^+][Fe^{2+}]}$

as $Q\uparrow \{[Ag^+]\downarrow, [Fe^{3+}]\uparrow\}, E\downarrow$

19. (b) Cell reaction :

$M + 3Ag^+(aq) \longrightarrow M^{3+} + 3Ag(s)$

$$E = E^0 - \frac{0.0591}{n}\log\frac{[\text{Product}]}{[\text{Reactant}]}$$

$$0.421 = E^0 - \frac{0.0591}{3}\log\frac{0.001}{(0.01)^3}$$

$E^0 = 0.48$

$$E^0 = E^0_{Ag^+/Ag} - E^0_{M^{3+}/M}$$

$$E^0_{M^{3+}/M} = 0.8V - 0.48V = 0.32 \text{ volt}$$

**20. (b)** $\Delta G = -nEF$

For 1 mole of Al, n = 3

$\therefore$ for $\frac{4}{3}$ mole of Al, $n = 3 \times \frac{4}{3} = 4$

According to question,

$-827 \times 1000 = -4 \times E \times 96500$

$$E = \frac{827 \times 1000}{4 \times 96500} = 2.14\text{ V}$$

$\therefore$ Minimum e.m.f. required = 2.14 V

**21. (c)** $\Lambda_m = \frac{\kappa}{M} \times 1000; (x + y) = \frac{\kappa}{M} \times 1000$

$$\Rightarrow M = \frac{1000 \times \kappa}{(x + y)}$$

$$\text{Solubility (in gL}^{-1}) = \frac{\kappa \times 1000 \times 188}{x + y}$$

**22. (b)** Cell constant

$$= \frac{\ell}{A} = \frac{10}{100} = 0.1; \text{conductance} = 0.0001\text{S}$$

$V = 100 \times 10 = 1000\text{ cm}^3 = 1$ litre

$\kappa$ = cell constant × conductance

$= 0.1 \times 0.0001 = 10^{-5}$

$$\Lambda_m = \frac{\kappa \times 1000}{M}$$

$$= \frac{(0.1 \times 0.0001) \times 1000}{0.1} = 0.1\text{ Scm}^2\text{mol}^{-1}$$

**23. (b)** $\Lambda^{\infty}_{HCl} = 426.2$ ... (i)

$\Lambda^{\infty}_{AcONa} = 91.0$ ... (ii)

$\Lambda^{\infty}_{NaCl} = 126.5$ ... (iii)

$$\Lambda^{\infty}_{AcOH} = (i) + (ii) - (iii) = [426.2 + 91.0 - 126.5] = 390.7$$

**24. (a)** 27 g of Al is obtained by charge of 3 × 96500 C.

$\therefore$ 1 g of Al is obtained by charge of

$$3 \times \frac{96500}{27}\text{C.}$$

$\therefore$ $5.12 \times 10^3$ g of Al is obtained by charge of

$$= 3 \times \frac{96500}{27} \times 5.12 \times 1000 = 5.49 \times 10^7\text{C.}$$

**25. (c)** Total charge = 2

Number of equivalent of ion

$$= \frac{\text{Charge on the ion}}{\text{Total charge}}$$

$$\therefore \quad \text{Eq of} \begin{pmatrix} COO^- \\ | \\ COO^- \end{pmatrix} = \frac{2}{2} = 1$$

$$\text{Eq of } Na^+ = \frac{1}{2}, \text{ Eq of } K^+ = \frac{1}{2}$$

$$\therefore \quad \lambda^0_{eq}\begin{pmatrix} COONa \\ | \\ COOK \end{pmatrix}$$

$$= \lambda^0_{eq}\begin{pmatrix} COO^- \\ | \\ COO^- \end{pmatrix} + \frac{1}{2}\lambda^0 Na^+ + \frac{1}{2}\lambda^0 K^+$$

$$= 74 + \frac{50}{2} + \frac{73}{2} = 135.5\text{ ohm}^{-1}\text{ cm}^2\text{ eq}^{-1}$$

**26.** (d) $(\Lambda^0_m)_{NaBr} - (\Lambda^0_m)_{NaI}$

$= \Lambda^0_m \overset{+}{Na} + \Lambda^0_m Br^- - (\Lambda^0_m \overset{+}{Na} + \Lambda^0_m I^-)$

$= \Lambda^0_m \overset{+}{Na} + \Lambda^0_m Br^- - \Lambda^0_m \overset{+}{Na} - \Lambda^0_m I$

$= \Lambda^0_m Br^- + \Lambda^0_m I^- \; (\Lambda^0_m)_{KBr} - (\Lambda^0_m)_{NaBr}$

$= \Lambda^0_m K^+ + \Lambda^0_m Br^- - (\Lambda^0_m Na^+ + \Lambda^0_m Br^-)$

$= \Lambda^0_m K^+ + \Lambda^0_m Br^- - \Lambda^0_m \overset{+}{Na} - \Lambda^0_m Br^-$

$= \Lambda^0_m K^+ + \Lambda^0_m \overset{+}{Na}$

$\therefore (\Lambda^0_m)_{NaBr} - (\Lambda^0_m)_{NaI} \neq (\Lambda^0_m)_{KBr} - (\Lambda^0_m)_{NaBr}$

**27.** **(a)** Millimoles of $Au^+ = 0.1 \times 250 = 25$

$$\text{Mole of } Au^+ = \frac{25}{1000} = \frac{1}{40} = 0.025$$

Similarly, moles of $Ag^+ = 0.025$

Charge passed $= I \times t = 1 \times 15 \times 60 = 900$ C

$$\text{Moles of } e^- \text{ passed} = \frac{900}{96500} = 0.0093 \text{ mol.}$$

Species with higher value of SRP will get deposited first at cathode.

$$\underset{0.025}{Au^+(aq)} + \underset{0.0093}{e^-} \longrightarrow Au(s)$$

So, only Au will get deposited.

**28.** **(d)** For the concentration cell, $E^o_{cell} = 0$

**Anode :** $Cu(s) \longrightarrow Cu^{2+}(aq)_A$

**Cathode :** $Cu^{2+}(aq)_e \longrightarrow Cu(s)$

**Overall :** $\underset{(C_2M)}{Cu^{2+}(aq)_C} \longrightarrow \underset{(C_1M)}{Cu^{2+}(aq)_A}$

As $\Delta G = -nFE$

If $\Delta G = -ve$, then $E_{cell}$ is $+v_e$.

$$E_{cell} = E^o_{cell} - \frac{RT}{2F}\ln\frac{C_1}{C_2}$$

$$E_{cell} = 0 - \frac{RT}{2F}\ln\frac{C_1}{C_2}$$

$$E_{cell} = \frac{RT}{2F}\ln\frac{C_2}{C_1}$$

So, $C_2 > C_1$.

Thus, $C_2 = \sqrt{2}C_1$ relation is correct.

**29.** **(b)** $Cu^{2+} + 2e^- \longrightarrow Cu,$

$\Delta G_1^\circ = -2F(0.34)$ ...(i)

$Cu^+ + e^- \longrightarrow Cu,$

$\Delta G_2^\circ = -F(0.522)$ ...(ii)

Subtract (ii) from (i)

$Cu^{2+} + e^- \longrightarrow Cu^+, \quad \Delta G_3^\circ = -F(E^0)$

$\therefore \Delta G_1^\circ - \Delta G_2^\circ = G_3^\circ$

$\Rightarrow -FE^\circ = -2F(0.34) + F(0.522)$

$\Rightarrow E^\circ = 0.68 - 0.522 = 0.158$ V

**30.** **(c)** $Ag^+(aq) + Fe^{2+}(aq) \longrightarrow Fe^{3+}(aq) + Ag(s)$

$$E^0_{cell} = E^0_{Ag^+/Ag} - E^0_{Fe^{3+}/Fe^{2+}}$$

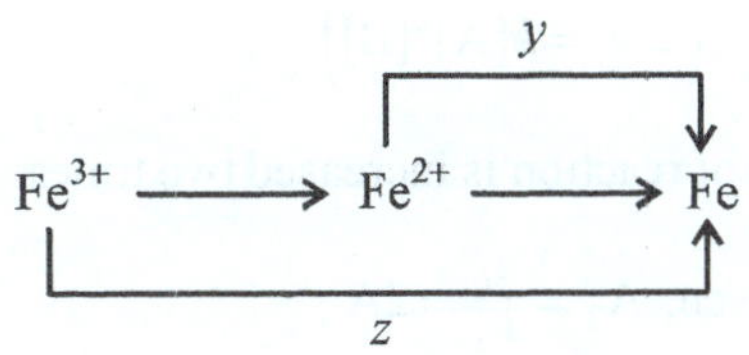


$E^0_{Fe^{3+}/Fe^{2+}} = 3z - 2y$

$E^0_{Ag^+/Ag} = x$ (given)

$\therefore E^0_{cell} = x - 3z + 2y$

# 18 Chemical Kinetics

1. **(d)** In the given options $-\frac{d[C]}{3.dt}$ will not represent the reaction rate. It should not have –ve sign as it is a product. $\frac{1}{3}\frac{d[C]}{dt}$ shows the rate of formation of product C.

2. **(a)** $2A + B \longrightarrow A_2B$

$r_1 = k[A]^2[B]$ ...(i)

When, $[A] = [2A]$, $[B] = \left[\frac{B}{2}\right]$

$r_2 = k[2A]^2\left[\frac{B}{2}\right]$

$r_2 = k\,4[A]^2\frac{[B]}{2}$

$r_2 = k\,2[A]^2[B]$

$r_2 = 2r_1 \quad (\because r_1 = k[A]^2[B])$

$\therefore$ Rate of reaction is increased two times.

3. **(d)** Given: $A_2 \underset{k_{-1}}{\overset{k_1}{\rightleftharpoons}} 2A$

Now, $-\frac{1}{2}\frac{d[A]}{dt} = k_{-1}[A]^2 - k_1[A_2]$

$\frac{d[A]}{dt} = -2k_{-1}[A]^2 + 2k_1[A_2]$

$\frac{d[A]}{dt} = 2k_1[A_2] - 2k_{-1}[A]^2$

4. **(c)** For the reaction $2X \longrightarrow B$, follow zeroth order

Rate equation is $kt = [A]_0 - [A]$

For the half-life; $t = t_{1/2}$ and $[A] = 0.1$

$k\,t_{1/2} = 0.2 - 0.1$

$\frac{0.2-0.1}{6} = \frac{0.1}{6}\,M\,h^{-1}$

time required to reach from 0.5 M to 0.2 M

$kt = [A]_0 - [A]$

$\frac{0.1}{6} \times t = (0.5 - 0.2)$; $t = 18$ hour

5. **(d)** Reaction is second order; $k = 10^{-4}\,L\,mol^{-1}\,min^{-1}$.

$\therefore \quad -\frac{1}{3}\frac{d[A]}{dt} = k[A]^2$

$-\frac{d[A]}{dt} = 10^{-4} \times 3 \times (0.5)^2$

$= 7.5 \times 10^{-5}\,M\,min^{-1}$

$= \frac{7.5 \times 10^{-5}}{60} = 1.25 \times 10^{-6}\,Ms^{-1}$

6. **(b)** $A \rightarrow B$ For a first order reaction

Given $a = 0.8$ mol, $(a - x) = 0.8 - 0.6 = 0.2$

$k = \frac{2.303}{1}\log\frac{0.8}{0.2}$ or $k = 2.303 \log 4$

again $a = 0.9$, $a - x = 0.9 - 0.675 = 0.225$

$k = \frac{2.303}{t}\log\frac{0.9}{0.225}$

$$2.303\log 4 = \frac{2.303}{t}\log 4$$

Hence $t = 1$ hour

**7.** **(a)** Rate constant of decomposition of $X = 0.05$ mg/year.

Unit of rate constant confirms that the decomposition of $X$ is a zero order reaction.

For zero order kinetics,

$$[X] = [X]_0 - kt$$

$$kt = [X]_0 - [X]$$

$$t = \frac{[X]_0 - [X]}{k}$$

$$\Rightarrow \quad t = \frac{5 - 2.5}{0.05}$$

$$= \frac{2.5}{0.05} = 50 \text{ years}$$

**8.** **(c)** As we know that, units of rate constant.

$= (\text{unit of conc.})^{1-n}\ (\text{unit of time})^{-1}$

$= (\text{mol L}^{-1})^{1-n}\ (\text{sec})^{-1}$

On comparing these units with the given units of rate constant, we get

$(\text{mol L}^{-1})^{1-n}\ (\text{sec})^{-1} = \text{L mol}^{-1}\ \text{sec}^{-1}$

$\Rightarrow \text{L}^{n-1}\ \text{mol}^{1-n}\ \text{sec}^{-1} = \text{L mol}^{-1}\ \text{sec}^{-1}$

On comparing the powers, we get

$n - 1 = 1 \Rightarrow n = 2$

So, reaction is of second order.

**9.** **(a)**

$$C_4H_8 \longrightarrow 2C_2H_4$$

Moles at $t = 0$ $\quad a \quad\quad 0$

Moles at $t = t$ $\quad (a - x) \quad\quad 2x$

when $\dfrac{2x}{a - x} = 1$ then $x = \dfrac{a}{3}$

$$\therefore \quad t = \frac{2.303}{k}\log\frac{a}{(a - x)}$$

$$= \frac{2.303}{2.3 \times 10^{-4}}\log\frac{a}{a - \frac{a}{3}} = 1760 \text{ sec}$$

**10.** **(c)** $t_{1/4} = \dfrac{2.303}{k}\log\dfrac{1}{3/4} = \dfrac{2.303}{k}\log\dfrac{4}{3}$

$$= \frac{2.303}{k}(\log 4 - \log 3) = \frac{2.303}{k}(2\log 2 - \log 3)$$

$$= \frac{2.303}{k}(2 \times 0.301 - 0.4771) = \frac{0.29}{k}$$

**11.** **(c)** Given initial mass $= a$

Mass left after time $t = x = 0.875\,a$

$t = 40$ minutes.

$$k = \frac{2.303}{t}\log\frac{a}{a - x} = \frac{2.303}{40}\log\frac{a}{a - 0.875\,a}$$

$$= \frac{2.303}{40}\log 8 = 0.052 \text{ min}^{-1}$$

$$t_{1/2} = \frac{0.693}{k} = \frac{0.693}{0.052} = 13 \text{ minutes } 32 \text{ sec.}$$

**12.** **(b)** Exothermic reaction

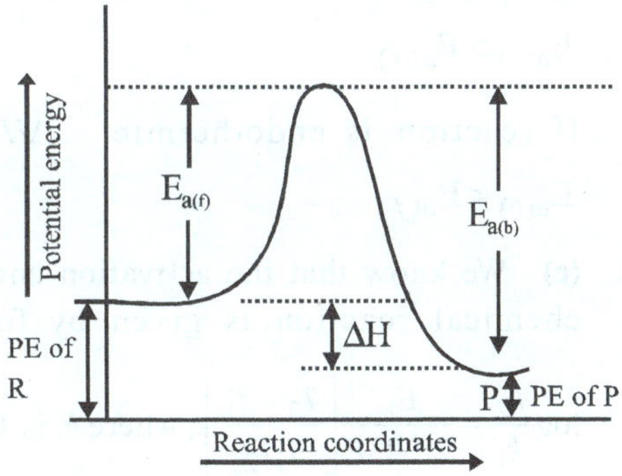


According to graph,

$$E_{a(b)} = E_{a(f)} + \Delta H$$

$$= 17 + 40$$

$$= 57 \text{ kJ mol}^{-1}$$

**13.** **(b)** From Arrhenius equation,

$$k = Ae^{-E_a/RT}$$

$$\ln k = \ln A - \frac{E_a}{RT}$$

slope = –y (given)

$$-y = -E_a \Rightarrow E_a = y$$

**14.** **(c)** $$\frac{k_2}{k_1} = \frac{Ae^{-E_{a_2}/RT}}{Ae^{-E_{a_1}/RT}} = e^{(E_{a_1}-E_{a_2})/RT}$$

$$2.303\log\frac{k_2}{k_1} = \frac{E_{a_1} - E_a}{RT} = \frac{(83.314-75)\times10^3}{8.314\times500} = 2$$

$$\log\frac{k_2}{k_1} = \frac{2}{2.303} = 0.868$$

Taking Antilog

$k_2 = 7.38\ k_1$

**15.** **(b)** $\Delta H = E_{a(f)} - E_{a(b)}$

Thus energy of activation for reverse reaction depends upon whether reaction is exothermic or endothermic.

If reaction is exothermic, $\Delta H = -ve$, $E_{a(b)} > E_{a(f)}$

If reaction is endothermic, $\Delta H = +ve$ $E_{a(b)} < E_{a(f)}$

**16.** **(c)** We know that the activation energy of chemical reaction is given by formula

$\log\frac{k_2}{k_1} = \frac{E_a}{2.303R}\left[\frac{T_2-T_1}{T_1T_2}\right]$, where $k_1$ is the rate constant at temperature $T_1$ and $k_2$ is the rate constant at temperature $T_2$ and $E_a$ is the activation energy. Therefore activation energy of chemical reaction is determined by evaluating rate constant at two different temperatures.

**17.** **(d)** Since the slow step is the rate determining step hence if we consider mechanism (A), we find

$$\text{Rate} = k[Cl_2][H_2S]$$

Now if we consider mechanism (B), we find

$$\text{Rate} = k[Cl_2][HS^-] \quad ...(1)$$

From equation (1) of mechanism (B)

$$k = \frac{[H^+][HS^-]}{H_2S}$$

or $$[HS^-] = \frac{k[H_2S]}{H^+}$$

Substituting this value in equation (1) we find

$$\text{Rate} = k[Cl_2]K\frac{[H_2S]}{H^+} = k'\frac{[Cl_2][H_2S]}{[H^+]}$$

hence only, mechanism (A) is consistent with the given rate equation.

**18.** **(b)** $2NO_2 \underset{k_2}{\overset{k_1}{\rightleftharpoons}} N_2O_4$,

For forward reaction rate $= -\frac{1}{2}\frac{dNO_2}{dt} = \frac{dN_2O_4}{dt}$
$= k_1[NO_2]^2$

For backward reaction

$$\text{Rate} = -\frac{dN_2O_4}{dt} = \frac{1}{2}\frac{dNO_2}{dt} = k_2[N_2O_4].$$

$$= 2k_1[NO_2]^2 - 2k_2[N_2O_4].$$

**19.** **(b)** $N_2 + 3H_2 \rightleftharpoons 2NH_3$

$$\frac{-\Delta[N_2]}{\Delta t} = -\frac{1}{3}\frac{\Delta[H_2]}{\Delta t} = \frac{1}{2}\frac{\Delta[NH_3]}{\Delta t}$$

$$\therefore \frac{-\Delta[H_2]}{\Delta t} = \frac{3}{2}\times\frac{\Delta[NH_3]}{\Delta t} = \frac{3}{2}\times2\times10^{-4}$$

$= 3 \times 10^{-4}$ mol litre$^{-1}$sec$^{-1}$

**20.** **(d)** Slow step is the rate determining step (RDS) and $(N_2O_2)$ is the reactive intermediate.

$\therefore r = k_2[N_2O_2][O_2]$

From reversible reaction, $[N_2O_2]$ is:

$$\frac{k_1}{k_{-1}} = \frac{[N_2O_2]}{[NO]^2}$$

Substitute $[N_2O_2]$ in Eq. (i),

$$r = k_2\left(\frac{k_1}{k_{-1}}\right)[NO]^2[O_2]$$

Hence, rate constant $= k_2\left(\frac{k_1}{k_{-1}}\right)$

**21.** **(c)** Unit of rate constant

$$= \frac{(\text{time})^{-1}}{(\text{concentration})^{n-1}} \text{ (when, } n = \text{order)}$$

$$\therefore \text{L mol}^{-1}\text{s}^{-1} = \frac{(\text{s})^{-1}}{(\text{mol L}^{-1})^{n-1}}$$

$$\therefore \text{L mol}^{-1}\text{s}^{-1} = \frac{(\text{s})^{-1}}{(\text{L mol}^{-1})^{1-n}} = (\text{s}^{-1})(\text{L mol}^{-1})^{n-1}$$

$1 = n - 1$

$n = 2,$

This is the unit for II[nd] order reaction.

**22.** **(c)** $t_{75\%} = 2t_{1/2}$

$$\therefore t_{1/2} = \frac{24\text{ min}}{2} = 12\text{ min}$$

$n$ = Number of half lives in 1 hr (60 min

$$= \frac{60}{12} = 5.$$

Amount of substance left after 5 half lives

$$= \left(\frac{1}{2}\right)^5 = \frac{1}{32}$$

$$\therefore \%\text{ of amount left} = \frac{100}{32} = 3.125\% \approx 3\%$$

**23.** **(c)** $kt = \frac{1}{n-1}\left[\frac{1}{A_t^{\,n-1}} - \frac{1}{A_0^{\,n-1}}\right]$

$$kt_{0.5} = kt = \frac{1}{n-1}\left[\frac{1}{\left(\frac{A_0}{2}\right)^{n-1}} - \frac{1}{A_0^{n-1}}\right] = \frac{1}{n-1}\left[\frac{2^{n-1}-1}{A_0^{\,n-1}}\right]$$

$$kt_{0.875} = \frac{1}{n-1}\left[\frac{1}{\left(\frac{A_0}{8}\right)^{n-1}} - \frac{1}{A_0^{n-1}}\right] = \frac{1}{n-1}\left[\frac{8^{n-1}-1}{A_0^{\,n-1}}\right]$$

$$\frac{t_{0.875}}{t_{0.5}} = \frac{8^{n-1}-1}{2^{n-1}-1}$$

**24.** **(c)** Given, $k = 6.909\text{ min}^{-1}$

For a first order reaction;

$$k = \frac{2.303}{t}\log\left(\frac{a}{a-x}\right)$$

$$6.909 = \frac{2.303}{t}\log\left(\frac{100}{100-75}\right) = \frac{2.303}{t}\log\left(\frac{100}{25}\right)$$

$$\Rightarrow t = \frac{2.303}{6.909}\log 4 \Rightarrow t = \frac{1}{3}\log(2^2) = \frac{2}{3}\log 2.$$

**25.** **(d)** From 1[st] and 2[nd] sets of data - no change in rate is observed with the change in concentration of 'C'. So the order with respect to 'C' is zero.

From 1[st] and 4[th] sets of data

Dividing eq. (4) by eq. (1)

$$\frac{1.25\times10^{-3}}{5.0\times10^{-3}} = \left[\frac{0.005}{0.010}\right]^x$$

or $0.25 = (0.5)^x$ or $(0.5)^2 = (0.5)^x$

$\therefore x = 2$

The order with respect to 'A' is 2

From the 1[st] and 3[rd] sets of data Dividing eq. (1) by eq. (3)

$$\frac{5.0\times10^{-3}}{1.0\times10^{-2}}=\left[\frac{0.005}{0.010}\right]^y$$

or $(0.5)^1=(0.5)^y \Rightarrow y=1$

The order with respect to 'B' is 1

So the order with respect to the reactants A, B and C is 2, 1 and 0.

**26.** **(b)** $k=\frac{0.693}{t_{1/2}}=\frac{0.693}{45}\,\text{min}^{-1}$

$$k=\frac{2.303}{t_{99.9\%}}\log\frac{a}{a-0.999a}$$

or $t_{99.9\%}=\frac{2.303\times45}{0.693}\log10^3$

$= 448.6$ min $\approx 7.5$ hrs

**27.** **(d)** Given, $k_1=10^{16}.e^{-\frac{2000}{T}}$

and $k_2=10^{15}.e^{-\frac{1000}{T}}$

when $k_1$ and $k_2$ are equal at any temperature T,

we have $10^{16}.e^{-\frac{2000}{T}}=10^{15}.e^{-\frac{1000}{T}}$

or $10\times10^{15}.e^{-\frac{2000}{T}}=10^{15}.e^{-\frac{1000}{T}}$

or $10.e^{-\frac{2000}{T}}=e^{-\frac{1000}{T}}$

or $\ln 10-\frac{2000}{T}=-\frac{1000}{T}$

or $\ln 10=\frac{2000}{T}-\frac{1000}{T}$

or $2.303\log 10=\frac{1000}{T}$

or $2.303\times1\times T=1000$ $\quad[\because \log 10=1]$

or $T=\frac{1000}{2.303}$ K

**28.** **(a)** Use Arrhenius equation

$T_1=273+14=287$ K,

$T_2=273+30=303$ K

$$\log\frac{k_2}{k_1}=\frac{E_a}{2.303R}\left[\frac{T_2-T_1}{T_1\times T_2}\right]$$

$$\log\frac{2.2\times10^{-5}}{2.0\times10^{-6}}=\frac{E_a}{2.303\times2\times10^{-3}}\left(\frac{16}{287\times303}\right)$$

$$E_a=\frac{\log(11)\times2.303\times2\times10^{-3}\times287\times303}{16}$$

$$=\frac{1.0414\times2.303\times2\times287\times303}{16000}$$

$\approx 26$ kcal mol$^{-1}$

**29.** **(c)** $k=Ae^{-E_a/RT}$

If $k_1=k_2$

$$A_1e^{-E_{a_1}/RT}=A_2e^{-E_{a_2}/RT}$$

$$\frac{A_2}{A_1}=e^{(E_{a_2}-E_{a_1})/RT}$$

$$\frac{10^{10}}{10^9}=e^{(1800-1200)/RT}$$

$10=\text{Exp}\left(\frac{600}{RT}\right)$, R = 2 cal/K-mol

$$\ell n\,10=\frac{600}{2T}$$

$$T=\frac{300}{2.303}\text{K}$$

**30. (a)**

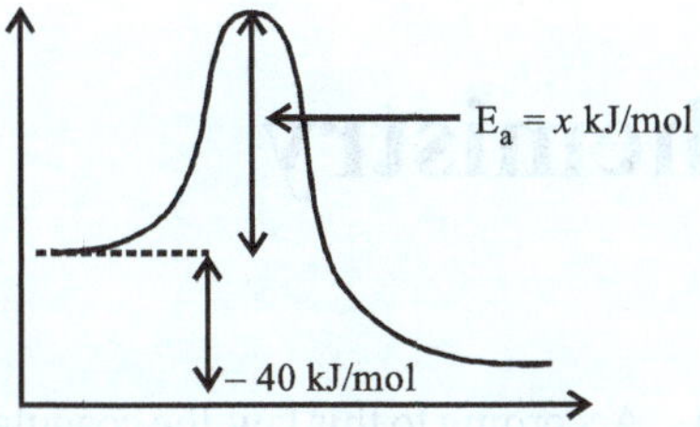


$$\left(\frac{\underset{(A\rightarrow B)}{E_{forward}}}{\underset{(B\rightarrow A)}{E_{backward}}}\right) = \frac{2}{3} = \frac{x}{-40+x}$$

$$\Rightarrow -80 + 2x = 3x$$

$$\Rightarrow x = -80 \text{ kJ/mol for forward}$$

For backward $= -40 + (-80) = -120$ kJ/mol

Because activation energy cannot be negative so, for forward reaction $E_a = 80$ kJ/mol

for backward reaction $E_a = 120$ kJ/mol

# 19 Surface Chemistry

1. (c) Van der Waal force ↑ adsorption ↑
2. (d) Surface area ↑ rate of adsorption ↑
3. (a) Hardness of water is due to carbonate or sulphate of $Ca^{2+}$ and $Mg^{2+}$ ions. When sodium aluminium silicate is added $Na^+$ replaces $Ca^{2+}$ and $Mg^{2+}$ by adsorption, and hence water becomes soft.
4. (d) The characteristics given suggests that this should be physical adsorption.

   Physical adsorption usually takes place at low temperature and decreases with increase in temperature. The force of attraction holding the adsorbate are van der Waal's forces. Heat of adsorption is low. It is reversible and forms multilayer. It does not require any energy of activation.
5. (b) $C + O_2 \longrightarrow CO_2$ No catalyst is required

   In Ostwald process, Haber's process and hydrogenation of vegetable oils, catalyst (solid)
   such as Pt/Rh, Fe and Ni are used.
6. (a)

| Solution | Particle size |
|---|---|
| True solution | Size < 1 nm |
| Colloidal solution | 1 nm < size < 1000 nm |
| Suspension | Size > 1000 nm |

7. (b)

| | Dispersed phase | Dispersion medium |
|---|---|---|
| Cheese liquid in solid (C) | liquid | solid |
| Milk liquid in liquid (M) | liquid | liquid |
| Smoke solid in gas (S) | solid | gas |

8. (c) According to this law, the coagulating effect of an ion on dispersed phase of opposite charge increases with the increase in valency of the ion. The precipitating power of $Al^{3+}$, $Ba^{2+}$, and $Na^+$ ions is in order $Al^{3+} > Ba^{2+} > Na^+$.
9. (a) Lower is the gold number, higher will be the protective power. Thus, gelatin has maximum protective power.
10. (d) $Al(OH)_3$ is positively charged sol. $K_3PO_4$ has greater negative charge. Hence, it is most effective in coagulation of $Al(OH)_3$ sol.
11. (c) Temp↑ Extent of adsorption ↓
12. (b) Mass of acetic acid adsorbed by 2 g charcoal

    $$= 100 \times 10^{-3} \times (0.6 - 0.5) \times 60 = 0.6 \text{ g}$$

    amount of acetic acid adsorbed per gram of carbon $\left(\frac{x}{m}\right) = \frac{0.6}{2} = 0.3$
13. (c) Adsorption is an exothermic process, hence $\Delta H$ will always be negative.
14. (c) After equivalence point, the AgCl particles adsorb $Ag^+$ ions (present in slight excess) and then fluorescein anion. The precipitate particles turn reddish pink due to the complex formation between $Ag^+$ and fluorescein anion.
15. (c) Hydrolysis of urea can be represented as follows

    $$H_2N-\underset{\underset{O}{\|}}{C}-NH_2 + H_2O \xrightarrow[\text{(enzyme)}]{\text{Urease}} 2NH_3 + CO_2$$

    Since it involves biological catalyst (enzyme), so it is an example of biochemical catalysis.
16. (b) $m$ moles of $AgNO_3 = 50 \times 0.1 = 5$

    $m$ moles of $KI = 50 \times 0.2 = 10$

    KI is in excess so $I^-$ is absorbed on AgI sol.

**17.** **(c)** The sols obtained in the two cases will be oppositely charged so coagulate each other.

**18.** **(b)** Colour of dye appear in patches in o/w emulsion.

**19.** **(d)** Sulphur solution is multimolecular and hydrophobic in nature.

**20.** **(c)** According to Hardy-Schulze rule "The amount of electrolyte required to coagulate a fixed amount of a sol depends upon the sign of charge and valency of the flocculating ion."

Thus, the coagulating power vary in the order.

$Al^{3+} > Zn^{++} > Na^{+}$

**21.** **(b)** When oppositely charged sols are mixed their charges are neutralised. Both sols may be partially or completely precipitated.

**22.** **(a)**

**23.** **(c)** $\dfrac{\text{Coagulation power of } AlCl_3}{\text{Coagulation power of NaCl}}$

$$= \frac{\text{Coagulation value of NaCl}}{\text{Coagulation value of } AlCl_3}$$

$$= \frac{52}{0.093} = 559.13 \approx 560$$

**24.** **(a)** Colloid of liquid in liquid is called emulsion. Colloid of liquid in solid is gel.

**25.** **(d)**

# 20 General Principles and Processes of Isolation of Elements

1. (c) Cuprite : $Cu_2O$; Chalcocite : $Cu_2S$; Chalcopyrite : $CuFeS_2$; Malachite: $Cu(OH)_2.CuCO_3$.

2. (a) $ZnCO_3$ is calamine.

3. (c) Carborundum - SiC

   Epsomite or Epsom salt - $MgSO_4.7H_2O$

   Cassiterite - $SnO_2$

   Spodumene - Ore of lithium

4. (c) Cr metal is commercially extracted by Al-reduction method.

5. (b)

6. (a)

7. (b)

8. (a) Electric furnaces are lined with magnesia so that furnace material can withstand high temperature.

9. (b) In Hall-Heroult process, steel vessel with lining of carbon acts as cathode and graphite is used as anode.

10. (b) Highly electropositive elements are obtained by electrolytic reduction.

11. (d)

12. (a) $MgCl_2 \rightarrow Mg^{2+} + 2Cl^-$

    At cathode $Mg^{2+} + 2e^- \longrightarrow Mg$,

    At anode $2Cl^- \longrightarrow Cl_2 \uparrow + 2e^-$

13. (a) When impure metal has impurity of its own metal oxide, then poling process is used, e.g., impure Cu and Sn are purified by this method.

14. (a)

$$Ti + 2I_2 \xrightarrow{523K} \underset{\text{Volatile stable compound}}{TiI_4} \xrightarrow{1700K} \underset{\text{Pure metal}}{Ti + 2I_2}$$

15. (d)

16. (c) Extraction of Zn from zinc blends is achieved by roasting followed by reduction with carbon. Reactions involved are :

$$2ZnS + 3O_2 \xrightarrow{heat} 2ZnO + 2SO_2 \text{ (Roasting)}$$

$$ZnO + \underset{\text{(Coke)}}{C} \xrightarrow{heat} Zn + CO \text{ (Reduction)}$$

17. (d)

18. (b) Refractories are the substances which can withstand very high temperature without melting or becoming soft.

19. (b)

20. (b)

# 21 The p-Block Elements (Group 15, 16, 17 & 18)

1. **(d)** Due to high N—F bond strength, $NF_3$ is highly stable and hence inert towards hydrolysis.

2. **(a)** $2NH_3 + 5/2\,O_2 \xrightarrow[\Delta]{Pt} 2NO + 3H_2O$

3. **(a)**

4. **(c)** Urea (46.6%N). percentage of N in other compounds are $(NH_4)_2SO_4 : 21.2\%$;

   $CaCN_2 : 35.0\%$ and $NH_4NO_3 : 35.0\%$

5. **(b)** $PCl_3 + H_2O \longrightarrow POCl_3 + 2HCl$

   $POCl_3 + 3H_2O \longrightarrow H_3PO_4 + 3HCl$

6. **(a)** Oxide in which central atom has higher charge and more electronegativity, is more acidic, i.e. $N_2O_5 > N_2O_4 > P_2O_5 > As_2O_3$.

7. **(a)** $PH_4I + NaOH \rightarrow NaI + PH_3 + H_2O$

8. **(d)** $P_2O_5 + 3H_2O \xrightarrow{\Delta} 2H_3PO_4$

9. **(d)** $NO_2$ is reddish brown coloured gas. Rest of the oxides are colourless.

10. **(c)** In cyclic metaphosporic acid, number of P–O–P bonds is three.

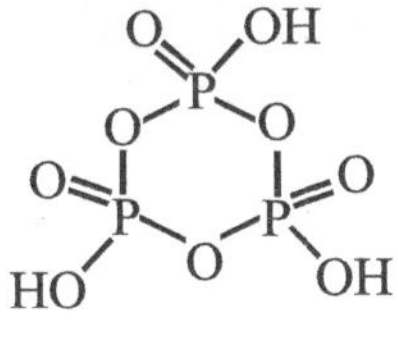


11. **(a)**

12. **(c)** The ignition temperature of black phosphorus is highest among all its allotropes, hence it is most stable.

13. **(a)**

$$\underset{\text{white phosphorus}}{P_4} + 8SOCl_2 \longrightarrow 4PCl_3 + 4SO_2 + 2S_2Cl_2$$

14. **(c)** Air is liquified by making use of the Joule-Thompson effect (cooling by expansion of the gas). Water vapour and $CO_2$ are removed by solidification. The remaining major constituents of liquid air i.e., liquid oxygen and liquid nitrogen are separated by means of fractional distillation (b.p. of $O_2 = -183$ °C : b. p. of $N_2 = -195.8$ °C)

15. **(a)** $\underset{\text{Thiosulphate}}{2S_2O_3^{-2}} + I_2 \rightarrow \underset{\text{Tetrathionate}}{S_4O_6^{-2}} + 2I^-$

16. **(d)** Hypo ($Na_2S_2O_3$) is used in photography. It is used during fixing of image. It dissolves AgBr that has not been affected by light during exposure leaving metallic silver (Ag) as such

$$AgBr + \underset{\text{Hypo}}{2Na_2S_2O_3} \longrightarrow \underset{\text{Soluble complex}}{Na_3[Ag(S_2O_3)_2]} + NaBr$$

17. **(c)** $SO_2$ is highly soluble in water and therefore cannot be collected over water.

18. **(c)** In $KMnO_4$, manganese is already present in its highest possible oxidation state i.e. +7. So no further oxidation is possible for $KMnO_4$.

19. **(c)** In liquid state $BrF_3$ dissociates into $BrF_2^+$ and $BrF_4^-$ ions most easily.

20. **(c)** The bond energy of interhalogen compounds is less than the bond energy of halogens.

21. **(c)** $2AgClO_3 + Cl_2(dry) \xrightarrow{90\,°C} 2AgCl + 2ClO_2 + O_2$

22. **(d)** $XeF_6 + H_2O \xrightarrow{\text{Partial}} XeOF_4 + 2HF$

$XeF_6 + 2H_2O \xrightarrow{\text{Partial}} XeO_2F_2 + 4HF$

$XeF_6 + 3H_2O \xrightarrow{\text{Complete}} XeO_3 + 6HF$

23. **(b)** In $XeOF_4$, xenon is $sp^3d^2$ hybridised and has one lone pair of electrons.

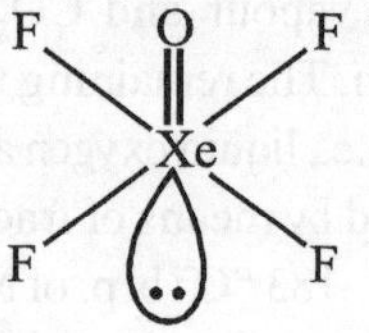


24. **(a)** Rn, because it is radioactive element obtained by the disintegration of Radium

$^{226}_{88}Ra \longrightarrow {}^{222}_{86}Rn + {}^{4}_{2}He$

25. **(d)** $XeO_2F_2$ has trigonal bipyramidal geometry, but due to presence of lone pair of electrons on equitorial position, its actual shape is *see-saw.*

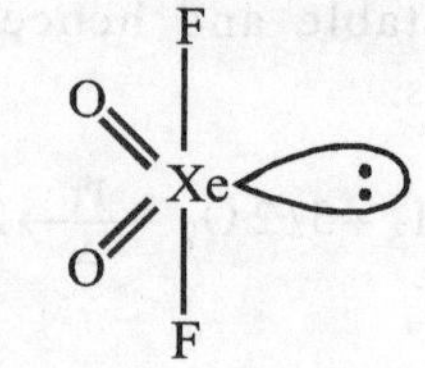

# 22 The d- and f-Block Elements

1. **(c)** Sc shows oxidation state of +3 only.
2. **(d)** $Sc^{3+}$ : $1s^2\ 2s^2p^6\ 3s^2p^6d^0\ 4s^0$; no unpaired electron.

   $Cu^+$ : $1s^2\ 2s^2p^6\ 3s^2p^6d^{10}\ 4s^0$; no unpaired electron.

   $Ni^{2+}$: $1s^2\ 2s^2p^6\ 3s^2p^6d^8\ 4s^0$; unpaired electrons are present.

   $Ti^{3+}$ : $1s^2\ 2s^2p^6\ 3s^2p^6d^1\ 4s^0$; unpaired electron is present.

   $Co^{2+}$ : $1s^2\ 2s^2p^6\ 3s^2p^6d^7\ 4s^0$; unpaired electrons are present.

   So from the given options the only correct combination is $Ni^{2+}$ and $Ti^{3+}$.
3. **(c)** A ruby is a crystal of alumina, aluminum oxide ($Al_2O_3$) containing a trace of chromium (III) ions replacing some of the aluminum ions. In ruby, each $Al^{3+}$ ion and $Cr^{3+}$ ion is surrounded by six oxide ions in an octahedral arrangement. The origin of the color of emeralds is similar to that of the color of rubies. However, the bulk of an emerald crystal is composed of beryl, beryllium aluminum silicate ($Be_3Al_2(SiO_3)_6$) instead of the alumina which forms rubies. The color is produced by chromium (III) ions, which replace some of the aluminum ions in the crystal. In emeralds, the $Cr^{3+}$ is surrounded by six silicate ions, rather than the six oxide ions in ruby. Therefore, the color (green) of emeralds is different from that of ruby.
4. **(d)** Manganese exhibits the large number of oxidation states. The most common oxidation states of Mn are +2, +3, + 4, + 6 and +7.
5. **(c)** Magnetic moment $\mu = \sqrt{n(n+2)}$ BM

   $1.73 = \sqrt{n(n+2)}\ \therefore n = 1$, it has one unpaired electron hence electronic configuration is $[Ar]3d^1$ and electronic configuration for Ti(Z= 22) is $[Ar]3d^2 4s^2$. Hence charge on Ti is +3.
6. **(a)** $Mn^{2+}$ – 5 unpaired electrons

   $Fe^{2+}$ – 4 unpaired electrons

   $Ti^{2+}$ – 2 unpaired electrons

   $Cr^{2+}$ – 4 unpaired electrons

   Hence maximum number of unpaired electron is present in $Mn^{2+}$.

   Magnetic moment $\propto$ number of unpaired electrons.
7. **(b)** $V^+ = 3d^3 4s^1, Cr^+ = 3d^5, Mn^+ = 3d^5 4s^1, Fe^+ = 3d^6 4s^1$

   Clearly, $IE_2$ of Cr will be highest as $Cr^+$ has exactly half filled *d*-subshell.
8. **(c)** (a), (b) and (d) are correct statements.
9. **(d)** $Ti^+$ does not exist, $Cu^+$ does not dissolve in water, $Cr^{2+}$ is less stable than $Cr^{3+}$ (both do not exist in aqueous solution) O.S. of V in $VO^{2+}$ is +6.
10. **(b)** $H_2$ is not a very strong reducing agent.
11. **(a)** AgCl is called Horn silver or Worm silver. $Ag_2S$ is called Argentite or silver glance.
12. **(c)**
13. **(a)** It is due to very high IE which results in weak metallic bonding.
14. **(a)** Wilkinson's catalyst is $[RhCl](PPh_3)_3]$, Red-violet in colour and has square planar structure. It is used for selective hydrogenation of organic molecules at room temperature and pressure.

    $TiCl_4 + (C_2H_5)_3Al$ is Zeigler Natta catalyst.

$(C_2H_5)_4$ Pb is an *anti*-knocking agent.
*cis*-platin is used as an anti-cancer agent.

**15.** **(b)** Interstitial compound $Fe_3C$ (cementite) is formed.

**16.** **(c)** Solid potassium dichromate when heated with concentrated sulphuric acid and a soluble chloride gives orange red vapours of a volatile oily liquid $CrO_2Cl_2$.

$$K_2Cr_2O_7 + 4NaCl + 6H_2SO_4 \longrightarrow 2KHSO_4 + 4NaHSO_4 + \underset{\text{chromyl chloride}}{2CrO_2Cl_2} + 3H_2O$$

**17.** **(c)** $I^-$ ion is a stronger reducing agent than $Cl^-$ ion. It reduces $Cu^{2+}$ ion to $Cu^+$ ion. Thus, $CuI_2$ is reduced to CuI and the species $(CuI_4)^{2-}$ does not exist.

**18.** **(a)** $Cr_2O_7^{2-} + 2OH^- \longrightarrow 2CrO_4^{2-} + H_2O$

**19.** **(a)** $2K_2CrO_4 + 2HNO_3 \longrightarrow K_2Cr_2O_7 + 2KNO_3 + H_2O$

**20.** **(b)** $2Cu + H_2O + CO_2 + O_2 \longrightarrow CuCO_3.Cu(OH)_2$ (green coloured basic carbonate of copper is formed)

**21.** **(c)** Gun metal is an alloy of Cu, Zn and Sn. It contains 88% Cu, 10% Sn and 2% Zn.

**22.** **(b)** $3Cu + (\text{dil.})\ 8HNO_3 \rightarrow 3Cu(NO_3)_2 + 2NO + 4H_2O$

**23.** **(d)** The chief ore of mercury is HgS (cinnabar)

**24.** **(b)** In $MnO_4^{2-}$ manganese is in +6 oxidation state which is having highest stability.

$MnO_4^{2-}$ disproportionates in neutral or acidic solution.

$$3MnO_4^{2-} + 4H^+ \longrightarrow 2MnO_4^- + MnO_2 + 2H_2O$$

**25.** **(a)** Ionic radii decrease across lanthanide series due to lanthanide contraction. As all ions are in +3 O.S., ionic radii will follow the trend of atomic radii.

$$\therefore \underset{(Z=57)}{La^{3+}} > \underset{(Z=58)}{Ce^{3+}} > \underset{(Z=61)}{Pm^{3+}} > \underset{(Z=70)}{Yb^{3+}}$$

**26.** **(b)**

**27.** **(d)**

**28.** **(b)** Pm is obtained by synthetic method.

**29.** **(d)** We know that lanthanides La, Gd shows +3, oxidation state, while Eu shows oxidation state of +2 and + 3. Am shows +3, +4, +5 and +6 oxidation states. Therefore Americium (Am) has maximum number of oxidation states.

**30.** **(d)** Atomic radii follows the order

| Eu | > | Ce | > | Ho |
|---|---|---|---|---|
| 199 pm | | 183 pm | | 176 pm |

# 23 Coordination Compounds

1. (b) $[Co(NO)_2(NH_3)_5]Cl_2$

pentaammine nitrito-N-cobalt (III) chloride

2. (c)

3. (d) More equivalents of $AgNO_3$ aqueous solution will be consumed if complex will furnish more $Cl^-$ ions in solution. Hence complex $[Cr(H_2O)_6]Cl_3$ will consume more equivalents of aqueous solution of $AgNO_3$.

4. (b)

| | $Ni(CO)_4$ | $[Ni(PPh_3)_2]Cl_2$ |
|---|---|---|
| O.S. | $Ni^0$ | $Ni^{2+}$ |
| E.C. | $[Ar]3d^84s^2$ | $[Ar]3d^84s^0$ |
| | Pairing of $e^-$ | No pairing of $e^-$ |
| Hybridization | $sp^3$ (tetrahedral) | square planar |

5. (c) (a) Ionization isomerism

(b) Co-ordination isomerism

(c) No isomerism

(d) Linkage isomerism

6. (d) $[Co(NH_3)_5Br]SO_4$ gives white precipitate of $BaSO_4$ with $BaCl_2(aq)$ whereas $[Co(NH_3)_5SO_4]Br$ gives yellow precipitate of AgBr with $AgNO_3(aq)$.

7. (b) The trans isomer and its mirror image are superim posable.

8. (d) (a) square planar - *cis* and trans isomers

(b) square planar - 3 isomers (while $NH_3$ at position 1, groups $NH_2OH$, $NO_2$ and $C_6H_5N$ can occupy position 3.

(c) 2 isomers (*cis* and *trans*)

9. (d) ⇒ $[Co(ox)(H_2O)_3(NH_3)]Br$ : Does not exhibit structural and optical isomerism but it can exhibit geometrical isomerism.

⇒ $[Cr(SCN)(H_2O)_3(en)](C_2O_4)$ : It can exhibit linkage and geometrical isomerism.

⇒ $[ZnBr(CN)(SCN)(NH_3)]^-$ : It exhibit optical isomerism.

⇒ $[Co(BrCl)(H_2O)_4][Ag(CN)_2]$ : and $[CoCl(CN)(H_2O)_4][AgBr(CN)]$ are co-ordination isomers.

10. (a) The compound shows linkage isomerism because the ligand in the compound is an ambidenate ligand that can bond at more than one atomic site.

*i.e.*, $NCS^-$ and $SCN^-$

11. (b) Non-superimposable mirror images are called optical isomers and may be described as "chiral'. They are also called enantiomers and rotate plane polarised light in opposite directions.

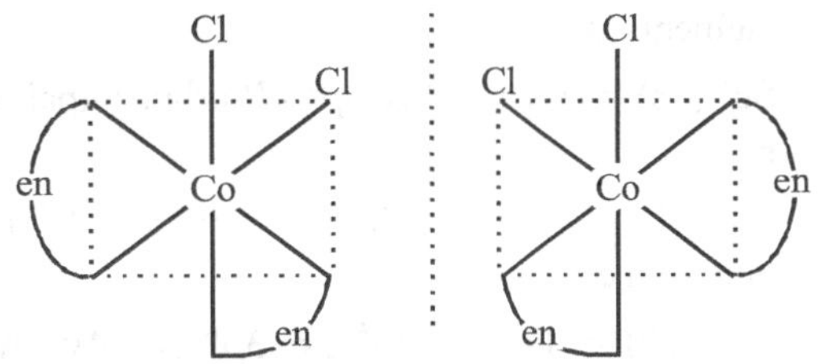


*dextro* *laevo*

12. (a) $MA_3B_3 - 2$ geometrical isomers

$MA_2B_4 - 2$ geometrical isomers

$MA_4B_2 - 2$ geometrical isomers

The complexes of general formula $MA_6$ and $MA_5B$ having octahedral geometry do not show geometrical isomerism.

13. (c) Diaminodichloroplatinum (II) commonly known as *cis* - platin is found to have anticancer property.

14. (c)

**15.** **(b)** Ionisation isomer of $[Cr(H_2O)_4Cl(NO_2)]Cl$ is $[Cr(H_2O)_4Cl_2]NO_2$.

**16.** **(d)** $Ni(CO)_4$; number of unpaired electrons = 0

$[Co(NH_3)_4(NO_2)_2]^+$; number of unpaired electrons = 0

$[Ag(CN_2)]$; number of unpaired electrons = 0

$[CuBr_4]^{2-}$; number of unpaired electrons = 1.0

**17.** **(a)** $t_2$ orbitals have higher energy by $(2/5)\Delta_t$.

**18.** **(d)** $Cr^{3+}$ has $3d^3 4s^0$ electronic configuration with 3 unpaired electrons, hence paramagnetic. In other cases pairing of *d*-electrons take place in presence of strong field ligands such as CO or $CN^-$.

In $Cr(CO)_6$ molecule, 12 electrons are contributed by CO group and it contains no odd electron.

**19.** **(c)** The absorption of visible light and hence coloured nature of the transition metal cation is due to the promotion of one or more unpaired - *d* - electron from a lower to higher level within same *d*-subshell. Hence higher will be the number of unpaired electron higher will be the absorpion in visible light.

The electronic configuration of the given elements is

$Sc^{3+}(18) = 1s^2 2s^2 2p^6 3s^2 3p^6 3d^0 4s^0$-no unpaired $e^-$.

$Ti^{4+}$ (18) = $1s^2\ 2s^2\ 2p^6\ 3s^2\ 3p^6\ 3d^0\ 4s^0$-no unpaired $e^-$.

$V^{3+}$ (20) = $1s^2\ 2s^2\ 2p^6\ 3s^2\ 3p^6\ 3d^2\ 4s^0$-two unpaired $e^-$.

$Zn^{2+}$ (28) = $1s^2\ 2s^2\ 2p^6\ 3s^2\ 3p^6\ 3d^{10}\ 4s^0$-no unpaired $e^-$.

hence $[V(NH_3)_6]^{3+}$ will most likely absorb visible light.

**20.** **(c)**

(a) High spin with $d^6$ configuration

$t_{2g}^4$ and $e_g^2$ CFSE $= -0.4\Delta_0$

(b) Low spin with $d^4$ configuration

$t_{2g}^4$ and $e_g^\circ$ CFSE $= -1.6\Delta_0$

(c) Low spin with $d^5$ configuration

$t_{2g}^5$ and $e_g^\circ$ CFSE $= -2.0\Delta_0$

(d) High spin with $d^7$ configuration

$t_{2g}^5$ and $e_g^2$ CFSE $= -0.8\Delta_0$

**21.** **(c)**

| $Mn^{2+}$ | $Cu^{3+}$ | $Co^{3+}$ | $Co^{2+}$ |
|---|---|---|---|
| $[Ar]3d^5$ | $[Ar]3d^8$ | $[Ar]3d^6$ | $[Ar]3d^7$ |
| No pairing of $e^-$ | No pairing of $e^-$ | Pairing of $e^-$ | No pairing of $e^-$ |
| Paramagnetic | Paramagnetic | Diamagnetic | Paramagnetic |

**22.** **(b)** Correct order is : $CN^- > en > NCS^- > Cl^-$

**23.** **(d)** $Cr(CN)_6]^{3-}$ : Hybridization : $d^2sp^3$ High or low spin is not defined because $Cr^{3+}$ is an example of $d^3$ system of configuration.

**24.** **(b)** $\mu = \sqrt{n(n+2)}$

$3.83 = \sqrt{n(n+2)}$

On solving, $n = 3$

Thus, it has three unpaired electrons.

$\therefore$ Cr : $1s^2\ 2s^2\ 2p^6\ 3s^2\ 3p^6\ 3d^4\ 4s^2$

$Cr^{3+}$ : $1s^2\ 2s^2\ 2p^6\ 3s^2\ 3p^6\ 3d^3$

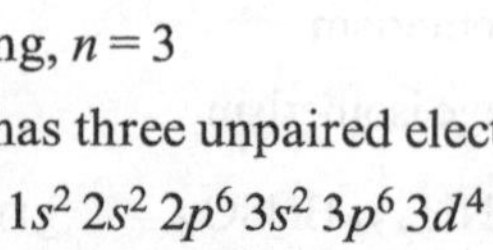


**25.** **(a)** Sc = [Ar] $3d^1, 4s^2$

Oxidation state of Sc in $[Sc(H_2O)_6]^{3+}$ is $Sc^{3+}$

$Sc^{3+}$ = [Ar] $3d^0, 4s^0$.

Thus $Sc^{3+}$ does not have unpaired electron, hence it is diamagnetic and colourless.

**26.** **(a)** $Cl^-$ is a weak field ligand.

**27.** **(b)** $[NiCl_4]^{2-}$, O.S. of Ni = +2

Ni(28) = $3d^8 4s^2$

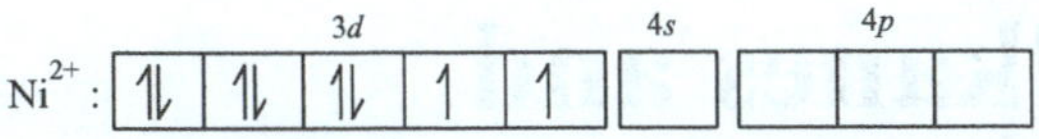

$Cl^-$ being weak ligand it cannot pair up the two electrons present in 3*d* orbital

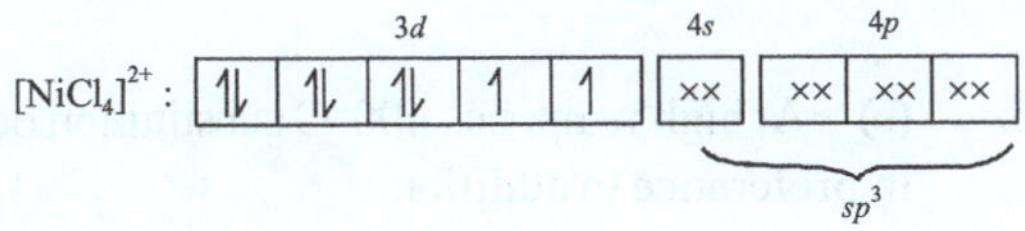

No. of unpaired electrons = 2

Magnetic moment, $\mu = 2.82$ BM.

**28.** **(d)** Hybridisation

$$\underset{d^2sp^3}{[Fe(CN)_6]^{4-}}, \underset{d^2sp^3}{[Mn(CN)_6]^{4-}},$$

$$\underset{d^2sp^3}{[Co(NH_3]^{3+}}, \underset{sp^3d^2}{[Ni(NH_3)_6]^{2+}}$$

Hence $[Ni(NH_3)_6]^{2+}$ is an outer orbital complex.

**29.** **(b)** A square planar complex is formed by hybridisation of

$s, p_x, p_y$ and $d_{x^2-y^2}$ atomic orbitals.

**30.** **(b)** Mole of AgCl $= \frac{1.435}{143.5} = 0.01$; 50 mL of 0.2 M complex $\equiv 0.01$ mole

$$[Co(NH_3)_4Cl_2]Cl \rightarrow [CoNH_3)_4Cl_2]^+ + Cl^-$$

# 24 Haloalkanes and Haloarenes

1. **(a)** $C_4H_7Cl$ is a monochloro derivative of $C_4H_8$ which itself exists in three acyclic isomeric forms.

$$\overset{4}{C}H_3\overset{3}{C}H_2\overset{2}{C}H=\overset{1}{C}H_2 \qquad \overset{1}{C}H_3\overset{2}{C}H=\overset{2}{C}H\overset{1}{C}H_3$$

I (Its has 4 types of carbon) II (It has 2 types of carbon)

$$\overset{1}{C}H_3-\underset{|}{\overset{}{C}}(\overset{1}{C}H_3)=\overset{2}{C}H_2$$

III (It has 2 types of carbon)

Following monochloro derivatives of I and II exist in two stereoisomeric forms each

$$CH_3CH_2CH=CHCl; \quad CH_3\overset{Cl}{\overset{|}{C}}=CHCH_3;$$

From I (*cis* - and *trans*-) From II (*cis* - and *trans*)

$$ClCH_2CH=CHCH_3$$

From II (*cis* and *trans*)

Grand total of acyclic isomers

$$=\underbrace{3+2}_{\text{From I}}+\underbrace{2+2}_{\text{From II}}+\underbrace{2}_{\text{From III}}=11$$

2. **(d)** *a*, *b* and *c* mainly undergo $S_N1$ reaction

3. **(d)** $Cl_3C-CH_2CH_3+KOH \longrightarrow (OH)_3C-CH_2CH_3+3KCl \xrightarrow{(-H_2O)} CH_3CH_2\overset{O}{\overset{||}{C}}-OH$

4. **(d)** $CCl_4$ has lowest (zero) dipole moment. This is due to its symmetrical tetrahedral structure. Due to which dipole moment of one bond is cancelled by opposite dipole moment of the other three bonds.

5. **(b)** At high temp. i.e., 400°C substitution occurs in preference to addition.

$$CH_3CH=CH_2 \xrightarrow[-HCl]{Cl_2,\,400^\circ C} ClCH_2CH=CH_2$$

6. **(c)** Potassium ethoxide is a strong base, and 2-bromopentane is a 2° bromide, so elimination reaction predominates

$$CH_3CH(Br)CH_2CH_2CH_3 \xrightarrow{OC_2H_5^-}$$

$$\underset{\text{Pentene - 2(major)}}{CH_3CH=CHCH_2CH_3}+\underset{\text{Pentene–1(minor)}}{CH_2=CHCH_2CH_2CH_3}$$

Since *trans*- alkene is more stable than *cis*, thus *trans*-pentene -2 is the main product.

7. **(d)**

$$\underset{\text{Ethyl bromide}}{C_2H_5Br} \xrightarrow{AgCN} \underset{\text{Ethyl isocyanide (major)}}{C_2H_5NC} \xrightarrow{\text{Reduction}} \underset{\text{Ethylmethylamine}}{C_2H_5NHCH_3}$$

8. **(d)** $S_N2$ reaction is favoured by small groups on the carbon atom attached to halogen. So, the order of reactivity is

$$CH_3Cl > (CH_3)_2CHCl > (C_2H_5)_2CHCl > (CH_3)_3CCl$$

$S_N2$ reaction is shown to maximum extent by primary halides. The only primary halide given is $CH_3Cl$, so the correct answer is (d).

9. **(c)** $C_6H_5CHCH_3Br$ being an optically active secondary alkyl bromide undergoes $S_N2$ nucleophilic substitution reaction. Hence it undergoes complete inversion of configuration.

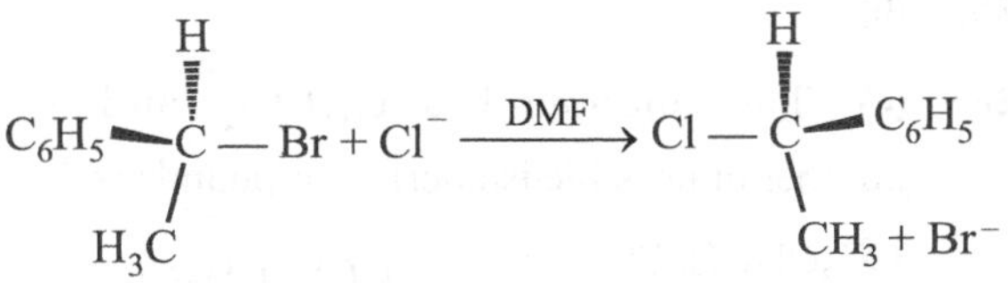

10. **(d)** $CH_3-\underset{\underset{Br}{|}}{C}H-CH_2-\underset{\underset{Br}{|}}{C}H-CH_2-CH_3$

$$\xrightarrow[E2]{KOH,\ CH_3OH\ \Delta}$$

$$\underset{\text{(Saytzeff product)}}{CH_3-CH=CH-CH=CH-CH_3}$$

11. **(b)**

$$C_2H_5I \xrightarrow{\text{alc. KOH}} CH_2=CH_2 \xrightarrow{Br_2}$$

$$BrCH_2-CH_2Br \xrightarrow{KCN} CNCH_2.CH_2CN$$

12. **(c)** $\underset{1^\circ\ \text{Carbocation}}{CH_3CH_2\overset{+}{C}H_2} \longrightarrow \underset{\substack{2^\circ\ \text{Carbocation} \\ \text{(more stable)}}}{CH_3\overset{+}{C}HCH_3}$

13. **(d)**

$$C_6H_5COOAg + Br_2 \xrightarrow{\text{Hunsdiecker reaction}}$$

$$C_6H_5Br + CO_2 + AgBr$$

14. **(b)** Reaction between alkyl halide, aryl halide and sodium in presence of ether is known as Wurtz Fittig reaction

$$C_6H_5Cl + 2Na + ClCH_3 \longrightarrow \underset{\text{Toluene}}{C_6H_5CH_3} + 2NaCl$$

15. **(a)**

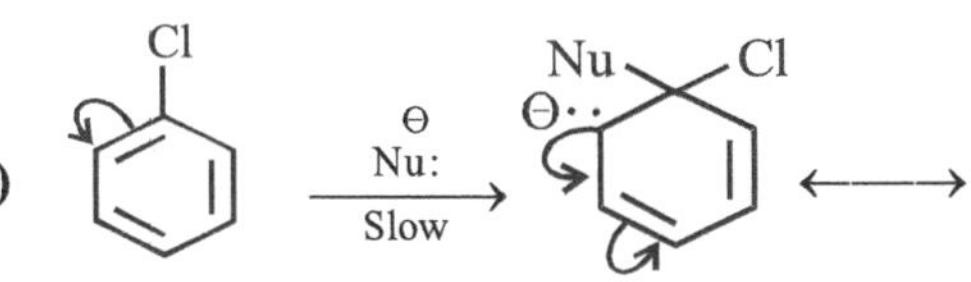

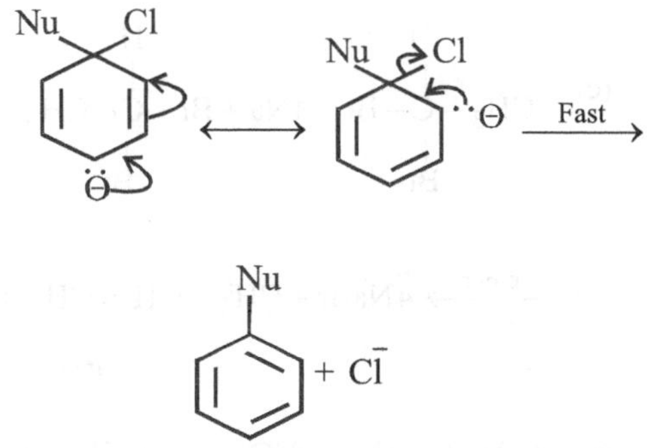

Rate $\propto$ $[C_6H_5Cl]\,[\bar{Nu}:]$

16. **(c)** Freons are chlorofluorocarbons.

17. **(d)** Carbonyl chloride ($COCl_2$).

18. **(a)** For a given alkyl group, the order of reactivity is

$$\xrightarrow[\text{increasing bond energy, decreasing halogen reactivity}]{R-I > R-Br > R-Cl > R-F}$$

19. **(b)** Weaker the base, better the leaving group. Hence

$$\xrightarrow{\text{Decreasing order of basicity}}$$

| OMe | OAc | $OSO_2Me$ | $OSO_2CF_3$ |
|---|---|---|---|
| (II) | (I) | (III) | (IV) |

$$\xleftarrow[\text{Decreasing order of leaving group}]{}$$

20. **(c)** $CH_3-\overset{\overset{Br}{|}}{C}H-CH_2-CH_3 \xrightarrow{\text{alc. KOH}}$

$$CH_3-CH=CH-CH_3 + HBr$$

The formation of 2-butene is in accordance to Saytzeff's rule. The more substituted alkene is formed in major quantity.

21. **(b)** 3° Alkyl halides on reaction with strong base ($CH_3O^-$) undergo elimination reaction and form alkene as major product.

$$\underset{\text{ter-Butyl bromide}}{CH_3-\underset{\underset{CH_3}{|}}{\overset{\overset{CH_3}{|}}{C}}-Br} \xrightarrow[\text{Strong base}]{CH_3O^-} \underset{\text{Isobutylene}}{CH_3-\underset{\underset{CH_3}{|}}{\overset{\overset{CH_2}{||}}{C}}} + HBr$$

**22.** **(c)**

$$CH_3-\underset{Br}{\overset{H}{C}}-Br+4Na+Br-\underset{Br}{\overset{H}{C}}-CH_3 \xrightarrow{\text{ether}} 4NaBr+\underset{\text{2-Butene}}{CH_3-CH=CH-CH_3}$$

**23.** **(d)** $C_2H_5Br + \text{alc. } AgNO_2 \longrightarrow \underset{\text{Nitroethane}}{C_2H_5NO_2}$

**24.** **(a)**

$$C_2H_6 \text{ (excess)} + Cl_2 \xrightarrow{\text{UV light}} C_2H_5Cl + HCl$$

**25.** **(b)**

**26.** **(c)** The compound is $C_3H_6Cl_2$ and the number of possible isomeric compounds is 5

$\underset{Cl}{CH_3CHCH_2Cl}$ I, II (*d* and *l*-)  $ClCH_2CH_2CH_2Cl$ III

$CH_3CH_2CHCl_2$ IV  $CH_3C(Cl_2)CH_3$ V

**27.** **(b)** The reaction proceeds via free radical mechanism.

As 2° free radical is more stable than 1°, so $CH_3CH_2CH(Br)CH_3$ would be formed.

**28.** **(a)**

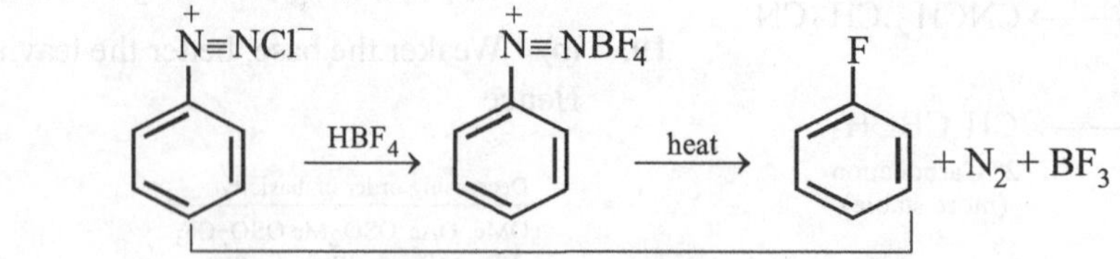


Balz–Schiemann reaction

**29.** **(a)**

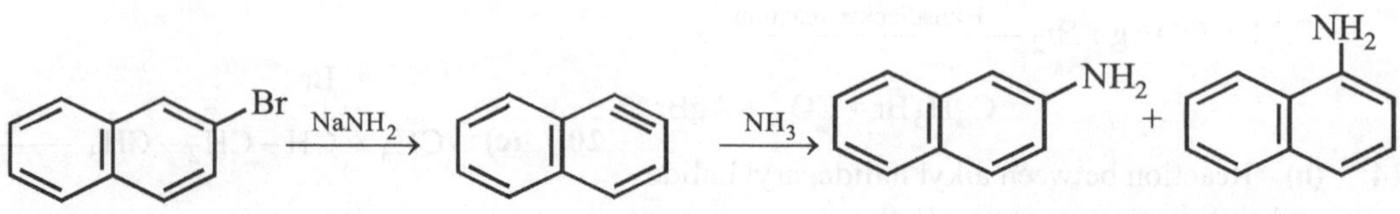


β–and α–Naphthylamines

**30.** **(b)**

# 25 Alcohols, Phenols and Ethers

1. **(a)** $2°$ Alcohols are more easily oxidised than $3°$ alcohols.

2. **(a)** More stable the carbocation more is the rate towards HBr (acid). $-OCH_3$ group exerts + M effect, hence stabilisers the carbocation, while – Br and $-NO_2$ extert – I effect hence destabilise the cabocation.

3. **(a)**

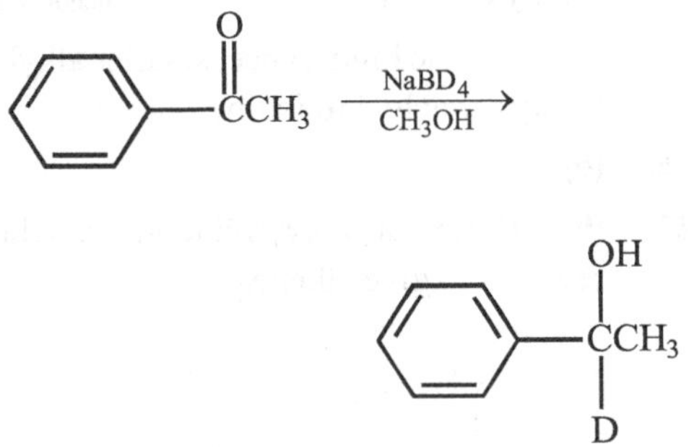

During reduction of carbonyl gp. by $NaBH_4$, hydride ion is supplied by $NaBH_4$.

4. **(d)**

$$CH_3-\underset{\displaystyle CH_3}{\underset{|}{CH}}-O-H \xrightarrow{CH_3MgBr} CH_4 \text{ (Major product)}$$

Acid-base reaction takes place.

5. **(b)** $CrO_3$ / pyridine is mild oxidising agent and oxidises

$1°$ Alcohol $\rightarrow$ Aldehyde

$2°$ Alcohol $\rightarrow$ Ketone

6. **(a)** Hydration via hydroboration - oxidation occurs accordring to *anti*-Markovnikoff's rule.

7. **(b)** This behaviour is related to the relative stabilities of carbocations ($3° > 2° > 1° > \overset{+}{C}H_3$).

8. **(b)** Greater the stability of the intermediate carbocation, more reactive is the alcohol. Since 2-methylpropan-2-ol generates $3°$ carbocation, therefore, it reacts fastest with HBr.

9. **(a)** $$\underset{1°\text{ Alcohol}}{RCH_2OH} \xrightarrow[300°C]{Cu} \underset{\text{Aldehyde}}{RCHO} + H_2$$

10. **(b)** Conc. HCl, HBr and conc. HCl + $ZnCl_2$ all are nucleophiles, thus convert alcohols to alkyl halides. However, conc. $H_3PO_4$ is a good dehydrating agent which converts an alcohol to an alkene.

11. **(d)** $C_6H_5CH_2OH$ has neither $CH_3CO-$ group nor $CH_3\underset{\displaystyle R}{\underset{|}{C}}HOH$ group.

12. **(c)** Because of larger number of intermolecular hydrogen bonding (three per molecule) in case of glycerol ($CH_2OH - CHOH - CH_2OH$ ) as compared to ethanol ($CH_3CH_2OH$), the attraction between molecules of glycerol is more than that between molecules of ethanol. Due to this glycerol is more viscous than ethanol.

13. **(a)** *o*-Nitrophenol has low b.p. due to chelation.

14. **(c)** $-COCH_3$ exerts – I and – M effects which stabilise the phenoxide ion; $-CH_2CH_3$ exerts + I effect which destabilise the phenoxide ion, $-OCH_3$ exerts + M effect which is more powerful than the + I effect of $-CH_2CH_3$ group.

15. **(a)**

16. **(c)** Due to strong electron-donating effect due to + M effect of the OH group, the electron density in phenol is much higher than that in toluene, benzene and chlorobenzene and hence phenol is readily attacked by the electrophile.

17. (d)

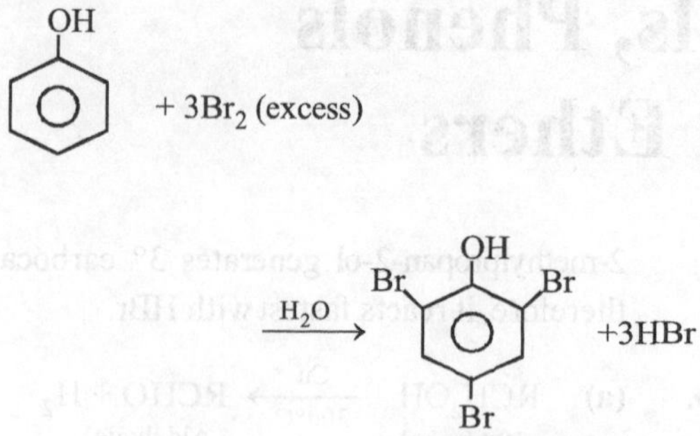

2, 4, 6-Tribromophenol

18. (c)

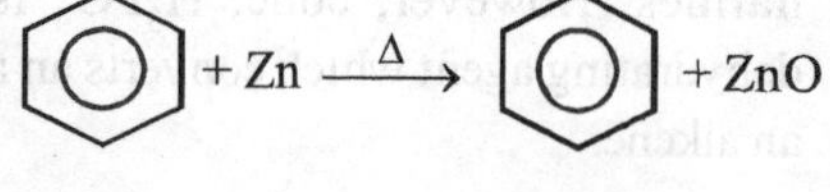

Phenol Benzene

19. (c)

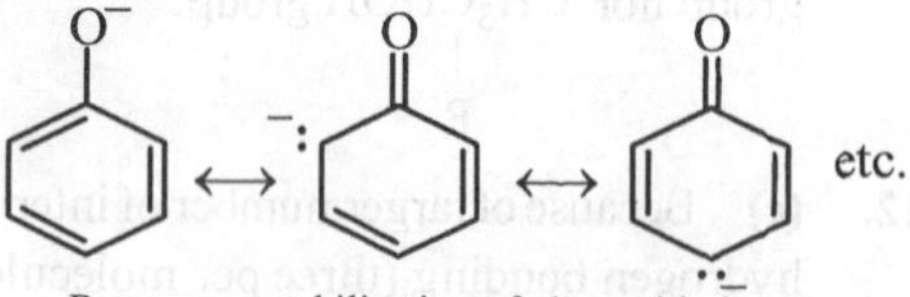

Resonance stabilisation of phenoxide ion (conjugate base of phenol)

Conjugate base of ethyl alcohol, i.e., $C_2H_5O^-$ does not show resonance.

20. (a)

21. (a)

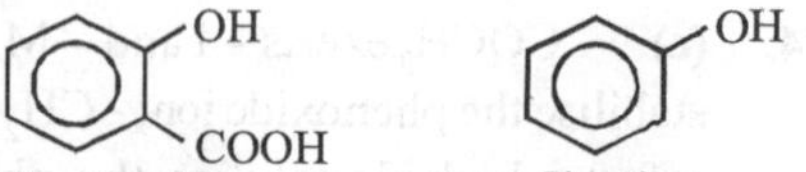

Salicylic acid (evolves $CO_2$ with $NaHCO_3$) Phenol (No reaction with $NaHCO_3$)

22. (a)

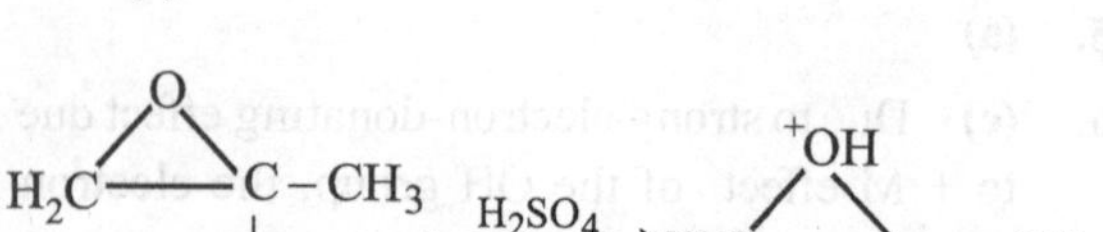

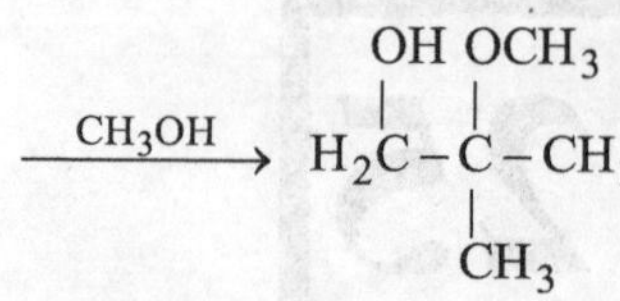

23. (b) Williamson's synthesis -

$$CH_3-CH_2-ONa+Br-CH_2-CH_3 \rightarrow$$

$$CH_3-CH_2-O-CH_2-CH_3$$

24. (b) Only alkyl aryl ethers e.g., $C_6H_5OCH_3$ undergo electrophilic substitution reactions.

25. (d) $R-O-Ar+HI \longrightarrow Ar-OH + RI$

Aryl-alkyl ether Phenol Alkyl iodide

Due to steric hinderance, smaller alkyl group is always attached to iodine.

26. (d)

27. (b) The tertiary alkyl halide undergo elimination reaction to give alkenes

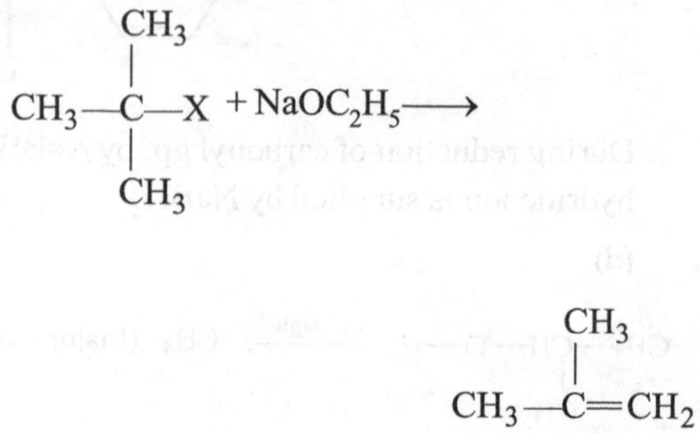

2-Methyl propene

28. (c) **Cannizzaro reaction** is given by aldehydes having no α-hydrogen atom to form a mixture of alcohol and sodium salt of the acid. It is a disproportionation reaction in which half of the aldehyde molecules are oxidised and other half reduced in presence of NaOH.

$$2C_6H_5CHO \xrightarrow{NaOH} C_6H_5CH_2OH + C_6H_5COONa$$

29. (c)

30. (d)

# 26 Aldehydes, Ketones and Carboxylic Acids

1. **(d)** Wolff-Kishner reduction is carried out in basic condition whereas Clemmensen reduction is carried out in acidic condition. Epoxides are unstable in both acidic and basic medium.

2. **(c)** $CH_3CHO \xrightarrow[\text{(ii)}\,\Delta]{\text{(i) NaOH}} CH_3-CH=CH-CHO$

$\xrightarrow{H_2/Ni} \underset{\text{(A)}}{CH_3-CH_2-CH_2-CH_2-OH}$

3. **(b)** Compounds having $-\overset{\overset{O}{\|}}{C}-CH_3$ group show positive iodoform.

Hence, $CH_3-CH_2-CH_2-\overset{\overset{O}{\|}}{C}-CH_3$ (pentanone-2) gives this test.

4. **(c)** Only acetaldehyde and methyl ketones react with $I_2$ and alkali to give iodoform.

5. **(b)**

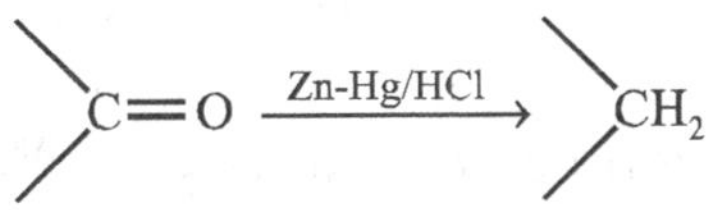

Ketone Alkane

6. **(d)** 2

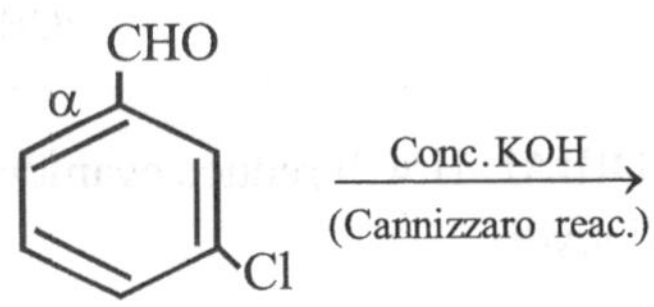

*m*-Chlorobenzaldehyde

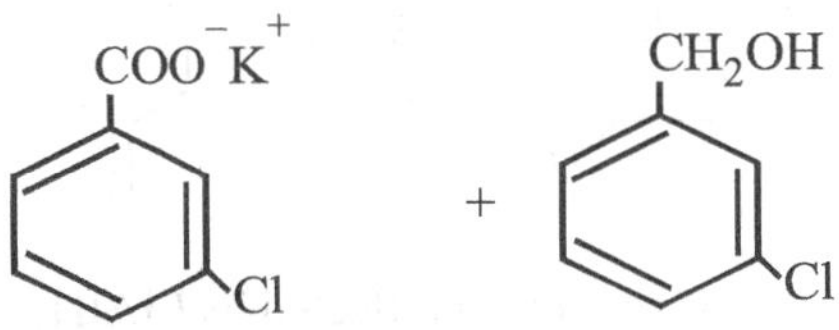

Pot. *m*-chlorobenzoate *m*-Chlorobenzyl alcohol

7. **(d)** Aldehydes which contain a $\alpha$-hydrogen on a saturated carbon, i.e., $CH_3CH_2CHO$ undergo aldol condensation.

$$\underset{\text{Propanal (2 molecules)}}{CH_3CH_2-\overset{H}{\overset{|}{C}}=O} + H-\overset{CH_3}{\overset{|}{C}}\underset{\overset{|\alpha}{H}}{}-CHO$$

$$\xrightarrow{OH^-} \underset{\text{3-Hydroxy-2-methylpentanal}}{CH_3CH_2-\overset{H}{\overset{\beta|}{\underset{\underset{OH}{|}}{C}}}-\overset{CH_3}{\overset{\alpha|}{C}}HCHO}$$

8. **(d)** Compounds having – CHO group reduce Tollen's reagent to silver mirror. It is called silver mirror test.

9. **(a)** In this reaction, one molecule is oxidised and other is reduced simultaneously.

10. **(b)** It is an example of Perken reaction.

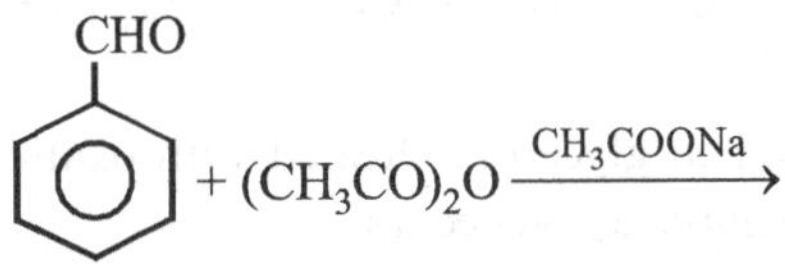

Benzaldehyde

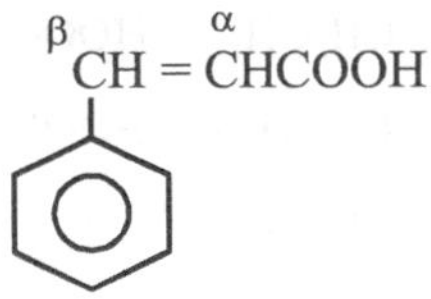

Cinnamic acid

11. **(d)** $C_6H_5CHO + KOH \longrightarrow C_6H_5CH_2OH + C_6H_5COOK$

No new C–C bond is formed in either of the products.

12. (b) β-Keto acid

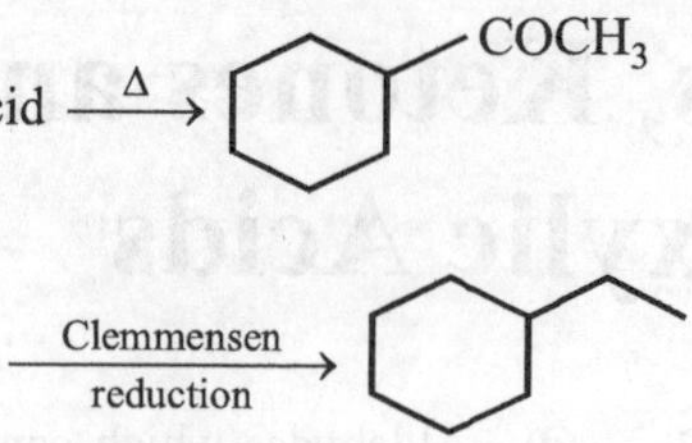

13. (b) $LiAlH_4$ reduces $>C=O \longrightarrow >CHOH$ group without affecting the double bond.

14. (b)

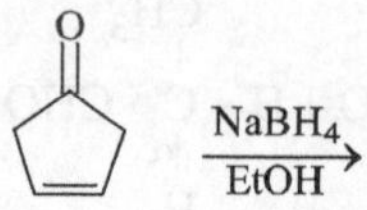

$NaBH_4$ does not reduce the double bond but can reduce keto group ( $>C=O$) into —OH group.

15. (a) Carboxylic acid is stronger acid than phenol. The presence of electron withdrawing group (e.g. Cl) increases acidic strength, while presence of electron donating group (e.g. $CH_3$) decreases acidic strength.

16. (a) Drugs which relieve pain are called analgesics. Aspirin (acetylsalicylic acid) is a non-narcotic analgesic.

17. (c) $C_6H_5COOH + SOCl_2 \longrightarrow C_6H_5COCl + SO_2 + HCl$

18. (c) When glycerol is heated with oxalic acid following reaction occurs.

$$\underset{\text{Glycerol}}{CH_2OH\text{–}CHOH\text{–}CH_2OH} + \underset{\text{Oxalic acid}}{HOOC\text{–}COOH} \xrightarrow[-H_2O]{100\text{–}110°C} CH_2OOC.COOH\text{–}CHOH\text{–}CH_2OH$$

$$\xrightarrow{-CO_2} CH_2COOH\text{–}CHOH\text{–}CH_2OH \xrightarrow{H_2O} CH_2OH\text{–}CHOH\text{–}CH_2OH + \underset{\text{Formic acid}}{HCOOH}$$

19. (a)

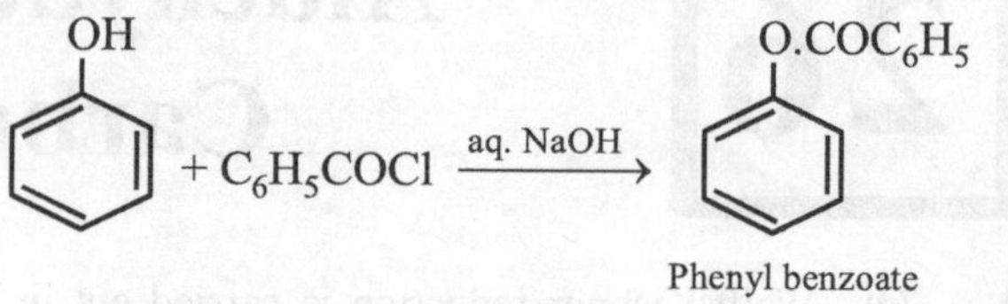

The function of NaOH is

(i) To convert phenol to more stronger nucleophile $PhO^-$.

(ii) To neutralize the acid formed.

20. (d)

$$RCOCl + AlCl_3 \longrightarrow \underset{\substack{\text{Acylium cation}\\ \text{(Electrophile)}}}{R\text{–}\overset{O}{\overset{\|}{C}}{}^{\oplus}} + AlCl_4^-$$

21. (c)

$$CH_3CH_2COOH \xrightarrow[\text{red P}]{Cl_2} \underset{A}{CH_3CHClCOOH}$$

$$\xrightarrow[-HCl]{\text{alc. KOH}} \underset{\text{Acrylic acid, B}}{CH_2=CHCOOH}$$

22. (d) $\underset{\text{Acetic anhydride}}{(CH_3CO)_2O} + \underset{\text{Diethyl ether}}{C_2H_5OC_2H_5} \xrightarrow{AlCl_3} \underset{\text{Ethyl acetate}}{2CH_3COOC_2H_5}$

23. (c) DIBAL-H will reduce cyanides and esters to aldehydes.

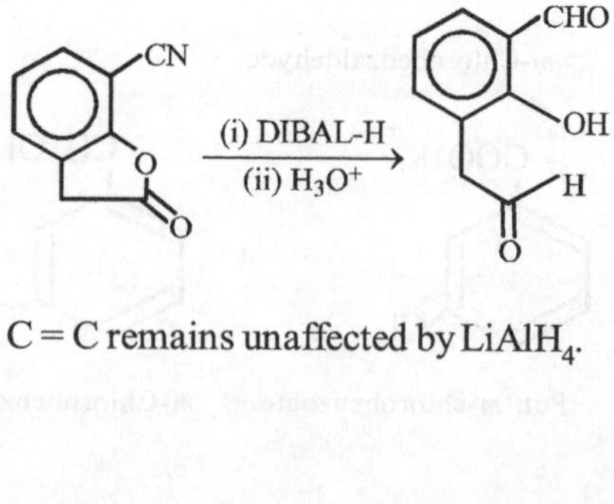

$C=C$ remains unaffected by $LiAlH_4$.

**24. (c)**

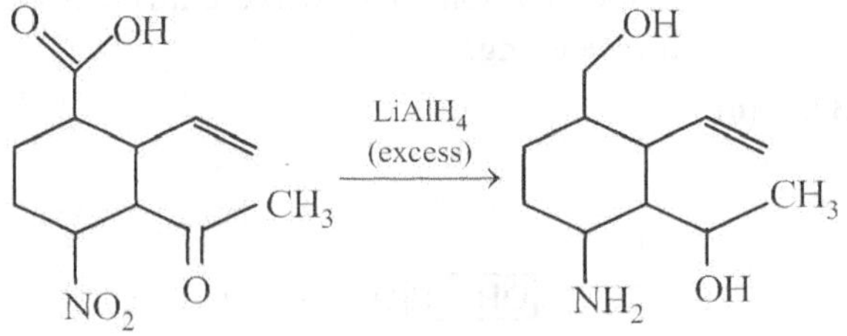

C = C remains unaffected by $LiAlH_4$.

**25. (c)**

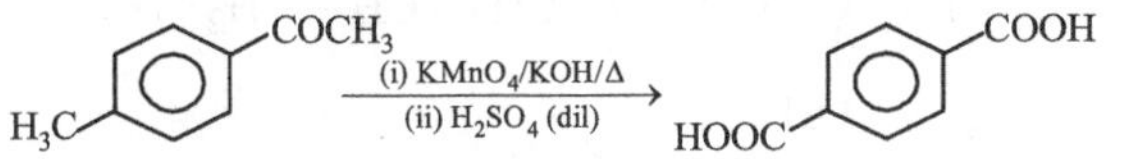

**26. (c)**

**27. (b)** β-Ketoacids undergo decarboxylation easily.

**28. (b)**

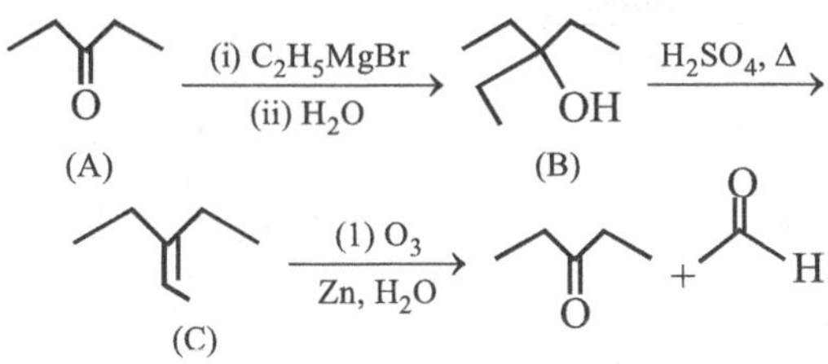

**29. (b)**

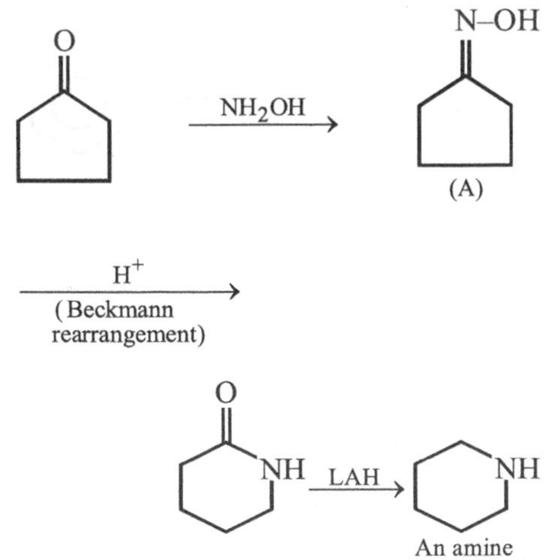

Amides on reduction with $LiAlH_4$ form amines, not alcohols.

**30. (a)**

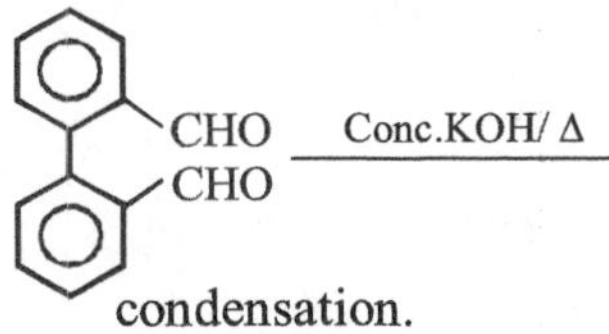

No α-H, condensation.
hence no aldol

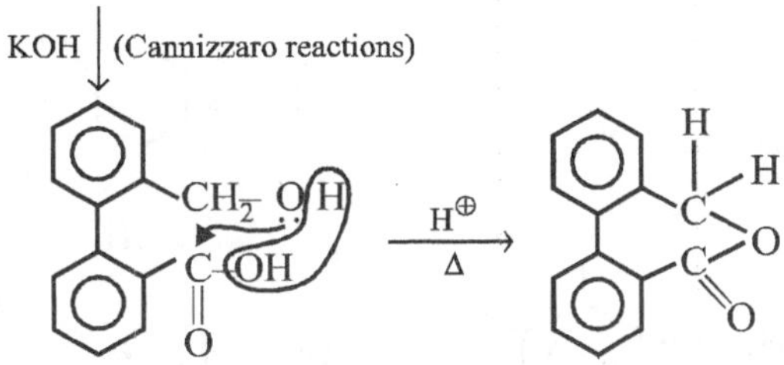

**31. (a)**

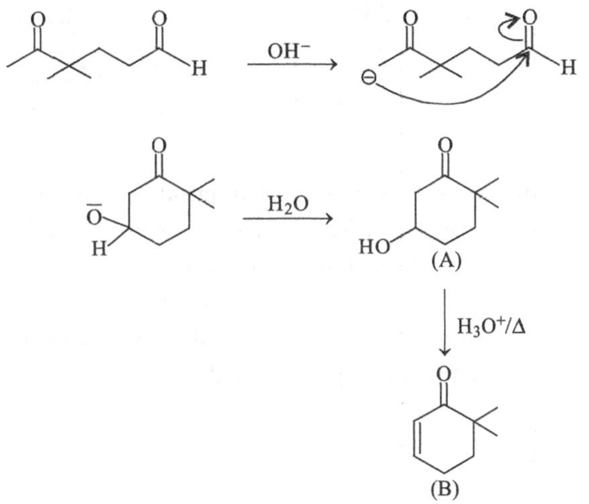

**32. (d)** Reaction involved:

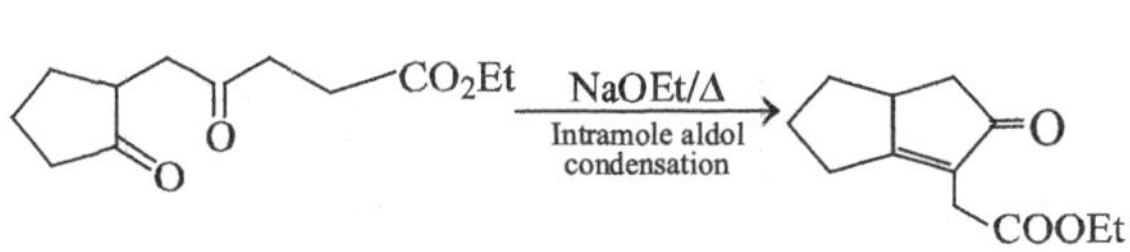

**33. (c)**

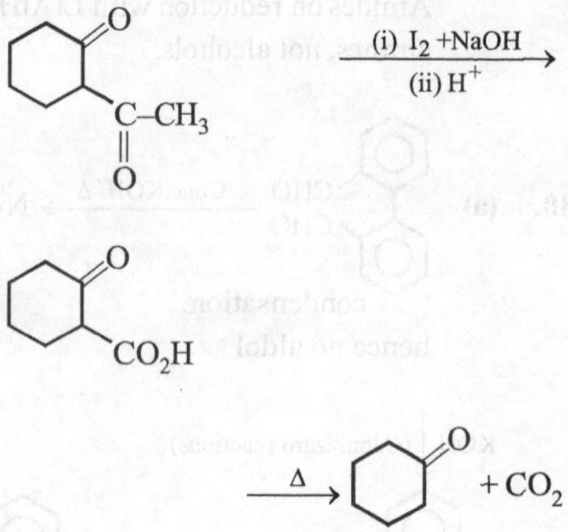

**34. (c)**

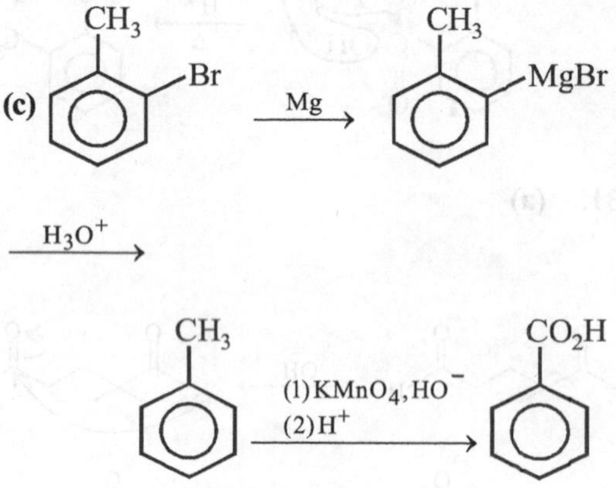

**35. (b)** It is an example of internal Cannizzaro reaction, where –CHO is oxidised while ketonic group of the same molecule is reduced. Since aldehyde group is more susceptible to oxidation, it is oxidised and ketonic group is reduced.

**36. (c)**

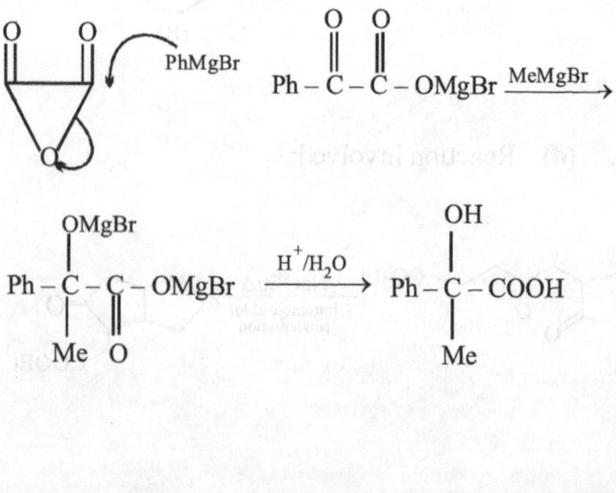

The ketonic group attached to phenyl group is more electron deficient due to delocalisation of positive charge over benzene ring.

**37. (b)**

$$CH_3-\underset{OH}{\overset{H}{C}}-CO\boxed{OH+H}O-CH_2-CH=CH_2$$

$$\downarrow$$

$$CH_3-\underset{OH}{\overset{H}{C}}-CO-O-CH_2-CH=CH_2+H_2O$$

X (Ester)

**38. (d)** $CH_3COOH \xrightarrow{SOCl_2} CH_3-\overset{O}{\overset{||}{C}}-Cl$ (A)

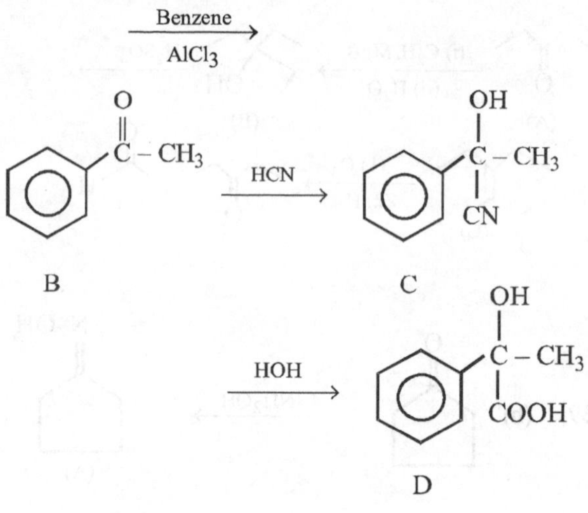

**39. (a)** (A)

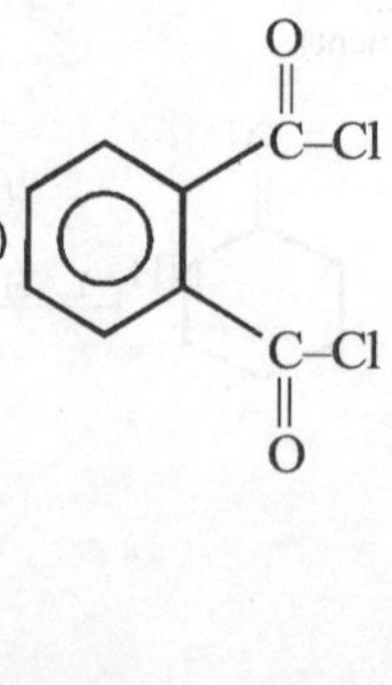

(B) 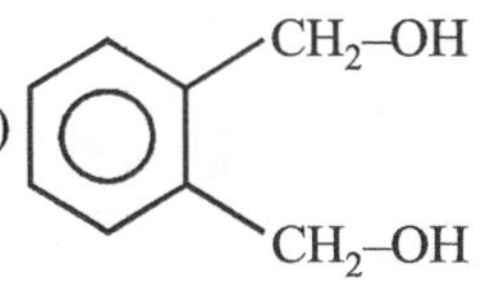

(C) 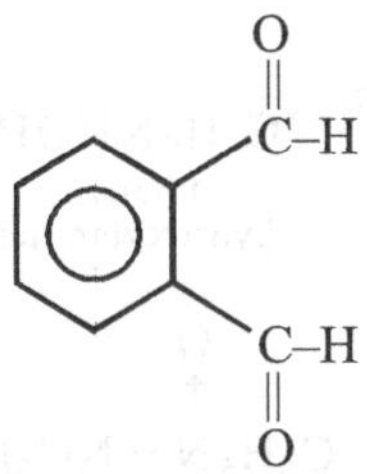

(D) 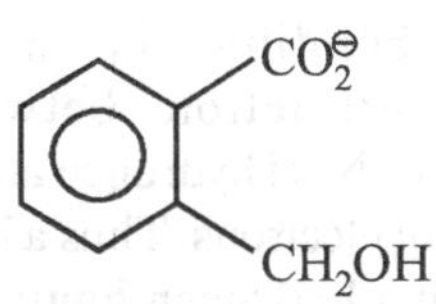

**40. (c)**

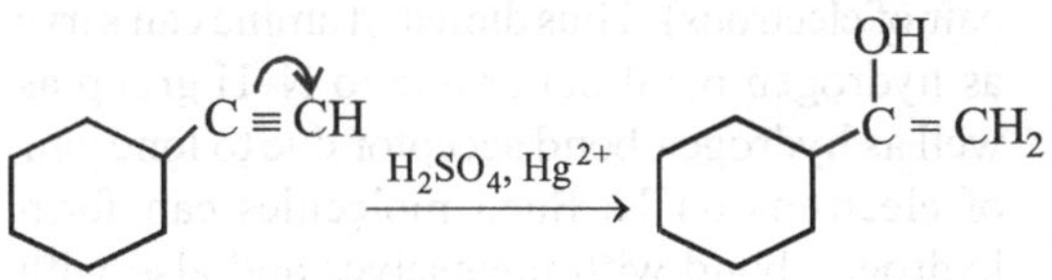

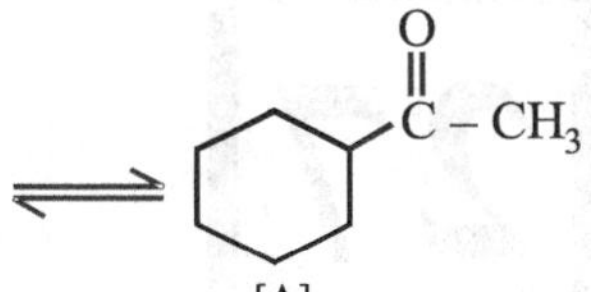

[A]

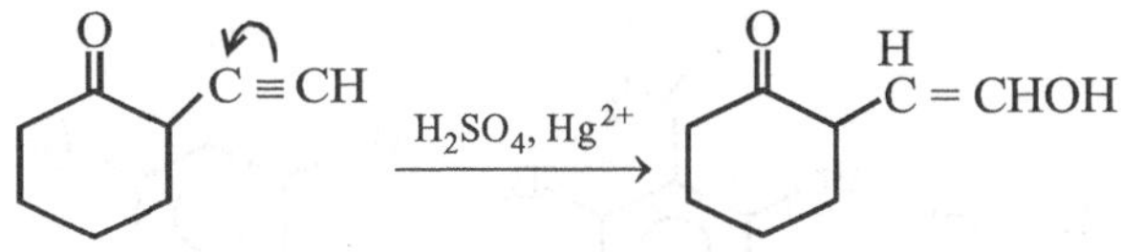

Due to electronegative nature of > C = O, π electrons are transferred toward ring

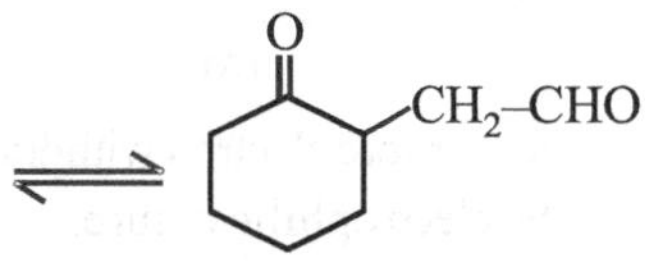

[B]

# 27 Amines

1. (b)

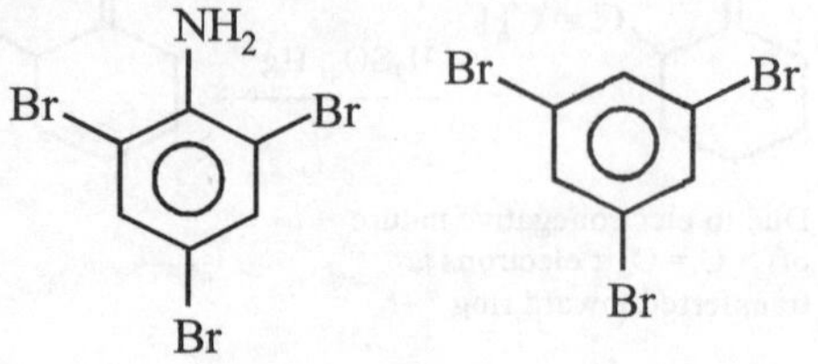

(A) (B)

2. (b) More electron withdrawing group, more will be electrophilic nature.

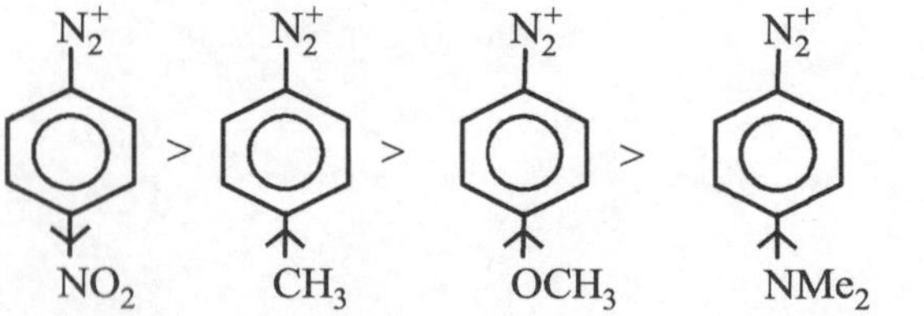



– I effect > + I effect > +M effect > More +M effect

3. (a) On reduction with Zn and HCl, $C_6H_5N_2Cl$ forms aniline as the final product.
4. (c) The first compound will give azo dye

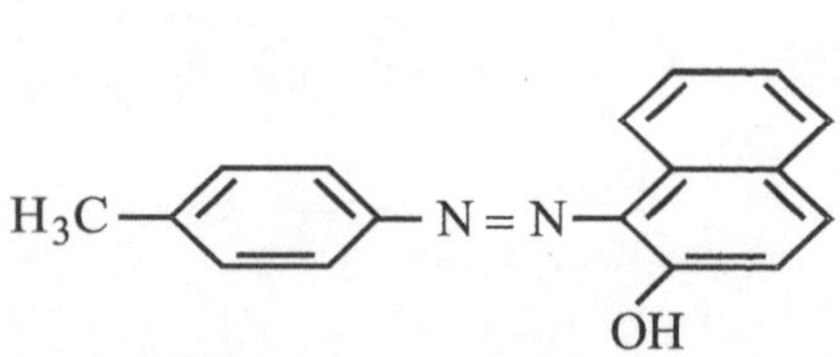



5. (c) When nitrobenzene is reduced in alkaline medium like $Na_3AsO_3$ / NaOH or glucose / NaOH, azoxybenzene is formed as the reduction product.

$$C_6H_5NO_2 \xrightarrow[-H_2O]{2H} C_6H_5NO \xrightarrow{2H} C_6H_5NHOH$$

$$\underset{\text{Nitroso benzene}}{C_6H_5NO} + \underset{\text{Phenyl hydroxylamine}}{C_6H_5NHOH} \longrightarrow \underset{\text{Azoxybenzene}}{C_6H_5\overset{\overset{O}{\uparrow}}{N} = NC_6H_5} + H_2O$$

6. (b) Hydrogen bonding is a strong intermolecular attraction between an electrophilic O–H or N–H hydrogen atom and a pair of non-bonding electrons. Thus a hydrogen bond requires both a **hydrogen bond donor** (a molecule having O–H or N–H group) and a **hydrogen bond acceptor** (a molecule having lone pair of electrons). Thus dimethyl amine can serve as hydrogen bond donor due to N–H group as well as hydrogen bond acceptor due to lone pair of electrons on N. Such molecules can form hydrogen bond with themselves and also with water (or other hydrogen bond donor). On the other hand, trimethyl amine can serve only as hydrogen bond acceptor since it has lone pair of electrons but not hydrogen on N. Hence it can form hydrogen bond with water but not with themselves.

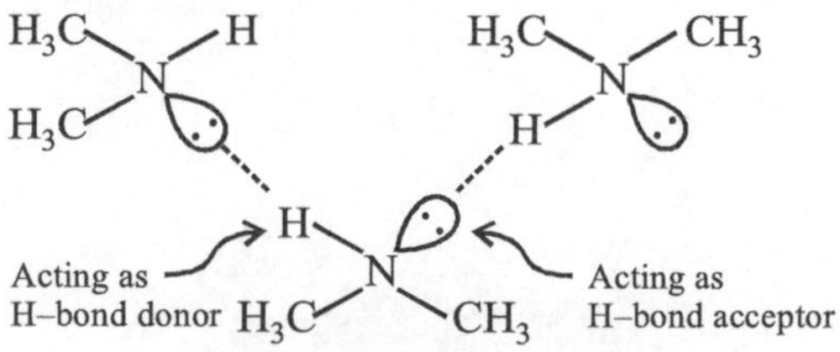



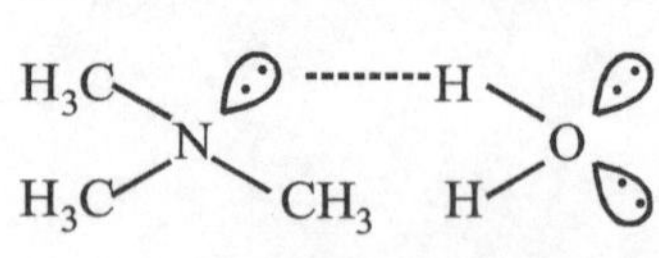

Trimethyl amine only as H– bond acceptor

7. (b)

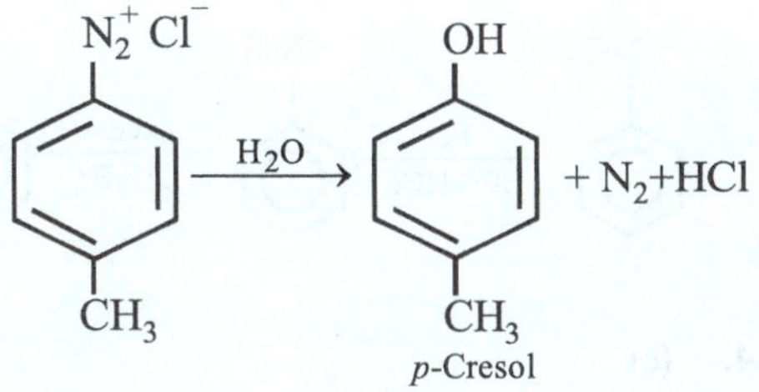

8. (a)

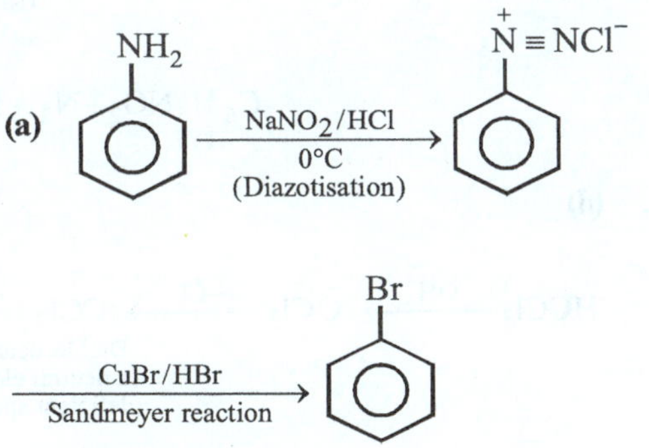

9. (d) $CH_3COONH_4 \xrightarrow{\Delta} \underset{(X)}{CH_3CONH_2}$

$\xrightarrow{\Delta/P_2O_5} \underset{(Y)}{CH_3CN} \xrightarrow{H_3O^{\oplus}} \underset{(Z)}{CH_3COOH}$

10. (a) $\begin{matrix} C_6H_5 \\ CH_3 \end{matrix}\!\!>C=O \xrightarrow{H_2NOH}$

$\underset{\text{Oxime}}{\begin{matrix} C_6H_5 \\ CH_3 \end{matrix}\!\!>C=NOH} \xrightarrow[\text{(Beckmann rearrangement)}]{PCl_5}$

$\underset{\text{Acetanilide}}{C_6H_5NHCOCH_3}$

11. (c) Reaction with nitrous acid at low temperature to give an oily nitrosoamine is characteristic of secondary aliphatic amines.

12. (a)

$CH_3-\underset{\underset{CH_2}{|}}{CH}-CH_3 \xrightarrow[H_2O]{HNO_2} CH_3-\underset{\underset{\text{OH}}{|}}{CH}-CH_3$ (A)

$\xrightarrow{[O]} CH_3-\underset{\underset{O}{\|}}{C}-CH_3 \xrightarrow[H^+/H_2O]{CH_3MgI}$

$CH_3-\overset{\overset{CH_3}{|}}{\underset{\underset{OH}{|}}{C}}-CH_3$

(C)

1,1–Dimethyl ethanol

13. (a) $\underset{\text{Ethyl amine}}{C_2H_5NH_2} + \underset{\text{Nitrous acid}}{HNO_2} \xrightarrow{273–278K}$

$\underset{\text{Ethanol}}{C_2H_5OH} + N_2 + H_2O$

14. (c) Completing the given reaction, we get

$CH_3CONH_2 \xrightarrow[\Delta]{P_2O_5} \underset{X}{CH_3C\equiv N} \xrightarrow{Sn/HCl} \underset{\text{Ethanamine, Y}}{CH_3CH_2NH_2}$

15. (b)

$\underset{\text{Ethyl amine}}{C_2H_5NH_2} \xrightarrow{HNO_2} \underset{\text{Ethyl alcohol, A}}{C_2H_5OH} \xrightarrow{PCl_5} \underset{B}{C_2H_5Cl}$

$\xrightarrow{NH_3} \underset{\text{Ethyl amine, C}}{C_2H_5NH_2}$

16. (c)

17. (d) Electron pair on N in $C_6H_5CH_2\ddot{N}H_2$ is localised.

18. (d) In acidic condition, protonation of $-NH_2$ group gives anilinium ion $(C_6H_5\overset{+}{N}H_3)$, which is deactivating and *m*-directing in nature.

**19. (b)**

$C_2H_5NH_2 > (CH_3)_2NH > CH_3NH_2 > (CH_3)_3N$

Strong + I; + I as well as solvation effect; + I effect; Solvation and steric factor

**20. (a)** 1° Amine is on reaction with HONO converted into alcohol.

**21. (b)**

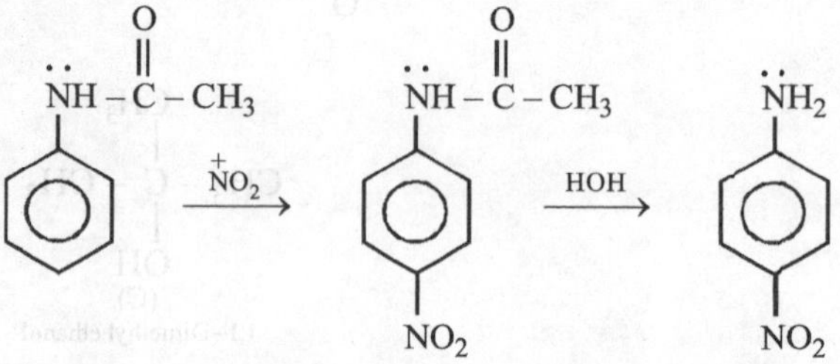

**22. (d)** The reaction involves the conversion of one $NO_2$ to $NH_2$ group (reduction) which occurs in presence of $NH_4HS$.

**23. (b)**

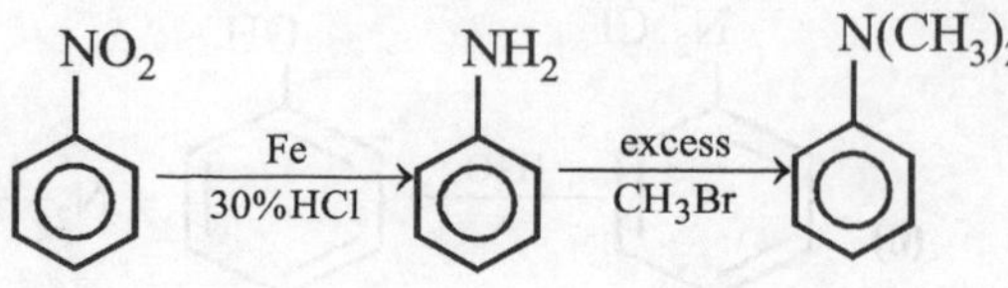

**24. (c)**

$$C_6H_5NH_2 \xrightarrow[0°C-5°C]{NaNO_2/HCl} \underset{(X)}{C_6H_5N_2^+Cl^-} \xrightarrow[H_2O]{HNO_2} \underset{(Y)}{C_6H_5NO_2} + N_2 + HCl$$

**25. (d)**

$$HCCl_3 \xrightarrow{OH^-} :\bar{C}Cl_3 \xrightarrow{-Cl^-} :CCl_2$$

Dichlorocarbene (a neutral electron deficient species)

# 28 Biomolecules

1. **(d)** We know that glucose reacts with one molecule of phenyl hydrazine to give phenyl hydrazone. When warmed with excess of phenylhydrazine, the secondary alcoholic group adjacent to the aldehyde group is oxidised by another molecule of phenylhydrazine to a ketonic group. With this ketonic group, the third molecule of phenylhydrazine condenses to glucosazone. Therefore the value of X is 3

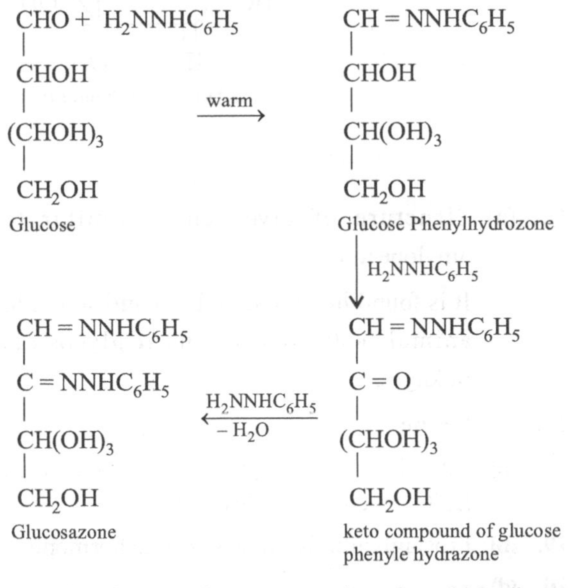


2. **(d)** Sucrose does not contain a free aldehydic or ketonic group hence it does not show mutarotation.

3. **(c)** In sucrose the two monosaccharides are held together by glycosidic linkage and not by peptide linkage.

4. **(a)** Due to resonance C — N bond in protein acquires double bond character and is smaller than usual C — N bond.

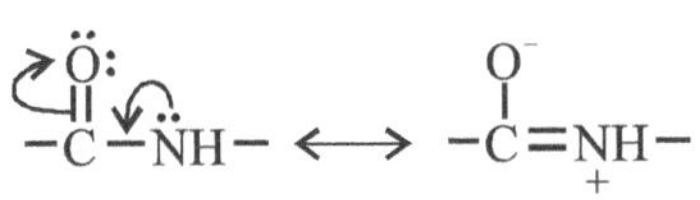

5. **(d)**

6. **(a)** Isoelectric point (pH)

$$= \frac{pK_{a_1} + pK_{a_2}}{2} = \frac{2.34 + 9.60}{2} = 5.97$$

7. **(d)** All are chiral

8. **(d)** Mg acts as a cofactor to the enzyme as it forms complex with phosphate group of ATP that is utilized in the transfer of ATP phosphate.

9. **(b)** DNA consists of two polynucleotide chains, each chain forms a right handed spiral with ten bases in one turn of the spiral. The two chains coil to double helix and run in opposite direction held together by hydrogen bonding.

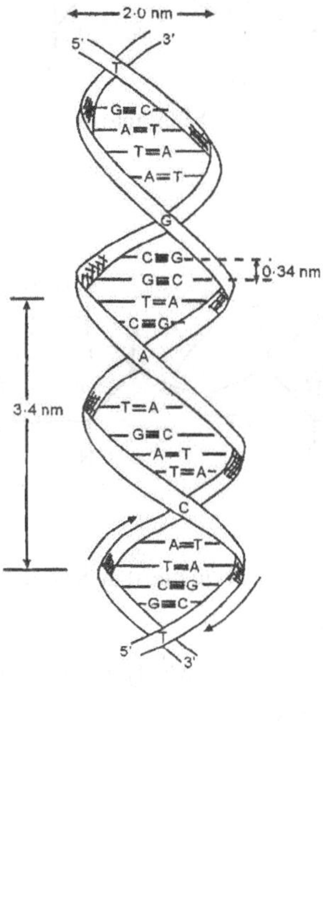

**10.** **(d)**

| Vitamin | Disease caused by deficiency |
|---|---|
| $B_6$ | Dermatitis |
| $B_1$ | Beri-beri |
| $B_2$ | Photophobia, glossitis |
| $B_{12}$ | Pernicious anaemia |

**11.** **(b)** Triglycerides are lipids, hence these are hydrolysed by *lipases* to glycerol and fatty acids.

**12.** **(c)** Vitamin A - Xerophthalmia

Vitamin $B_{12}$ - Pernicious anaemia

Vitamin C - Scurvy

Vitamin E - Sterility

**13.** **(a)** Lactose contains β -glycosidic linkage between $C_1$ of galactose and $C_4$ of glucose.

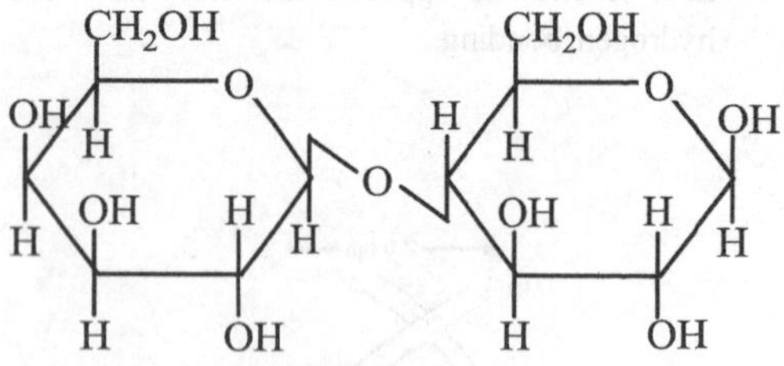

β -D-Galactose

**14.** **(c)**

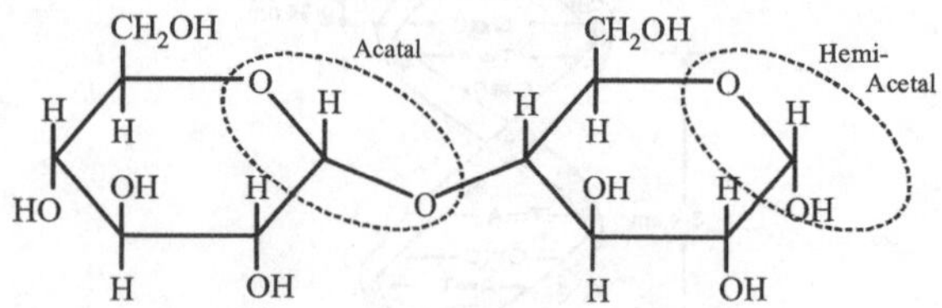


Maltose

One acetal and one hemi acetal group is present in maltose.

**15.** **(d)** Maltose on hydrolysis gives two moles of α-D-glucose.

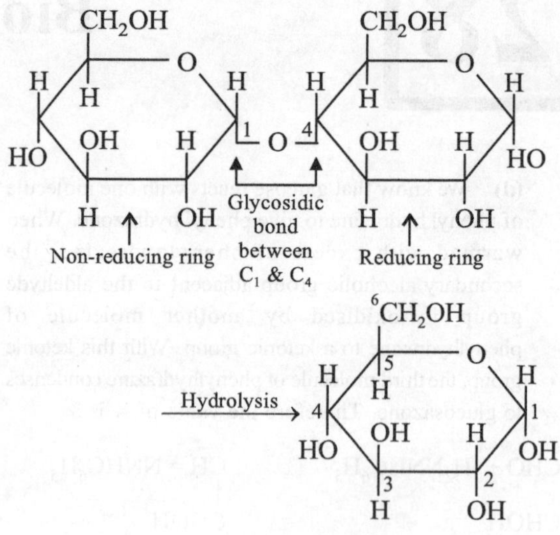


α-D-Glucose (2 moles)

**16.** **(a)** Structure of glycogen is similar to amylopectin.

It is found in yeast and fungi and stored in animal body. It contains α-glycosidic linkages.

**17.** **(b)** Lysine

**18.** **(a)** Vitamin $B_6$ is called pyridoxine. It is found in fruits, green-vegetables, milk, etc.

**19.** **(b)** Prostaglandin is a non-steroidal hormone.

**20.** **(d)**

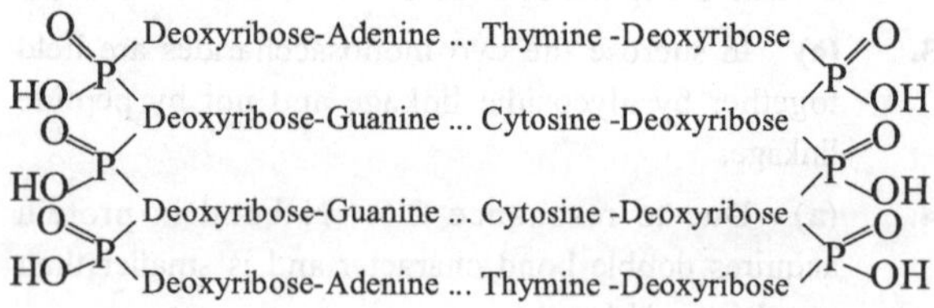

The hydrogen bonds (shown by dotted lines) are formed between the bases. Because of size and geometries of the bases, the only possible pairing in DNA is between G(Guanine) and C(Cytosine) through three H-bonds and between A (Adenine) and T (Thymine) through two H-bonds.

**21. (d)** Glucose being an aldose responds to Tollen's test, while fructose, although a ketose, undergoes rearrangement in presence of basic medium (provided by Tollen's reagent) to form glucose, which then responds to Tollen's test.

**22. (c)** Sucrose does not have free –CHO or –CO group, hence it does not reduce Benedict's solution. Remember that fructose has an α-hydroxy ketonic group, which is also reducing group (difference from ordinary ketonic group)

**23. (a)**

**24. (c)** Butyric acid (butanoic acid) is found in milk, and butter and is a product of anaerobic fermentation. It has an unpleasant smell and acrid taste.

**25. (a)**

# 29 Polymers

1. **(b)**

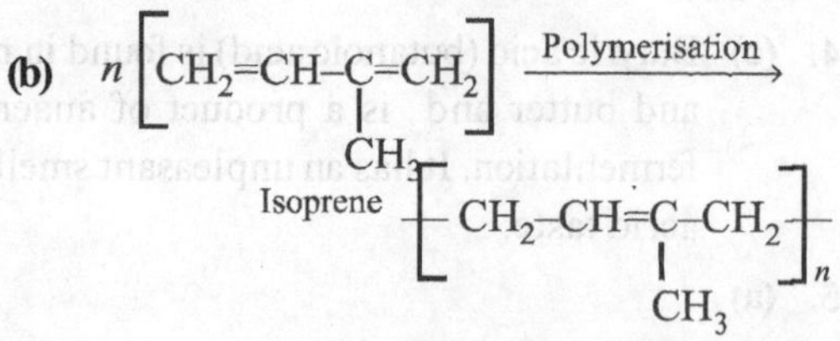


Polyisoprene (Natural rubber)

2. **(d)**
3. **(d)** These are characteristics of thermosets.
4. **(d)** All the given statements about fibres are correct.
5. **(b)**
6. **(b)** Perlon is nylon-6. It is prepared from a single monomer (caprolactam) having a potential amino group at one end and a potential carbonyl group at other end.
7. **(b)** $nCH_2 = CH - CH = CH_2 + n$

1, 3-Butadiene

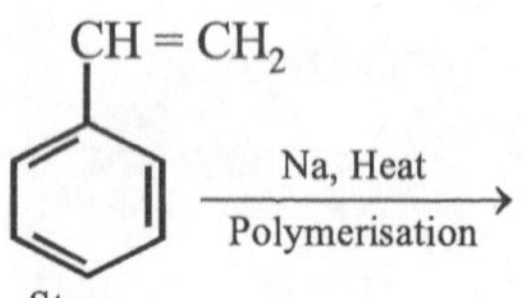


Styrene

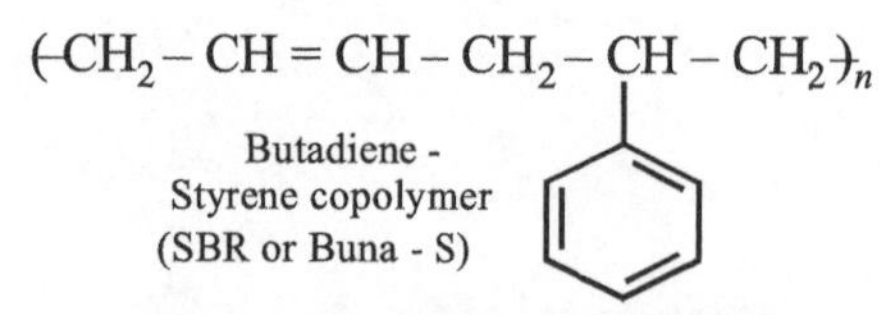

Butadiene - Styrene copolymer (SBR or Buna - S)

8. **(a)** Melamine plastic crockery is a copolymer of HCHO and melamine.
9. **(d)** Teflon or polytetrafluoroethene is an addition polymer and its monomer is alkene derivative ($CF_2{=}CF_2$), whereas terylene, melamine and nylon-6, 6 are condensation polymers.

10. **(d)** Phenol and formaldehyde undergo condensation polymerisation under two different conditions to give a cross linked polymer called bakelite.

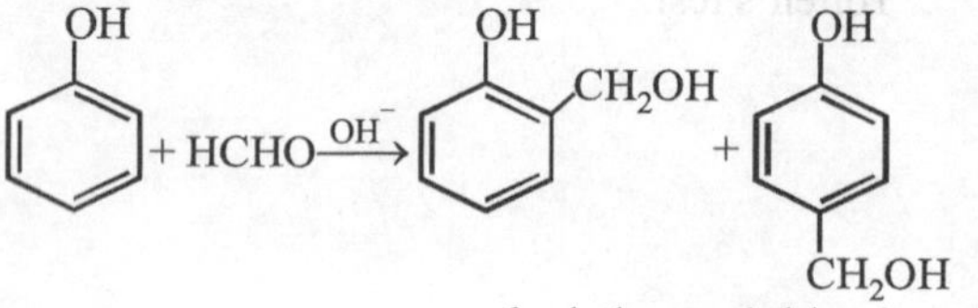

*o* & *p*-hydroxymethylphenol (intermediate)

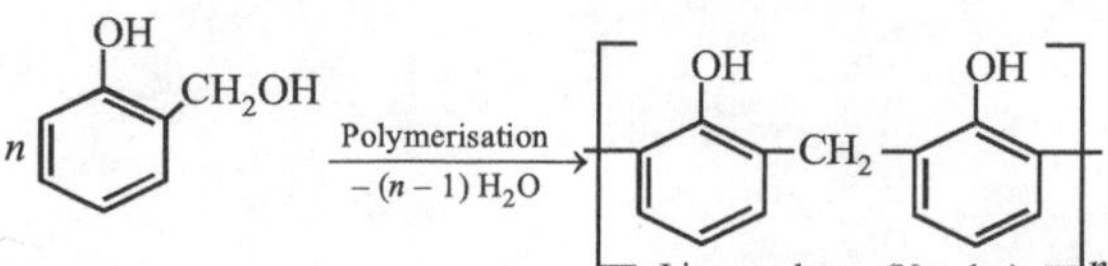


Linear polymer (Novalac)

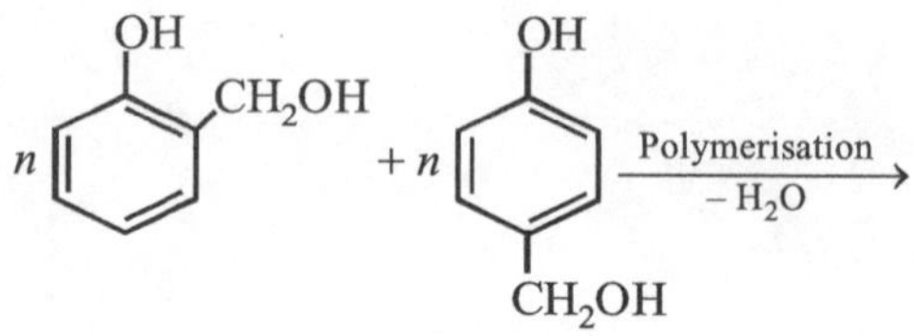


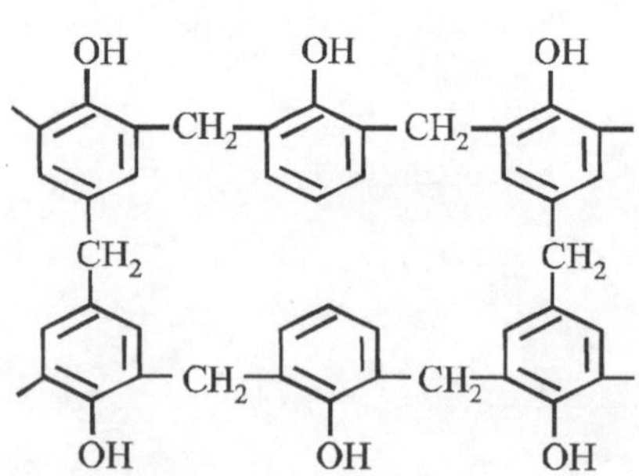

Bakelite

**11.** **(b)**

**12.** **(d)**

**13.** **(b)**

**14.** **(c)** Polythene is a linear polymer

**15.** **(c)** $\text{PDI} = \dfrac{\overline{M}_w}{\overline{M}_n}$

For synthetic polymer, PDI > 1

$\therefore \overline{M}_w > \overline{M}_n$

**16.** **(a)** Ethene on free radical polymerisation gives low density polythene.

**17.** **(d)** Polymethyl methacrylate (PMMA) is hard, fairly rigid. It is used for optical lenses.

**18.** **(a)** SARAN, a polymer of vinyl chloride ($CH_2$=CHCl) and vinylidene chloride, is used for making synthetic hair wigs.

**19.** **(d)** Nylon tyre cord is made from high tenacity continuous filament yarn by twisting and plying.

**20.** **(d)**

# 30 Chemistry in Everyday Life

1. (b) Paracetamol is an antipyretic
2. (a) Salol is phenyl salicylate used as antiseptic.
3. (d) Equanil is used in depression and hypertension.
4. (b) Terfenadine is commonly used as antihistamine.
5. (b)
6. (c) Sulphonamides act as antimicrobials.
7. (c) Paraldehyde is a hypnotic.
8. (d)
9. (d) Sulpha drugs (antibacterials and antibiotics) are group of drugs which are derivatives of sulphanilamide.
10. (c) Gammexane is an insecticide.
11. (b)
12. (c)
13. (d)
14. (d) Vitamin E is an antioxidant present in edible oils.
15. (c)
16. (d) Dettol (antiseptic) is a mixture of 4.8% chloroxylenol + 9.9% terpineol and absolute alcohol.
17. (a)
18. (a) 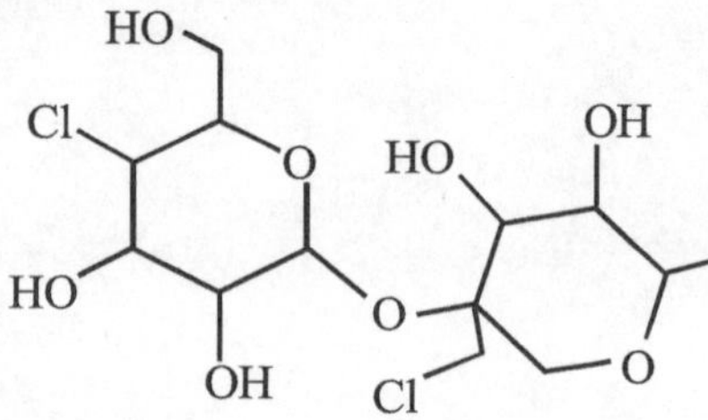 is



sucralose.

19. (d)
20. (b) A detergent molecule consists of a large hydrocarbon group that is non-ionic and a sulphonate ($SO_3^-Na^+$) or a sulphate ($SO_4^-Na^+$) group that is ionic. Examples of detergents are sodium-*n*-dodecyl benzene sulphonate, sodium dodecyl sulphate etc.

# 1 Mock Test -1

1. (d) $BF_3$ is planar triangular while $PF_3$ is pyramidal.

2. (b) Let the wt. of each gas mixed = x g

$\therefore$ mole of $SO_2 = \dfrac{x}{64}$

mole of $CH_4 = \dfrac{x}{16}$

mole of $O_2 = \dfrac{x}{32}$

Total number of moles of the three gases

$$= \frac{x}{64} + \frac{x}{16} + \frac{x}{32} = \frac{7x}{64}$$

Partial pressure exerted by a gas in the mixture of non-reacting gases (p) is given by

$$p = \frac{\text{moles of that gas}}{\text{total moles}} \times \text{Total pressure}$$

$$\therefore p_{CH_4} = \frac{x}{16} \times \frac{64}{7x} \times 2.1 = 1.2\,\text{atm}$$

3. (b) 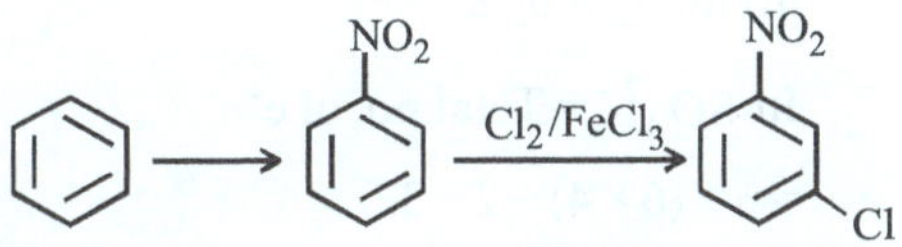


4. (d) Decomposition of carbonates and hydrated oxides.

5. (c) Chlorination of methane proceeds via free radical mechanism. Conversion of methyl chloride to methyl alcohol proceeds via nucleophilic substitution. Formation of ethylene from ethyl alcohol proceeds via dehydration reaction. Nitration of benzene is electrophilic substitution reaction.

6. (c) Benzene is non-polar and hence dissolves non-polar compounds (like dissolves like). Among the given compounds, only (c) is non-polar hence it dissolves in benzene.

7. (d) Ozone hole is reduction in ozone layer in stratosphere.

8. (a) In a period on moving from left to right ionic radii decreases.

(a) So order of cationic radii is

$Cr^{2+} > Mn^{2+} > Fe^{2+} > Ni^{2+}$ and

(b) Sc > Ti > Cr > Mn (correct order of atomic radii)

(c) For unpaired electrons

$$Mn^{2+}(\text{Five}) > Ni^{2+}(\text{Two})$$

$$< Co^{2+}(\text{Three}) < Fe^{2+}(\text{Four})$$

(d) For unpaired electrons

$$Fe^{2+}(\text{Four}) > Co^{2+}(\text{Three})$$

$$> Ni^{2+}(\text{Two}) > Cu^{2+}(\text{One})$$

9. (d) The reaction is an example of $S_N1$ reaction

$$CH_3-\underset{|}{\overset{CH_3}{CH}}-CH_2Br \xrightarrow{-Br^-} CH_3-\overset{CH_3}{\underset{|}{CH}}-\overset{+}{C}H_2 \quad (1^\circ\text{ carbocation})$$

$$\xrightarrow{\text{hydride shift}} CH_3-\overset{CH_3}{\overset{|}{C^+}}-CH_3 \quad (3^\circ\text{ carbocation})$$

$$\xrightarrow{^-OCH_3} CH_3-\underset{OCH_3}{\underset{|}{\overset{CH_3}{\overset{|}{C}}}}-CH_3$$

10. (a) According to the (n + l) rule the higher the value of (n + l), the higher is the energy. When (n + l) value is the same see value of n.

| | i | ii | iii | iv |
|---|---|---|---|---|
| (n + l) | (4 + 1) | (4 + 0) | (3 + 2) | (3 + 1) |
| | 5 | 4 | 5 | 4 |

$\therefore$ iv < ii < iii < i

11. (b) For adiabatic process, q = 0

12. (b) $Mn^{2+}$ $(3d^5)$ is more stable than $Mn^{3+}$ $(3d^4)$.

13. (c) In $NH_4NO_3$, there are two different N-atoms $(NH_4^+, NO_3^-)$ with different oxidation numbers, thus reaction is not disproportionation.

14. (c) In case of unsymmetrical ethers, the site of cleavage depends on the nature of alkyl group e.g.,

$$CH_3O-CH(CH_3)_2 + HI \xrightarrow{373K} \underset{\text{Methyl iodide}}{CH_3I} + \underset{\text{Isopropyl alcohol}}{(CH_3)_2CHOH}$$

The alkyl halide is always formed from the smaller alkyl group.

15. (d) $H_2(g) + Br_2(g) \rightleftharpoons 2HBr(g)$

Rate law, $R = k[H_2][Br_2]^{½}$

Order of reaction = 1 + ½ = 3/2

Molecularity of reaction = 2

The unit of $k = \dfrac{R}{[H_2][Br_2]^{½}}$

$= \dfrac{\text{mole. lit}^{-1}\text{s}^{-1}}{[\text{mole. lit}^{-1}][\text{mole. lit}^{-1}]^{½}}$

$= \text{mole}^{-½} . \text{lit}^{½} . \text{s}^{-1}$

16. (b) As the molecular weight of noble gas atoms increases down the group its polarity increases due to which van-der-waal's force between them increases. Due to increased polarity of heavier inert gas, its solubility in water also increases. So, most soluble gas will be Xe and least soluble will be He.

So correct order is Xe > Kr > Ar > Ne > He

17. (a) $\Delta x = \Delta v$

$$\Delta x . \Delta v = \frac{h}{4\pi m}$$

$$\Delta v^2 = \frac{h}{4\pi m}$$

$$\therefore \quad \Delta v = \sqrt{\frac{h}{4\pi m}}$$

$$\therefore \quad \Delta p = m.\Delta v = m\sqrt{\frac{h}{4\pi m}}$$

$$= \frac{1}{2}\sqrt{\frac{hm}{\pi}}$$

18. (c) In case two or more chains are of equal length, then the chain with greater number of side chains is selected as the principal chain.

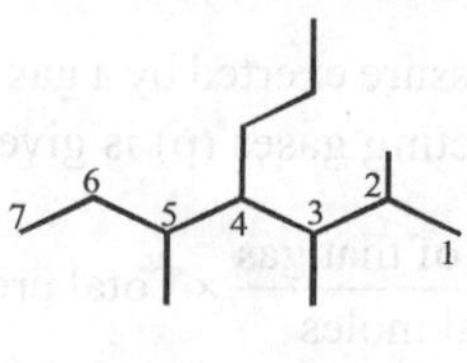

2, 3, 5-Trimethyl-4-propylheptane

19. (c) Hybridisation can be calculated by calculating the no of valence electron and dividing it by 8.

In $SO_4^{2-}$ = Total no. of $e^-$

$= 6 + (6 \times 4) + 2 = 32$

So, no. of hybrid orbitals $= \dfrac{32}{8} = 4$

$\therefore$ $sp^3$ hybridization.

Similarly, for $PO_4^{3-}$ ; no. of hybrid orbitals

$= \dfrac{5+24+3}{8} = \dfrac{32}{8} = 4$

Hybridisation = $sp^3$

Similarly, for $BF_4^-$, it is $sp^3$.

20. (d) $\begin{matrix} CH_2OH \\ | \\ CO \\ | \\ CH_2OH \end{matrix} \xrightarrow{HIO_4} 2CH_2O + CO_2$

21. (d) An ion exchange resin containing R–COOH group exchange cations like $Ca^{2+}$, $Mg^{2+}$, $Na^+$, $Fe^{2+}$ with $H^+$ when hard water is passed through it. This resin is called cation exchange resin.

22. (b) KI reacts with $CuSO_4$ solution to produce cuprous iodide (white precipitate) and $I_2$ (which gives brown colour) Iodine reacts with hypo ($Na_2S_2O_3 5H_2O$) solution. Decolourisaiton of solution shows the appearance of white precipitate.

$$2CuSO_4 + 4KI \rightarrow 2K_2SO_4 + \underset{\text{Cuprous iodide (White ppt.)}}{2CuI} + \underset{\text{(Brown colour in solution)}}{I_2}$$

$$2Na_2S_2O_3 + I_2 \longrightarrow \underset{\text{Sod. tetrathionate (coloourless)}}{Na_2S_4O_6} + 2NaI$$

23. (d) This reaction shows the formation of $H_2O$, and the $X_2$ represents the enthalpy of formation of $H_2O$ because as the definition suggests that the enthalpy of formation is the heat evolved or absorbed when one mole of substance is formed from its constituent atoms.

24. (c) $\overset{sp^2}{CH_2} = \overset{sp}{C} = \overset{sp^2}{CH_2}$

25. (b) The balloon would burst when V > 20 L

$P_1V_1 = P_2V_2$

$1 \times 10 = P_2 \times 20$

$P_2 = 0.5$ atm (no bursting)

Thus, a pressure below 0.5 atm, it would burst.

26. (b) Complex $Co(en)(NH_3)_2Cl_2]Cl$ will have four different isomcrs.

(i) **Geometrical isomers**

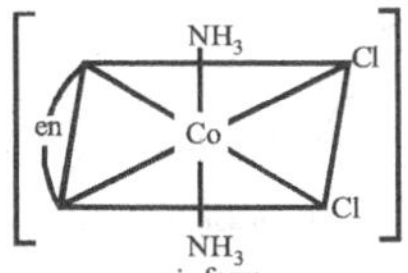
*cis*-form

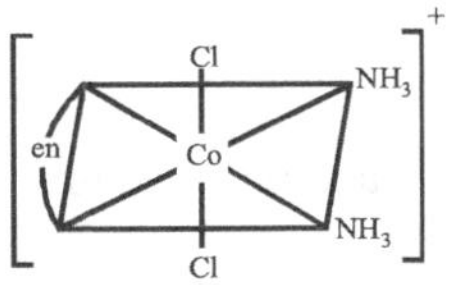
*trans*-form

(ii) **Optical isomers**

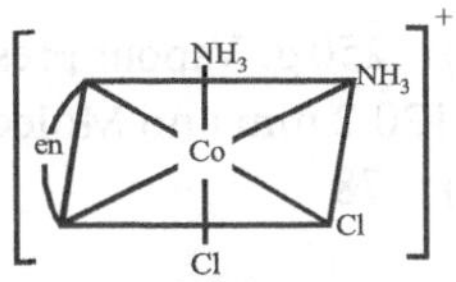
*cis*-form

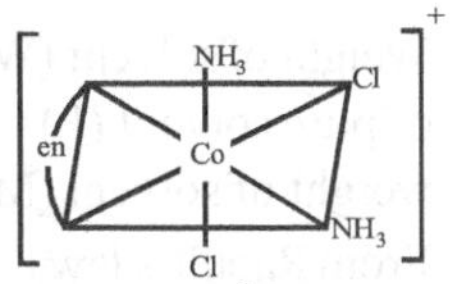
*trans*-form

27. (c) $AB \rightleftharpoons A^+B^-$

$$K_{sp} = \frac{[A^+][B^-]}{[AB]}$$

Salt will precipitate if ionic conc. > $K_{sp}$

$[A^+][B^-] > 1 \times 10^{-8}$

$(1 \times 10^{-3})[B^-] > 1 \times 10^{-8}$

$$[B^-] > \frac{1 \times 10^{-8}}{1 \times 10^{-3}} \text{ or } 1 \times 10^{-5}$$

28. (c) The hydrolysis of sucrose by boiling with mineral acid or by enzyme invertase or sucrase produces a mixture of equal molecules of D(+) glucose and D(–) Fructose.

$$\underset{\substack{\text{sucrose} \\ [\alpha_D] = +66.5^\circ}}{C_{12}H_{22}O_{11}} + H_2O \xrightarrow{HCl} \underbrace{\underset{\substack{\text{D-glu cose} \\ [\alpha_D] = +52.5^\circ}}{C_6H_{12}O_6} + \underset{\substack{\text{D-Fructose} \\ [\alpha_D] = -92^\circ}}{C_6H_{12}O_6}}_{\text{Invert sugar}, [\alpha_D] = -20^\circ}$$

29. (d) In $CO_2$ we have 22 (6 + 8 + 8 = 22) electrons. In ($CN_2^{2-}$), we have 22 (6 + 7 + 7 + 2 = 22) electrons. Both $CO_2$ and ($CN_2^{2-}$) have linear structures. Thus, statement (a) is correct.

$$Mg_2C_3 + 4H_2O \longrightarrow$$
$$2Mg(OH)_2 + \underset{\text{Propyne}}{CH_3C \equiv CH}$$

i.e., statement (b) is also correct.

The structure of $CaC_2$ is of NaCl type

i.e., statement (c) is also correct.

30. (a) Due to resonance C — N bond in protein acquires double bond character and is smaller than usual C — N bond.

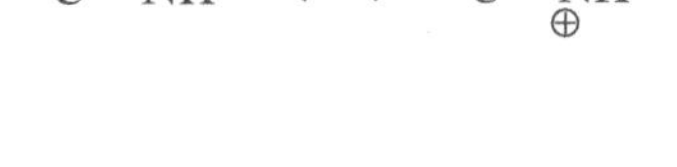

31. (a) Given vapour pressure of pure solute $(P^0) = 121.8$ mm; Weight of solute (w) = 15 g
Weight of solvent (W) = 250 g; Vapour pressure of pure solvent (P) = 120.2 mm and Molecular weight of solvent (M) = 78
From Raoult's law

$$= \frac{P^o - P}{P^o} = \frac{w}{m} \times \frac{M}{W} = \frac{121.8 - 120.2}{121.8} = \frac{15}{m} \times \frac{78}{250}$$

$$\text{or } m = \frac{15 \times 78}{250} \times \frac{121.8}{1.6} = 356.2$$

32. (b) With the decrease in the electronegativity of central atom the bond angle decreases

33. (b) When the concentration of reactant is reduced to half its initial value, the rate is reduced by $\frac{2.4}{0.6} = 4$ times
It means, rate $\propto$ [reactant]$^2$
So, order of reaction = 2

34. (b) *p-p* overlap between B and F is maximum due to identical size and energy of *p*- orbitals, so electron deficiency in boron of $BF_3$ is neutralized partially to the maximum extent by back donation.
Hence $BF_3$ is least acidic.

35. (a) Following generalization can be easily derived for various types of lattice arrangements in cubic cells between the edge length (a) of the cell and r the radius of the sphere.

For simple cubic : $a = 2r$ or $r = \frac{a}{2}$

For body centred cubic :

$$a = \frac{4}{\sqrt{3}} r \text{ or } r = \frac{\sqrt{3}}{4} a$$

For face centred cubic :

$$a = 2\sqrt{2} r \text{ or } r = \frac{1}{2\sqrt{2}} a$$

Thus the ratio of radii of spheres for these will be

simple : bcc : fcc

$$= \frac{a}{2} : \frac{\sqrt{3}}{4} a : \frac{1}{2\sqrt{2}} a$$

i.e. option (a) is correct answer.

36. (b) Recall that presence of electron-withdrawing group increases, while presence of electron-releasing group decreases the acidity of carboxylic acids.

$$\underset{\text{(electron-withdrawing gp.)}}{ClCH_2COOH} > \underset{\text{(Electron-releasing character increasing from left to right)}}{H-\overset{\overset{O}{\|}}{C}-OH > CH_3-\overset{\overset{O}{\|}}{C}-OH >}$$

$$C_2H_5-\overset{\overset{O}{\|}}{C}-OH$$

37. (d) Penicillin is an antibiotic which was first obtained from a fungus, penicillium notatum by the scientist, Flemming.

38. (a) Slow step is rate determining step
$\therefore$ Rate law = k $[NOBr_2][NO]$, $[NOBr_2]$ is the intermediate

For the fast reaction, $K = \frac{[NOBr_2]}{[NO][Br_2]}$

$\therefore \quad [NOBr_2] = K[NO][Br_2]$
$\therefore \quad$ Rate law = K k $[NO]^2[Br_2]$
$= K'[NO]^2[Br_2]$

39. (d) Various products are formed when nitroarenes are reduced. These are given below for $C_6H_5NO_2$.

| Medium | Main product |
|---|---|
| In acidic medium (metal/HCl) | Aniline ($C_6H_5NH_2$) |
| In neutral medium ($Zn/NH_4Cl$) | Phenyl hydroxylamine, 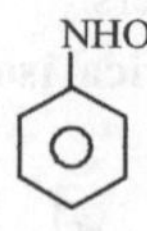 |
| In alkaline medium | 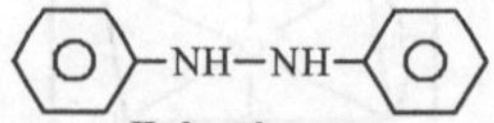 Hydrazobenzene |

Thus, Aniline will be main product in case of (d).

40. (c) Reaction used in fuel cell is

$$2H_2(g) + O_2(g) \longrightarrow 2H_2O(\ell)$$

At anode : $[H_2 \longrightarrow 2H^+ + 2e] \times 2$

At cathode : $O_2 + 2H_2O + 4e \longrightarrow 4OH^-$

41. (c) Carbon cannot expand its coordination number beyond four due to the absence of d-orbitals, hence it cannot form $[CCl_6]^{2-}$ ion

42. (b) *i* remains unchanged when number of ions before and after complex ion remains constant.

| | Solute | y | Complex | y |
|---|---|---|---|---|
| (a) | $PtCl_4$ | 5 | $K_2[PtCl_6]$ | 3 |
| (b) | $ZnCl_2$ | 3 | $Zn[(NH_3)_4]Cl_2$ | 3 |

43. (d) The equivalent conductivity of a solution,

$$\Lambda_{eq} = \frac{1000}{C} \times \kappa$$

Where,

$\kappa$ = specific conductance = Unit $ohm^{-1} cm^{-1}$

C = normality of the solution unit gm eq/$cm^3$

Hence, the unit of $\Lambda_{eq}$ is $Ohm^{-1}.cm^2$ (gm equivalent)$^{-1}$.

44. (c) Nylon-6 is also called as perlon. It is a polymer of caprolactam.

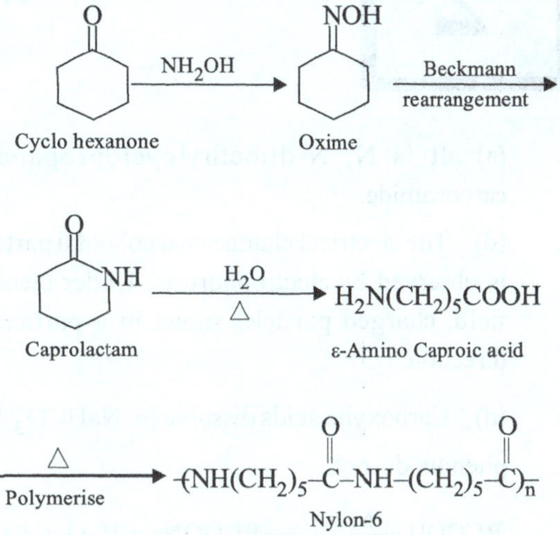


45. (b) Tertiary nitro compound do not have α hydrogen atom therefore they did not show tautomerism.

2

# Mock Test -2

1. (a) It is N, N-dimethylcyclopropane – carboxamide.

2. (d) The electrical change on a colloidal particle is observed by electrophoresis. Under electric field, charged particles move in a particular direction.

3. (d) Carboxylic acids dissolve in $NaHCO_3$ but phenols do not.

$$RCOOH \xrightarrow{NaHCO_3} RCOONa + H_2O + CO_2$$

by evolving $CO_2$ gas.

4. (d) Zinc and lead in molten state are immiscible and form separate layers, further Zn, being ligher, forms upper layer. Silver is soluble in both Zn and Pb, and hence all statements are correct.

5. (a) The order of all photochemical reactions is zero as it does not depend upon the concentration of reactants.

6. (a) The correct reaction is

$$3O_2(g) \underset{\substack{\text{Electric}\\\text{discharge}}}{\overset{\text{Silent}}{\rightleftharpoons}} 2O_3(g);\ \Delta H = +284.5\text{ kJ}.$$

7. (b) A set of question number is valid when $l < n$ and $m_1$ lies between $-l$ to $+l$. Thus sets I, II, IV are valid, III, V invalid.

8. (d) Ionic compounds are dissociated in solution state and form ions. Ions are good carrier of charge. So it makes solution conducting.

9. (d) $Br_2$ in $CCl_4$ (a), $Br_2$ in $CH_3COOH$ (b) and alk. $KMnO_4$ (c) will react with all unsaturated compounds, i.e., 1, 3 and 4 while ammonical $AgNO_3$ (d) reacts only with terminal alkynes, i.e., 3 and hence compund 3 can be distinguished from 1, 2 and 4 by. ammonical $AgNO_3$ (d).

10. (a) $N_2 = 3H_2 = 6H$

$$\therefore\quad 1H = \frac{N_2}{6}$$

Thus, equivalent weight of $N_2$

$$= \frac{\text{molar mass}}{6} = \frac{28}{6} = 4.67$$

11. (c) CO and oxides of Nitrogen are poisnous gases present in automobile exhaust gases.

12. (b) For spontaneous reaction $E^0_{cell}$ must be positive.

$$Zn^{2+} \longrightarrow Zn;\ E^0 = -0.76\text{V}$$

$$Cu^{2+} \longrightarrow Cu;\ E^0 = -0.34\text{V}$$

Here Cu acts as cathode and zinc acts as anode.

$$E^{\circ}_{cell} = E^{\circ}_C - E^{\circ}_A = (-0.34) - (-0.76)$$

$$= 0.42\text{ V.}$$

13. (a) The smaller is the size of cation, the more is heat of hydration. Since hydration is exothermic process, thus heat evolves and hence system having lower energy are stable.

14. (a) For a cubic structure,

$$\text{No. of X atoms} = 8 \times \frac{1}{8} = 1$$

$$\text{No. of Y atoms} = 6 \times \frac{1}{2} = 3$$

$\therefore$ Formula of the compound $= XY_3$

15. (d) 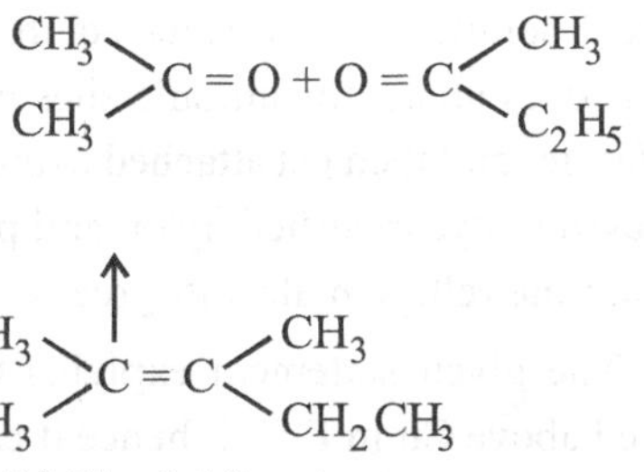

2,3-Dimethyl-2-pentene

16. (a) Vapour pressure of solution

$= p_A + p_B = p_A^o x_A + p_B^o x_B$

$= \frac{120 \times 2}{5} + \frac{180 \times 3}{5} = 156$ mm

17. (b) Since $Cr^{3+}$ in the complex has unpaired electrons in the d orbital, hence will be coloured

$Ti = [Ar]3d^2\,4s^2$; $\quad Ti^{4+} = 3d^0$

$Cr = [Ar]\,3d^5\,4s^1$; $\quad Cr^{3+} = 3d^3$

$Zn = [Ar]\,3d^{10}\,4s^2$; $\quad Zn^{2+} = 3d^{10}$

$Sc = [Ar]\,3d^1\,4s^2$; $\quad Sc^{3+} = 3d^0$

18. (a) According to the adsorption theory of catalysis, the activity of catalysis is due to the presence of free valencies on its surface due to which surface of catalyst has chemical force of altraction. When a gas comes in contact with this surface molecules get attached attached through these valencies. Further the rate of reaction is always increases by decreases in activation energy

When any of the reactants is strongly adsorbed on the surface of catalyst, the rate becomes inversely proportional to the concentration of that reaction. The reaction is then said to be inhibited by such reactant. The lowering of activation energy always leads to the increase in speed of reaction.

19. (a) On increasing pressure, the temperature is also increased. Thus in pressure cooker due to increase in pressure the b.p. of water increases.

20. (c) More stable the carbocation, more reactive will be the parent alkyl halide towards $S_{N^1}$ reaction.

3° > Benzyl > Allyl > 2° > 1° > methyl

21. (b) 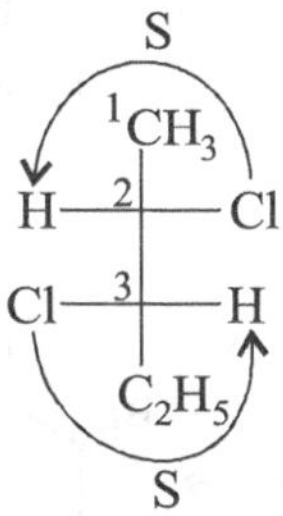

So compound is (2S, 3S)

22. (d) As the unit of rate constant is $sec^{-1}$, so the reaction is first order reaction. Hence

$$k = \frac{1}{t} = \log \frac{a}{(a-x)} \text{ or } kt = \log \frac{[N_2O_5]_0}{[N_2O_5]_t}$$

23. (d) Among 1, 2- and 1, 3- configurations, 1, 3- is more stable due to less repulsion.

Further among *cis* and *trans* isomers, *trans* is more stable due to less crowding.

24. (c) Option (a) is false as Coke is not found in nature. It is an artificial product. Option (d) is also false as $CO_2$ cannot be formed by dehydration of formic acid.

$$HCOOH \xrightarrow[H_2SO_4]{\text{Conc.}} CO + H_2O$$

Option (b) is also false as Producer gas is a mixture of CO and $N_2$.

25. (d) 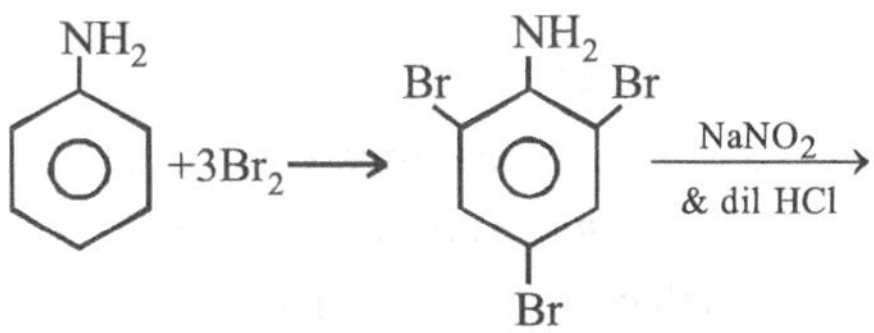

2, 4, 6 tribromoaniline

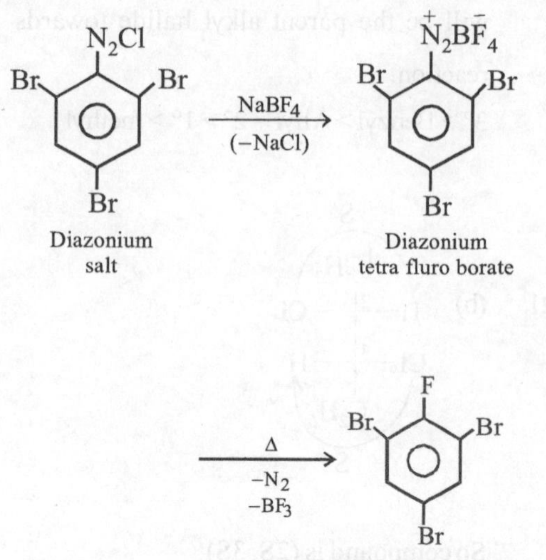

2,4,6 tribromofluorobenzene

26. (d) The semiconductors formed by the introduction of impurity atoms containing one elecron less than the parent atoms of insulators are termed as p-type semiconductors. Therefore silicon containing 14 electrons is to be doped with boron containing 13 electrons to give a p- type semi-conductor.

27. (c)

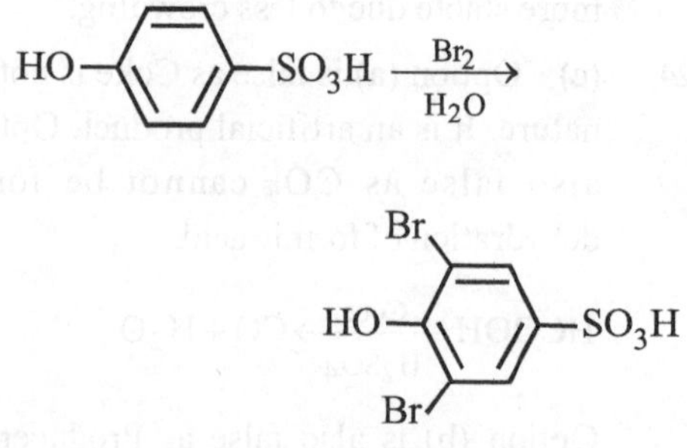


– OH group is highly activating. This is a type of electrophillic substitution reaction at ortho and para position.

28. (d) The appearance of colour in solid alkali metal halide is due to presence of F-centres found as defect in the crystal structure.

29. (b) Basic dyes have salts of amino or substituted amino group ($-NH_2$ or $-NR_2$) which in acid solution forms water soluble cations. These dyes attack the anionic sites present on the fabrics and then get attached to them. These are used to dye modified nylon and polyesters, e.g. aniline yellow, malachite green etc.

30. (b) The given statement explains that Al is placed above Cu in E.C.S. hence it can reduce Cu from its salt solution (reduction). Thus Al acts as a reducing agent now,

Given : electrode potential of copper

$(E^0_{cell}) = +0.34$ V

e.m.f of cell = 2 V

We know that,

emf of a galvanic cell $(E^0_{cell})$

= electrode potential of Cu (cathode) – electrode potential of Al (anode)

$2.0 = 0.34 - E^0_{Al}$

$E^0_{Al} = 0.34 - 2.00 = -1.66$ V

Hence, electrode potential of Al is – 1.66 V.

Option (b) is correct.

31. (a) $X \xrightarrow{PCC} Y \xrightarrow{I_2/\text{alkali}} CHI_3$

Compund Y must give iodoform test. Further since Y is obtained by the oxidation of X which must be an alcohol ($CH_3CH_2OH$) and thus Y is $CH_3CHO$.

32. (c) On losing two electrons from $1s^2, 2s^2 2p^6, 3s^2$ electronic configuration, becomes $1s^2, 2s^2 2p^6, 3s^0$, it is more stable than $1s^2, 2s^2 2p^6, 3s^2$. Since energy gap between $2p^6$ and $3s^2$ will be more due to changing of shell from $3s$ to $2p$. Therefore, the difference in values of IInd ionisation energy and IIIrd

ionisation energy of this configuration is more. Hence, option (c) is correct.

33. (a) Completing the given reaction.

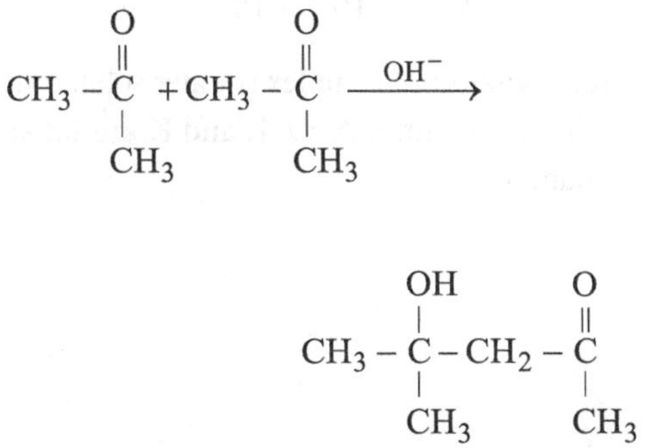

Diacetonyl alcohol

[Note: Carbonyl compounds having $\alpha-$H atom undergoes aldol condensation in presence of dilute base {e.g., NaOH, $Ba(OH)_2$ etc.} to form a class of compounds known as aldol].

34. (a) For exothermic reaction, the reaction goes in forward direction as temp. is lowered.

If high pressure is applied, reaction will go in that direction where number of moles is less (Le-Chatelier's principle).

35. (b) Heavy metal ions, particularly $Ag^+$, catalyse $S_N1$ reaction because of presence of empty orbital.

$$CH_3CH_2Br + Ag^+ \rightleftharpoons [CH_3CH_2 .... Br .... Ag]^+$$

$$\xrightarrow[(-AgBr)]{slow} CH_3\overset{+}{C}H_2 \xrightarrow[\text{from } H_2O]{OH^-} CH_3CH_2OH$$

36. (c) Calculating the oxidation states of I, we get

$H_5IO_6$ ; $5+x-12=0$ or $x=+7$

$H_3IO_5$; $3+x-10=0$ or $x=+7$

$HIO_4$ ; $1+x-8=0$ or $x=+7$

Thus, the correct answer is $+7, +7, +7$

37. (a) Starch is also know as amylum which occurs in all green plants. A molecule of starch $(C_6H_{10}O_5)_n$ is built of a large number of $\alpha$-glucose ring joined through oxygen-atom.

38. (d) The halide ions act as reducing agents . $F^-$ ion does not show any reducing nature but $Cl^-$ , $Br^-$ & $I^-$ ion act as reducing agents and their reducing nature is in increasing order

$$\xrightarrow[\text{Reducing nature increases}]{Cl^- \quad Br^- \quad I^-}$$

39. (a) Square Plannar Structure : $XeF_4$ and $[PtCl_4]^{2-}$

40. (a) Sodium silicate ($Na_2SiO_3$) is known as water glass. It is soluble in water. Just as plants grow in the soil, coloured crystals grow in the water glass.

41. (b)

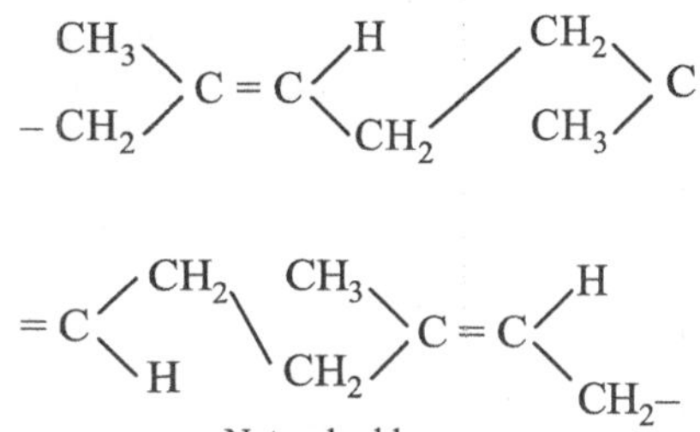

Natural rubber
(All cis configuration)

All statements except (b) are correct

42. (b) For a first order reaction the positive slope is obtained when we plot $-\log_e[A]$ vs $t$.

43. (d)

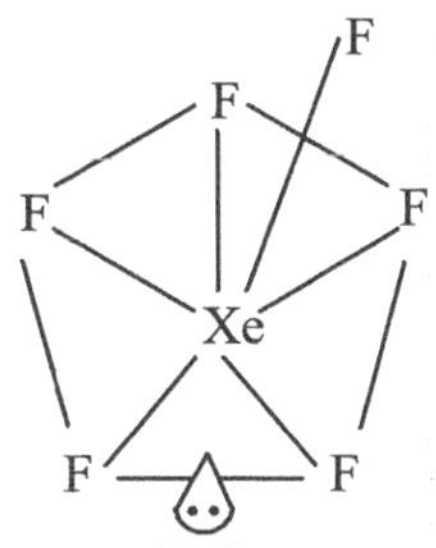

$XeF_6$

(Xe atom in 3rd excited state)

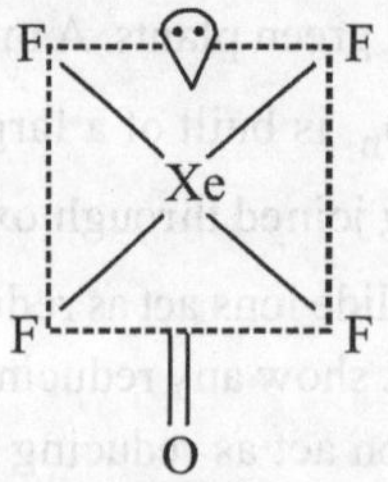


$XeOF_4$

(Xe in 3rd excited state)

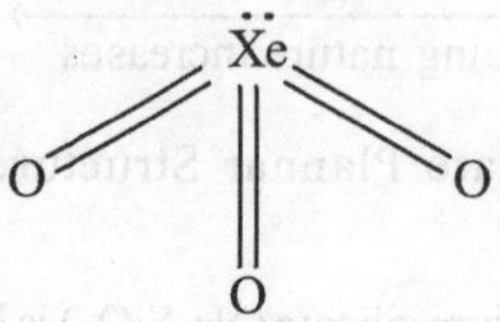


$XeO_3$

(Xe in 1st excited state)

Thus, all the three have same no. of lone pair of electrons i.e. one.

44. (d) $\lambda = \frac{h}{mc} = \frac{6.6 \times 10^{-34}}{10^{-6} \times 10} = 6.63 \times 10^{-29}\,\text{m}$

45 (a) Vitamin B complex is water soluble vitamin whereas vitamin A, D, E and K are fat soluble vitamin.

# 3 Mock Test -3

1. (a) As both the solutions are isotonic hence there is no net movement of the solvent through the semipermeable membrane between two solutions.

2. (d) $R\,COCl + AlCl_3 \longrightarrow \underset{\text{Electrophile}}{R-\overset{\overset{O}{\|}}{C}{}^{\oplus}} + AlCl_4^-$

3. (c) White lead is $2PbCO_3.Pb(OH)_2$ which is prepared by $Pb(NO_3)_2$ & $Na_2CO_3$. It is called as basic lead carbonate.

$3Pb(NO_3)_2 + 3Na_2CO_3 + H_2O \longrightarrow$

$Pb(OH)_2 + 2PbCO_3 + NaNO_3 + CO_2$

Basic lead carbonate

4. (d) Specific volume (volume of 1 gm) of cylindrical virus particle $= 6.02 \times 10^{-2}$ cc/gm

Radius of virus (r) $= 7\ \text{Å} = 7 \times 10^{-8}$ cm

Length of virus $= 10 \times 10^{-8}$ cm

Volume of virus

$\pi r^2 l = \frac{22}{7} \times (7 \times 10^{-8})^2 \times 10 \times 10^{-8} = 154 \times 10^{-23}$ cc

Wt. of one virus particle $= \frac{\text{volume}}{\text{specific volume}}$

$\therefore$ Mol. wt. of virus = Wt. of $N_A$ particle

$= \frac{154 \times 10^{-23}}{6.02 \times 10^{-2}} \times 6.02 \times 10^{23}$

$= 15400$ g/mol $= 15.4$ kg/mole

5. (a) $C_2H_5OH$

Mechanism :

(1) Protonation :

$$C_2H_5OH + H^{\oplus} \rightleftharpoons C_2H_5OH_2^{\oplus}$$

(2) $C_2H_5OH_2^+ \longrightarrow C_2H_5^{\oplus} + H_2O$

$$\xrightarrow{C_2H_5OH} C_2H_5-\overset{\overset{H}{|}}{\underset{\oplus}{O}}-C_2H_5$$

$$\downarrow\uparrow$$

$$H^{\oplus} + \underset{\text{Diethyl ether}}{C_2H_5-O-C_2H_5}$$

6. (c) The tendency of an atom in a compound to attract a pair of bonded electrons towards itself is known as electronegativity of the atom.

7. (a) $Cl_2 + OH^- \longrightarrow Cl^- + ClO^-$

$\frac{1}{2}\underset{0}{Cl_2} \longrightarrow \underset{-1}{Cl^-} + ClO^-$ oxidation change = 1

equivalent mass of $Cl_2$ in reduction half-reaction.

$$= \frac{\frac{1}{2}Cl_2}{1} = \frac{M}{2}$$

$\frac{1}{2}\underset{0}{Cl_2} \longrightarrow Cl^- + \underset{+1}{ClO^-}$ reduction change = 1 equivalent mass of $Cl_2$ in oxidation half-reaction.

$$= \frac{\frac{1}{2}Cl_2}{1} = \frac{M}{2}$$

Thus, equivalent mass in overall reaction

$$= \frac{M}{2} + \frac{M}{2} = M$$

8. (b) $BiF_5$ not possible.

Bi comes in nitrogen family down the group. Hence tendency to show + 5 (co-ordination state) decreases, due to larger size of orbitals, the vaccant d orbitals can not overlap with orbitals of fluorine.

9. (a) $Br_2 \longrightarrow BrO_3^-$

O.N. of Br 0 +5

Thus, it changes from 0 to + 5.

10. (c) Observe the relative stability of their corresponding conjugate bases.

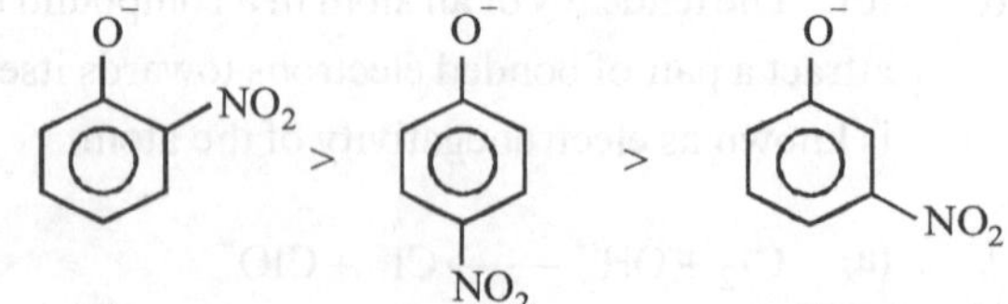

I — Stabilised by both –I and – R effects of the $-NO_2$ group

III — Stabilised by both –I and – R effects, but – I is less than in I

II — Stabilised only by –I effect

However, the acidity of the corresponding phenols will be different because of H–bonding in the ortho isomer.

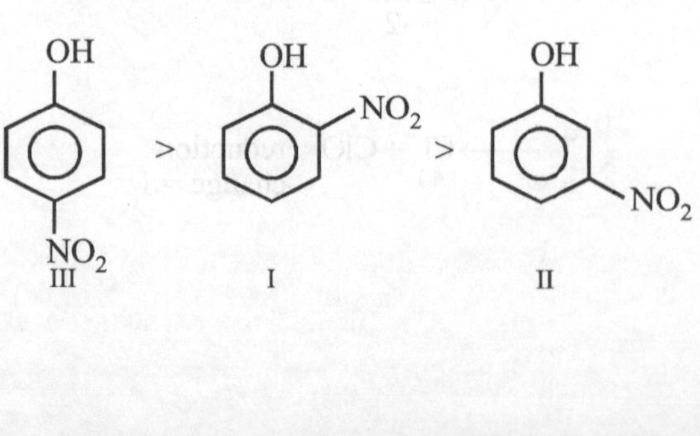

III I II

11. (d) Average molecular speed $= \sqrt{\frac{8RT}{\pi M}}$ is dependent on T and M. Thus, greater the value of $\sqrt{\frac{T}{M}}$, greater the molecular speed.

Thus, Gas $\sqrt{\frac{T}{M}}$

$O_2 \sqrt{\frac{560}{32}}$ 4.18

$Ne \sqrt{\frac{500}{20}}$ 5.0

$O_2 \sqrt{\frac{440}{44}}$ 3.16

$He \sqrt{\frac{140}{4}}$ 5.91

12. (d) Aniline when treated with acetic anhydride forms acetanilide (nucleophilic substitution)

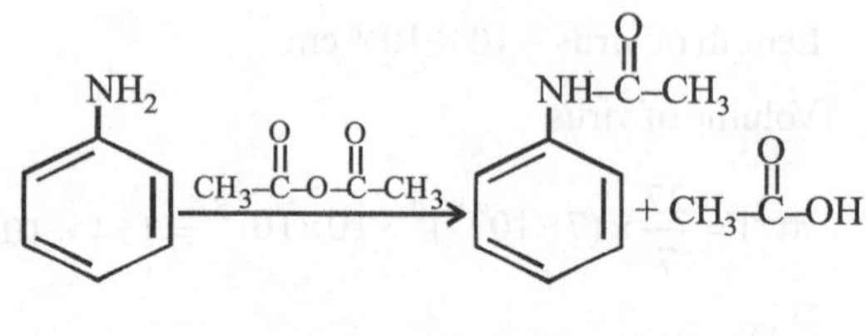

13. (a) Mohr's salt is $FeSO_4.(NH_4)_2SO_4.6H_2O$. $Fe^{2+}$ present in it is oxidized to $Fe^{3+}$.

So, we have, $Fe^{2+} \longrightarrow Fe^{3+} + e$

Thus, equivalent mass $= \frac{\text{Formula mass}}{1}$

$= 392$

14. (b) Domestic sewage constitute biodegradable pollutants.

15. (a) Langmuir adsorption isotherm is based on the assumption that every adsorption site is equivalent and the ability of a particle to bind there is independent of whether or not nearby sites are occupied.

16. (b) Thermosetting plastics consist of chain molecules which are chemically bonded, or cross-linked, with each other when heated. When thermosetting plastics cross-link, the molecules create a permanent, 3-D network that can be considered one giant molecule. Once cured, thermosetting plastic cannot be remelted, in the same way that cured concrete cannot be reset.

17. (a) From the graph we can see the correct order of pressures $p_1 > p_3 > p_2$

18. (a) $SiO_2$ is used for this purpose.

19. (c) The acid strength of oxyacids of the same halogen increases with increase in oxidation state of the halogen

$$\overset{+7}{HClO_4} > \overset{+5}{HClO_3} > \overset{+3}{HClO_2} > \overset{+1}{HClO}$$

Thus Cl in $HClO_4$ is in highest oxidation state (+7) and hence strongest acid, while HClO (Cl is in +1 oxidation state) is weakest.

20. (b) Concentration of $Na_2CO_3 = \frac{25.3}{106} \times \frac{1000}{250} =$

0.955 M

$[Na^+] = 2 \times 0.955 = 1.91$ M

$\left[CO_3^{2-}\right] = 0.955$ M

21. (a) $S_N2$ mechanism is favoured maximum in methyl chloride among all the given options. Difference in rates are related to the bulk of the substituents. As the number of substituents attached to carbon bearing the halogen is increased, the reactivity towards $S_N2$ substitution decreases. The order of reactivity towards $S_N2$ mechanism is

$CH_3Cl > CH_3CH_2Cl > (CH_3)_2CHCl > (CH_3)_3CCl$

22. (c) K decreases with increase in temperature. Thus, forward reaction is exothermic.

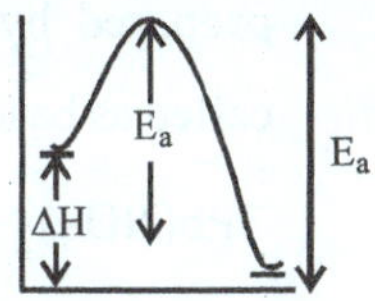


$E_a$ = activation energy of forward reaction

$E_a'$ = ... backward ...

$= (E_a + \Delta H)$

Thus, $E_a' > E_a$

23. (a) Hybridisation $= \frac{1}{2}$ [No. of valence electrons of central atom + no. of monovalent atoms attached to it –

Negative charge if any – positive charge if any]

$NO_2^-$ $H = \frac{1}{2}[5 + 0 + 1 - 0] = 3 = sp^2$

$NO_3^-$ $H = \frac{1}{2}[5 + 0 + 1 - 0] = 3 = sp^2$

$NH_2^-$ $H = \frac{1}{2}[5 + 2 + 1 + 0] = 4 = sp^3$

$NH_4^+$, $H = \frac{1}{2}[5 + 4 + 0 - 1] = 4 = sp^3$

$SCN^- = sp$

i.e., $NO_2^-$ and $NO_3^-$ have same hybridisation.

24. (a)

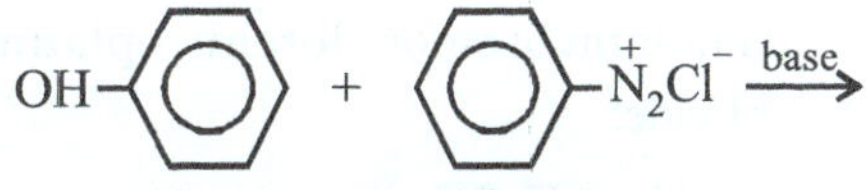


Phenol    Phenyldiazonium chloride

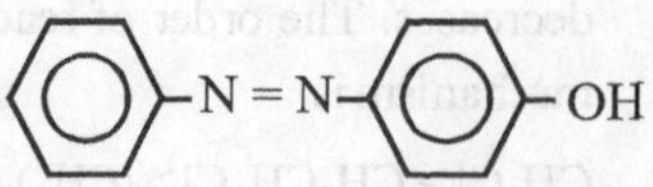

azo dye

25. (c) White lead is $2PbCO_3.Pb(OH)_2$ which is prepared by $Pb(NO_3)_2$ & $Na_2CO_3$. It is called as basic lead carbonate.

$$3Pb(NO_3)_2 + 3Na_2CO_3 + H_2O \longrightarrow$$

$$\underset{\text{Basic lead carbonate}}{Pb(OH)_2 + 2PbCO_3} + NaNO_3 + CO_2$$

26. (a) Most metals occur in their combined state. They have to be reduced to become free metals. The choice of reducing agent is decided by the factors of energetics and economics. In this regard C is the most common reducing agent used. Carbon can be used in the form of coal, coke, charcoal and carbon monoxide. e.g :-

$$SnO_2 + 2C \xrightarrow{1473-1573K} Sn + 2CO$$

$$ZnO + CO \xrightarrow{1600K} Zn + CO_2$$

$$Fe_2O_3 + CO \xrightarrow{823K} 2FeO + CO_2$$

$$FeO + CO \xrightarrow{1123K} Fe + CO_2$$

27. (d) The semiconductors formed by the introduction of impurity atoms containing one elecron less than the parent atoms of insulators are termed as p-type semiconductors. Therefore silicon containing 14 electrons is to be doped with boron containing 13 electrons to give a p- type semi-conductor.

28. (c) We know that IUPAC name of $[Pt(NH_3)_3 (Br) (NO_2)Cl]Cl$ is

triamminebromochloronitroplatinum (IV) chloride.

29. (c) Van't Hoff factor

$$= \frac{\text{Normal Molecular Mass}}{\text{Observed Molecular Mass}}$$

30. (d) Aldehydes which contain a $\alpha$-hydrogen on a saturated carbon, i.e., $CH_3CH_2CHO$ undergo aldol condensation.

$$\underset{\text{propanol}}{CH_3CH_2-\overset{\overset{H}{|}}{C}=O} + H-\underset{\alpha}{H\overset{\overset{CH_3}{|}}{C}}-CHO$$

$$\xrightarrow{OH^-} CH_3CH_2-\underset{\underset{OH}{|}}{\overset{\overset{CH_3}{\beta|}}{C}}-\overset{\overset{CH_3}{\alpha|}}{C}HCHO$$

3.hydroxy,2 methyl pentanal

31. (d) When there is simultaneously change in temperature and volume (or pressure)

$$\Delta S = nC_V \log_e\left(\frac{T_2}{T_1}\right) + nR\log_e\left(\frac{V_2}{V_1}\right)$$

$$= C_V \log_e\left(\frac{2}{1}\right) + R\log_e\left(\frac{1}{2}\right)$$

$$= C_V \log_e 2 - R\log_e 2$$

$$= (C_V - R)\log_e 2$$

32. (d) $\frac{x}{m} = p$

33. (a) $Zn + H_2SO_4 \rightarrow ZnSO_4 + H_2$

In bomb calorimeter, there is no expansion in volume, so, work done will be zero. This reaction is exothermic. So, some heat will be evolved which will result in lowering of internal energy. Hence,

$$\Delta U < 0 \;\&\; w = 0$$

34. (d) The reactivity of H-atoms depends upon the stability of free radicals follows the order :

Tertiary > secondary > primary, therefore, reactivity of H-atoms follows the same order, i.e., tertiary > secondary > primary.

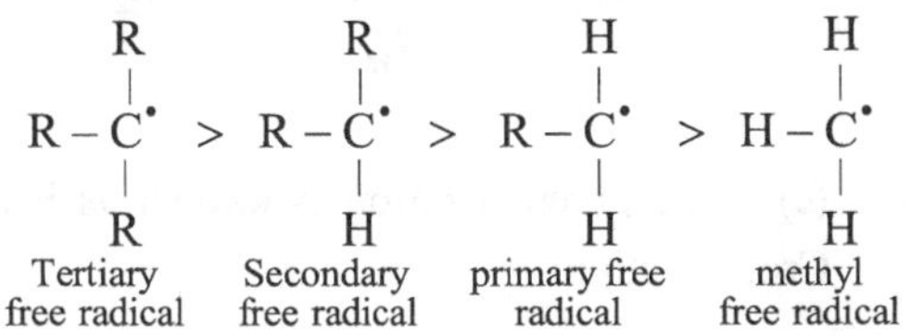


35. (b) For a 10 K rise in temperature, collision frequency increases merely by 1 to 2% but the number of effective collisions increases by 100 to 200%.

36. (d) Rotation around $\pi$ bond is not possible. If any attempt is made to rotate one of the carbon atoms, the lobes of $\pi$-orbital will no longer remain coplanar i.e no parallel overlap will be possible and thus $\pi$-bond will break . This is known as concept of restricted rotation. In other words the presence of $\pi$-bonds makes the position of two carbon atom.

37. (a) Molecular masses of polymers are best determined by osmotic pressure method . Firstly because other colligative properties give so low values that they cannot be measured accurately and secondly, osmotic pressure measurements can be made at room temperature and do not require heating which may change the nature of the polymer.

38. (d) All the properties mentioned in the question suggest that it is a benzene molecule. Since in benzene all carbons are $sp^2$–hybridized, therefore, C – C – C angle is 120°

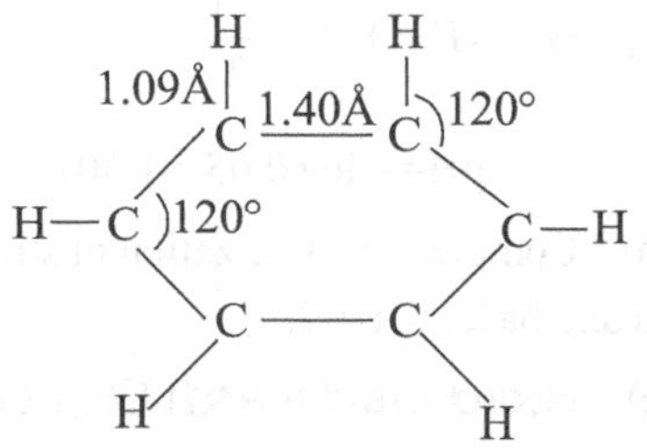


39. (c) C has highest boiling point, so, it should have maximum number of carbon atoms in its molecule, because weak intermolecular force of attraction in a covalent molecule is vander waal's force of attraction which is directly proportional to the number of carbon atoms in the molecule.

40. (a) Flocculating value $\propto \frac{1}{(z)}$, where z = valency of coagulating ion.

Since, $Fe(OH)_3$ is a positively charged sol so it will be coagulated by negative ions considering the valencies of various negative ions used i.e., $Cl^-$, $S^{2-}$, $PO_4^{3-}$ and $SO_4^{2-}$, we find that the valency of $Cl^-$ is least so it will have maximum flocculation value i.e., NaCl.

41. (a) In DNA, adenine faces thymine and guanine faces cytosine.

42. (c) Number of unpaired electrons in various species.

| | |
|---|---|
| $Mn^{2+}$ $3d^5$ | **5** |
| $Cr^{2+}$ $3d^4$ | **4** |
| $V^{2+}$ $3d^3$ | **3** |

Since, $\mu = \sqrt{n(n+2)}$

i.e., it increases with increase in number of unpaired electrons present in a species. Thus, the correct order is

$Mn^{2+} > Cr^{2+} > V^{2+}$.

43. (c) (a) $[H_3O^+] = \frac{0.1}{2} = 0.05$;

$$pH = -\log 0.05 = 1.301$$

(b) Complete neutralization of strong acid and strong base, pH = 7.

(c) Hydrolysis of the salt $CH_3COOK$, pH > 7 (salt of weak acid with strong base)

(d) Hydrolysis of the salt $NH_4NO_3$, pH < 7 (salt of strong acid with weak base)

44. (a)

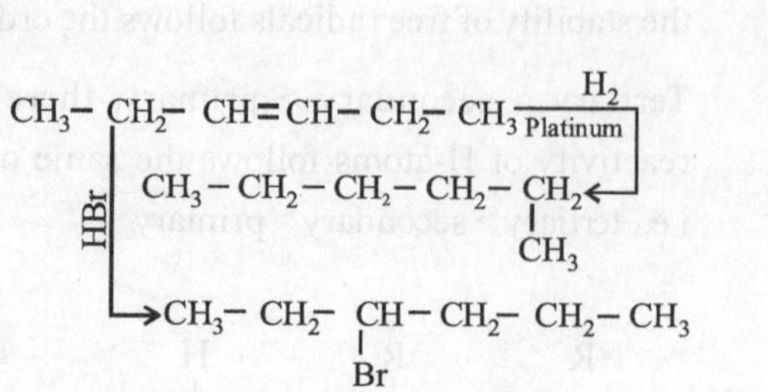

45. (c) The given reaction is known as Friedel-Craft reaction.